AMERICAN ACADEMY OF PEDIATRICS

Dedicated to the Health of All Children

EDITORS

Jeffrey P. Baker, MD, PhD, FAAP

Howard A. Pearson, MD, FAAP

AAP DEPARTMENT OF MARKETING AND PUBLICATIONS STAFF

Maureen DeRosa, MPA
Director, Department of Marketing and Publications

Mark Grimes
Director, Division of Product Development

Jeff Mahony
Manager, Product Development

Sandi King, MS
Director, Division of Publishing and Production Services

Kate Larson
Manager, Editorial Services

Leesa Levin-Doroba
Manager, Print Production Services

Linda Diamond
Manager, Graphic Design

Jill Ferguson
Director, Division of Marketing and Sales

Linda Smessaert
Manager, Publication and Program Marketing

Library of Congress Control Number: 2004102271
ISBN: 1-58110-140-6
MA0283

TABLE OF CONTENTS

FOREWORD

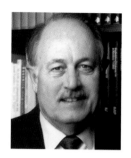

I hope you enjoy this wonderful book commemorating 75 years of child health and the accomplishments of the American Academy of Pediatrics (AAP). It has been the highlight of my professional career to serve as the AAP executive director from 1993 to 2004, and to have participated directly in some of the exciting times depicted herein. As our organization's logo indicates, the AAP is "dedicated to the health of all children," and I believe this theme rings loud and true as you read these fascinating accounts about many great efforts and achievements in pediatrics through the years.

I would like to offer my sincerest gratitude to the book's editors, Jeffrey P. Baker, MD, PhD, and Howard A. Pearson, MD, who have put forth a tremendous effort to make this book a truly wonderful keepsake to be cherished. I also would like to thank all the members of the AAP 75th Anniversary Project Advisory Committee chaired by Carden Johnston, MD, and Carol D. Berkowitz, MD, along with staff chair Maureen DeRosa, MPA, for their roles in planning the AAP 75th anniversary celebration.

Joe M. Sanders, Jr, MD, FAAP
Immediate Past Executive Director
American Academy of Pediatrics

PREFACE

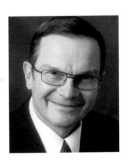

As the new executive director of the American Academy of Pediatrics (AAP), I am proud to serve the AAP in this, its 75th anniversary year. In looking back at all of the wonderful progress we have made in 75 years of caring for children, I cannot help but think of our continuing mission and ongoing responsibilities to the children of the world. We have accomplished so much, and yet there is still work to be done—new techniques to be learned, new ideas to be fostered, new initiatives to be cultivated, and new problems to be tackled.

In the years ahead, we will also need to continue our efforts to advocate for a more family-friendly society that is sensitive to the needs of our culturally diverse population. We will need to adapt our methods of practicing medicine to incorporate new technologies and advances. The mapping of the human genome will enable us to provide our patients with tailor-made medical care. While we cannot know exactly what the future will hold, one thing is certain—the AAP will be providing pediatricians with vital backup and support just as it has for the past 75 years. We also can count on the AAP to continue to be at the forefront in advocating for all infants, children, adolescents, and young adults to attain their optimal physical, mental, and social health and well-being. That is our mission, and our patients are the future.

I thank Jeffrey P. Baker, MD, PhD, and Howard A. Pearson, MD, for preparing this wonderful tribute to pediatricians, past and present, and to the children for whom they cared. May we, and future generations of pediatricians, be inspired to carry forth this honorable legacy that has been entrusted to us.

Errol R. Alden, MD, FAAP
Executive Director/CEO
American Academy of Pediatrics

PROLOGUE

The fifth year of the new millennium is the occasion of the 75th anniversary of the American Academy of Pediatrics (AAP). Milestones such as this often provide a rationale for historical reviews that look back on an organization's past activities and accomplishments, as well as an opportunity for looking ahead to guess what might transpire in the future. Yet, all too often, such histories can unduly focus on committee meetings and internal minutiae, losing sight of the more fundamental themes and issues that have shaped an association's vision over time.

We believe that the history of the AAP cannot be told apart from the broader history of child health and welfare over the course of the 300 years preceding the AAP, as well as the last 75 years. To that end, we have tried to construct more than a review of the internal history of the AAP. We hope that the reader will gain a sense of how science, politics, and social reform have transformed the health care of children and also have shaped the substance and content of pediatric practice in the United States during the last century. While acknowledging that many individuals and advocacy groups have contributed to this story, we do wish to highlight the particular contributions of AAP members and leaders on behalf of America's children.

The editors of this commemorative volume have been afforded a chance to review the personalities and social forces that led to the creation of the AAP in 1930, its role in the remarkable transformation of child health over the course of the 20th century, and its many accomplishments on behalf of children over the last 75 years. We make no claim to comprehensiveness, and acknowledge that, in some cases, our selection of certain individuals, accomplishments, or milestones over others has been difficult if not arbitrary. History must be selective if it is to be told as a story rather than a collection of tables and lists.

Although we believe that this volume provides an accurate historical account, we wanted to enliven it with the personal recollections and anecdotes of AAP members who lived these times and so are part of the history. In early 2002, we began to solicit personal accounts from the AAP members and we are grateful that a large number responded. We also had access to the rich resources of the oral histories compiled by the AAP Pediatric History Center. The anecdotes we collected have been woven into our historical account and we believe that they add insight, color, emotion, and sometimes humor to what might have otherwise been a rather sterile review. In addition, the early AAP history written by Marshall Carleton Pease, MD, in 1951 and the semicentennial AAP history written by James G. Hughes, MD, in 1980 (see Selected Reading) were of enormous value in our efforts.

This book would have been impossible without the contributions of many people. We are sincerely grateful for the contributions of all of

We believe in the inherent worth of all children;
they are our most enduring and vulnerable legacy.

the AAP members who provided submissions for this publication (and, regrettably, many more were received than could possibly be included). Without the wisdom and memories of these fine people, this book never could have been accomplished. In particular, we would like to call out the stellar efforts of James E. Strain, MD; David Annunziato, MD; William A. Silverman, MD; Seymour E. Wheelock, MD; Robert Grayson, MD; and Lewis A. Barness, MD.

The valuable contributions of the AAP staff in developing this book cannot be overstated. Jeff Mahony was crucial in coordinating our activities and the member submissions from all around the country; Susan Bolda Marshall, MALS; John F. Zwicky, PhD; and Chris D. Kwiat, MALS, provided historical support; Kate Simone and Jason Crase researched and organized the photographs that grace this volume; Holly Kaminski helped organize all of the submissions; Jackie Noyes, MA, provided important insights on legislative aspects of the history; and Maureen DeRosa, MPA, and Mark Grimes provided tireless support to this project from conception to production. Needless to say, even this lengthy list is too short, as many members of the AAP staff (in both Elk Grove Village, IL, and Washington, DC) can proudly say that they participated in helpful ways to the development of this book.

Finally, we want to thank our families for their forbearance and understanding during what has been a very time-consuming labor of love over the past 3 years.

Jeffrey P. Baker, MD, PhD, FAAP
Howard A. Pearson, MD, FAAP

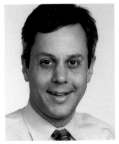

Jeffrey P. Baker, MD, PhD, FAAP

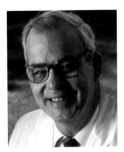

Howard A. Pearson, MD, FAAP

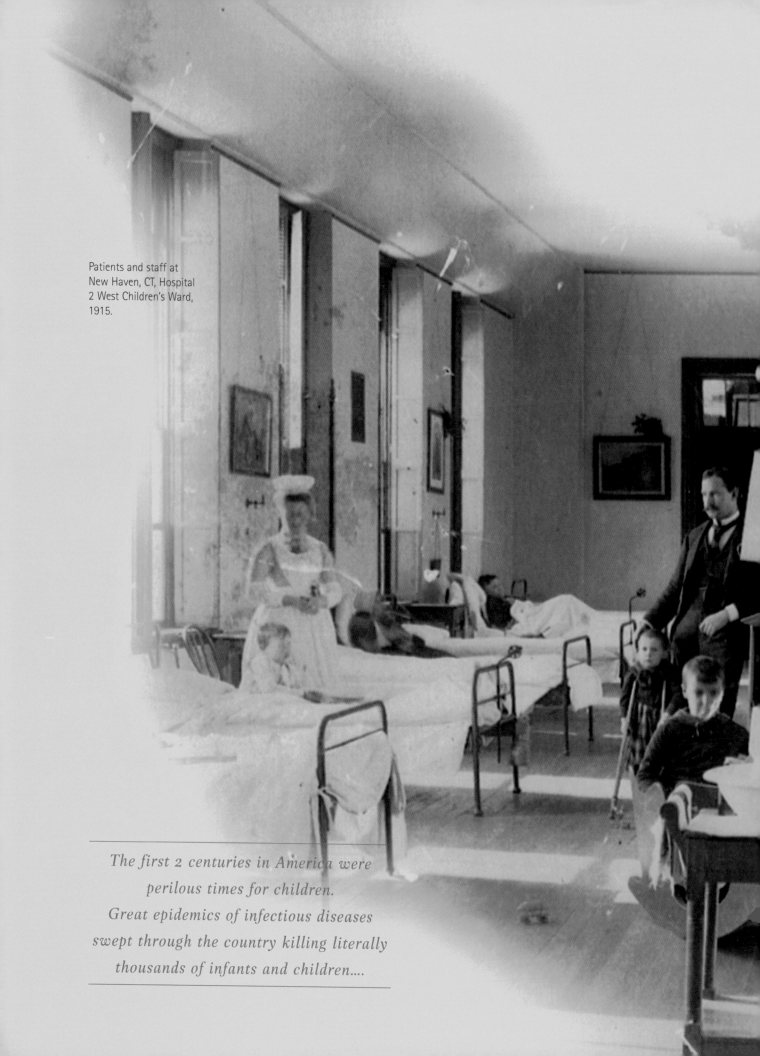

Patients and staff at
New Haven, CT, Hospital
2 West Children's Ward,
1915.

The first 2 centuries in America were
perilous times for children.
Great epidemics of infectious diseases
swept through the country killing literally
thousands of infants and children....

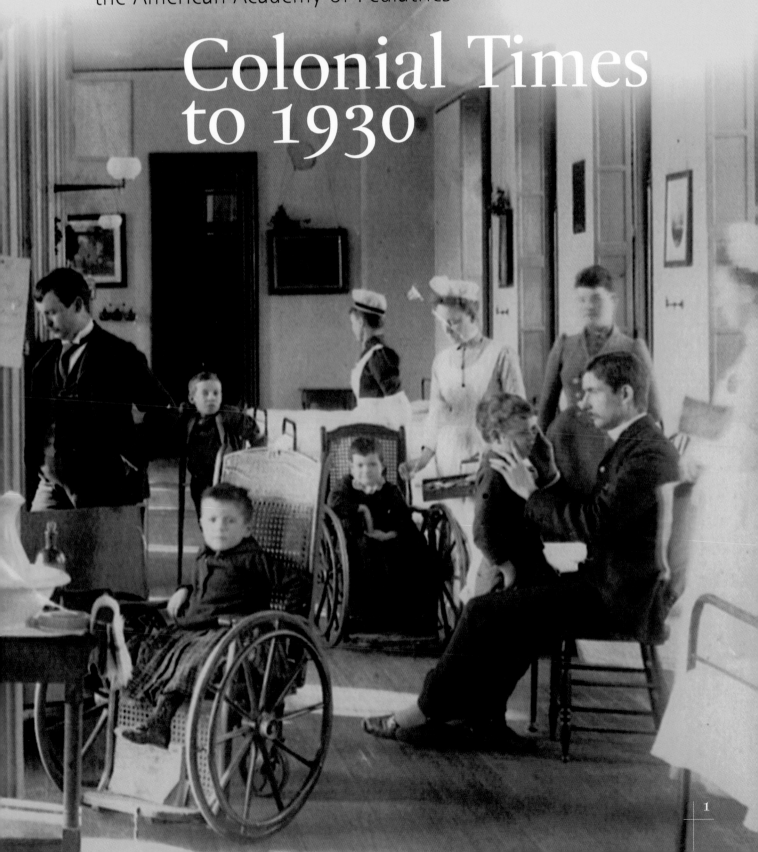

Chapter 1

Pediatrics in America Before the Founding of the American Academy of Pediatrics

Colonial Times to 1930

"Street Arabs at Night, Mulberry Street," a classic picture by photojournalist Jacob Riis, who was known for his gritty depictions of poor urban conditions in the late 19th century.

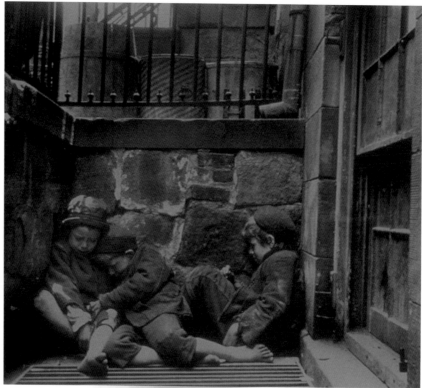

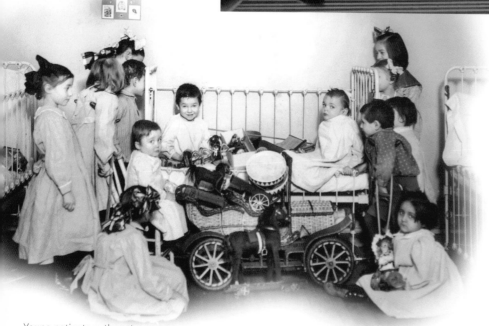

Young patients gather at a 1906 Christmas party at a home for disabled children in Chicago, IL.

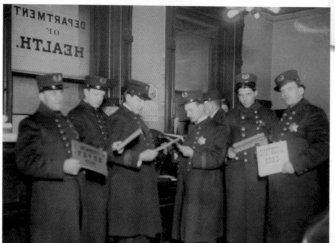

Septic SORE THROAT CONTAGIOUS KEEP OUT ORDER BOARD OF HEALTH

Left, policemen at the Chicago Department of Health hold signs about a scarlet fever epidemic (photo taken February 11, 1907); *above*, a sign posted on quarantined houses.

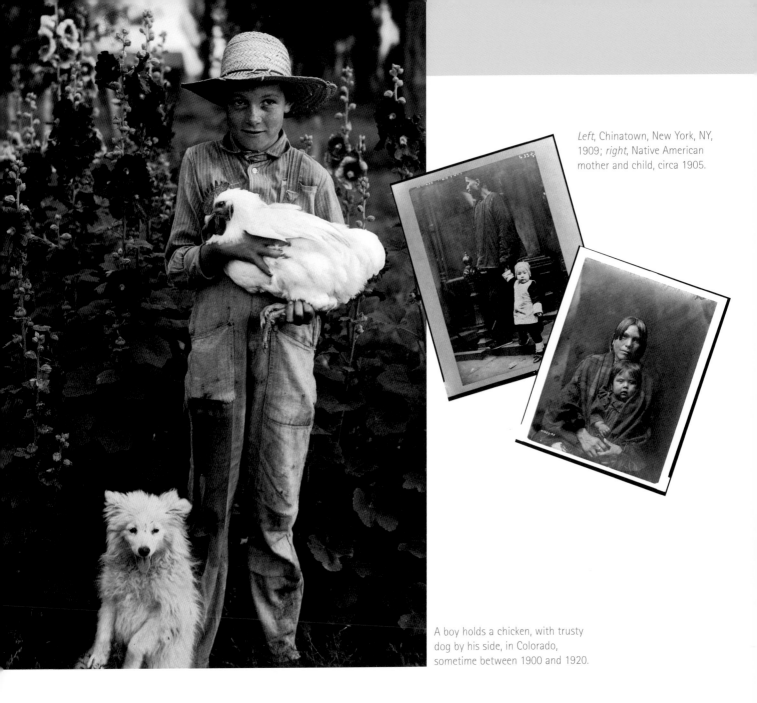

Left, Chinatown, New York, NY, 1909; *right*, Native American mother and child, circa 1905.

A boy holds a chicken, with trusty dog by his side, in Colorado, sometime between 1900 and 1920.

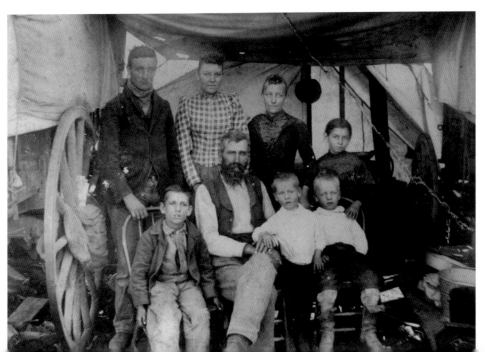

Portrait of the Henry Smith family in camp, at head of Lay Creek, Moffat County, CO, in September 1893. Henry Smith and his 7 children pose under a canvas awning stretched over 2 covered wagons.

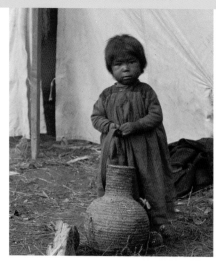
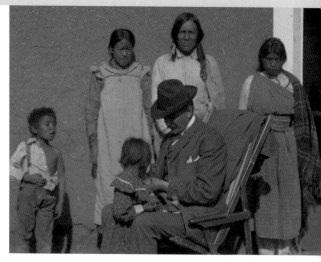

Left, a Native American (Ute) child holds a strap to a woven water basket in front of a tent, circa 1907 (probably in New Mexico); *right*, a physician vaccinates a young Native American (Tewa) girl in New Mexico, circa 1910.

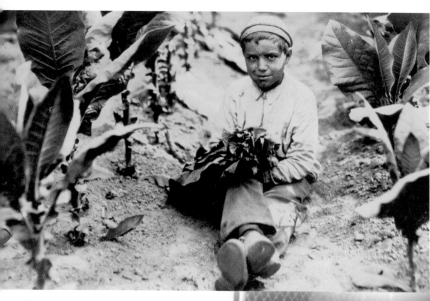

Immigrant families being sent by rail from Ellis Island, NY, in 1926.

Boy works in a tobacco field in Gildersleeve, CT, in 1917.

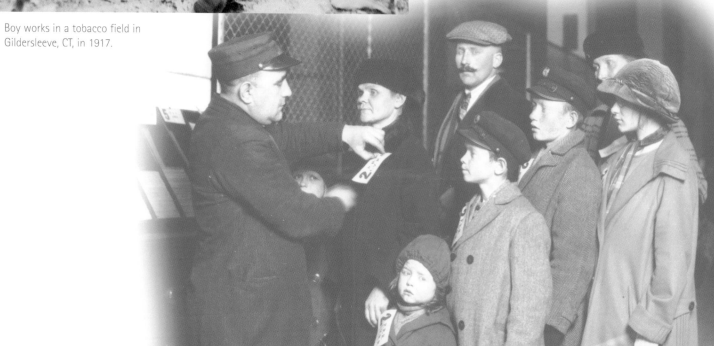

Cotton Mather's Measles Experiences in Colonial America

October 17, 1713

Increase Mather, fourteen years old, began to have symptoms of measles but recovered after being moderately sick.

October 27

Nibby, the nineteen-year-old daughter, was very ill with measles.

October 30

Mrs. Mather gave birth to twins. Katy, the twenty-four-year-old daughter, became sick but recovered after a very severe illness lasting thirteen days.

November 4

Mrs. Mather down with measles: Nanny, a sixteen-year-old daughter, sick; Lizzy, a nine-year-old daughter, very sick; daughter Jerusha, two and a half years old, became ill.

November 5

A son, Samuel, seven years old, taken with a case of average severity. The maid was very sick with measles.

November 7

"Not only are my children, with a servant, lying sick, but also my consort is in dangerous condition and can get no rest. Either Death, or Distraction is much feared for her."

November 9

Mrs. Mather, "My dear, dear, dear Friend expired." She died "between 3 and 4 in the afternoon."

November 14

The maid died with "malignant Feavor." "Tis a Satisfaction to me, that tho' she had been a wild, vain, airy Girl, yet since her coming into my Family, she became disposed unto serious Religion."

November 17

"Little Eleazor," one of the twins, died "about midnight"—eighteen days old.

November 20

"Little Martha," the other twin, died "about ten o'clock A.M."—twenty-one days old.

November 21

"My lovely Jerusha died on her 17th day of illness, between 9 h. and 10 h. at Night."

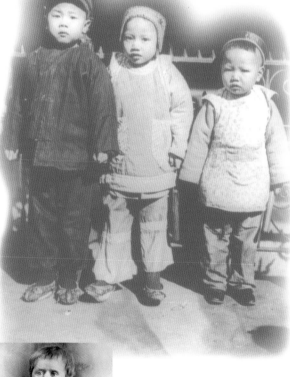

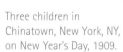

Afternoon tea at the Babies' Hospital of New York City, circa 1896.

Three children in Chinatown, New York, NY, on New Year's Day, 1909.

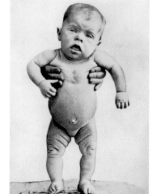

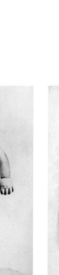

Left, a child with congenital hypothyroidism (cretin) shown at 17 months of age; *right*, the same child after 6 months' treatment (circa 1895).

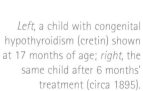

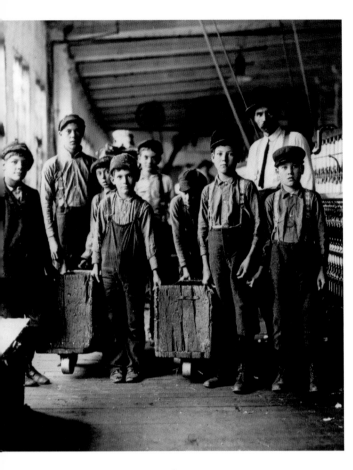

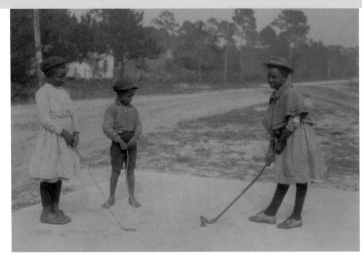

Children playing golf with clubs made of sticks, circa 1905.

Young children working at the
Catawba Cotton Mill, Newton,
NC, in 1908.

Vera Hill, 5 years old,
picking 25 pounds of
cotton a day (photo taken
October 11, 1916).

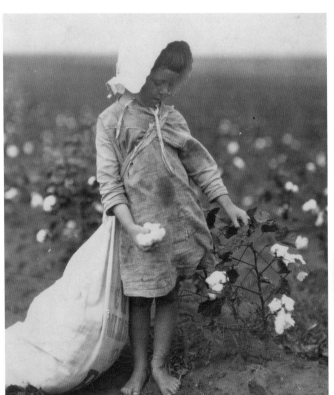

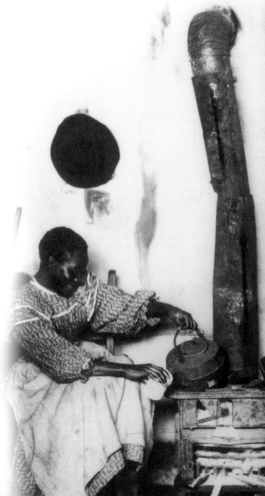

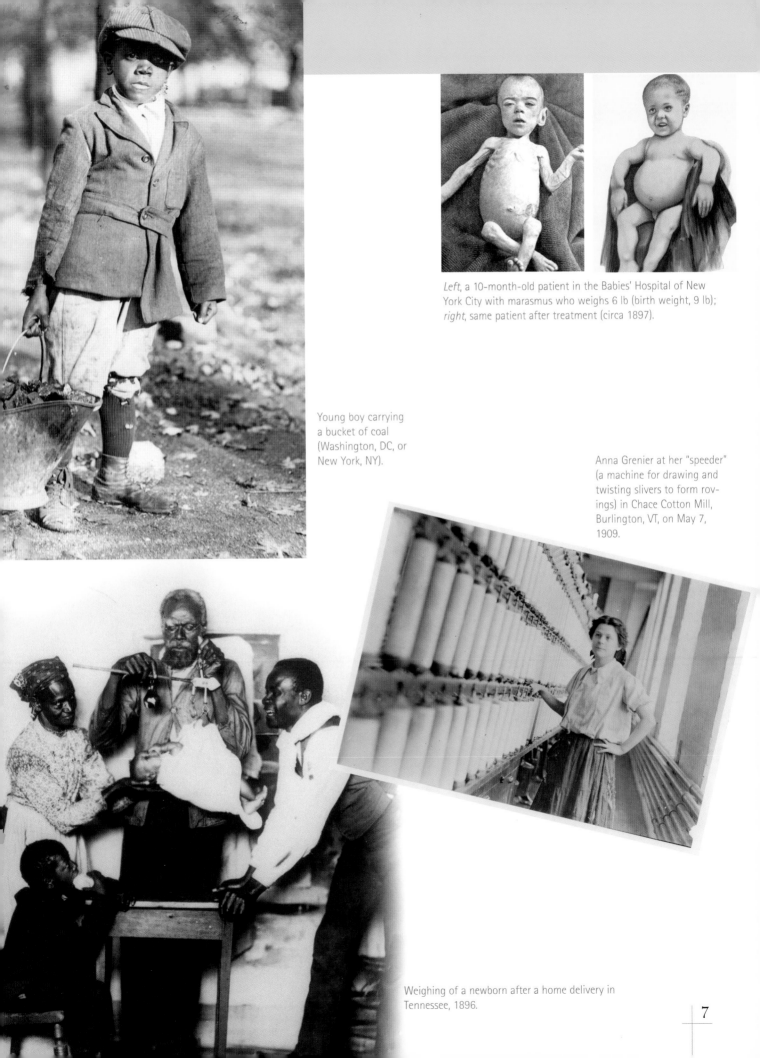

Left, a 10-month-old patient in the Babies' Hospital of New York City with marasmus who weighs 6 lb (birth weight, 9 lb); *right*, same patient after treatment (circa 1897).

Young boy carrying a bucket of coal (Washington, DC, or New York, NY).

Anna Grenier at her "speeder" (a machine for drawing and twisting slivers to form rovings) in Chace Cotton Mill, Burlington, VT, on May 7, 1909.

Weighing of a newborn after a home delivery in Tennessee, 1896.

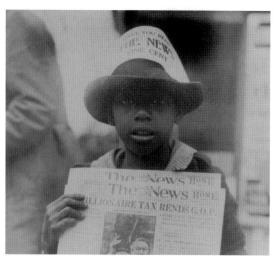

Boy selling *The Washington Daily News*,
November 8, 1921.

Description of an Influenza Epidemic from John Steinbeck's *Cannery Row*

All in all it was a terrific month and right in the middle of it the influenza epidemic had to break out. It came to the whole town. Mrs. Talbot and her daughter of the San Carlos Hotel had it. Tom Work had it. Benjamin Peabody and his wife had it. Excelentísima Maria Antonia Field had it. The whole Gross family came down with it.

The doctors of Monterey—and there were enough of them to take care of the ordinary diseases, accidents and neuroses—were running crazy. They had more business than they could do among clients who if they didn't pay their bills, at least had the money to pay them. Cannery Row which produces a tougher breed than the rest of the town was late in contracting it, but finally it got them too. The schools were closed. There wasn't a house that hadn't feverish children and sick parents. It was not a deadly disease as it was in 1917 but with children it had a tendency to go into the mastoids. The medical profession was very busy, and besides, Cannery Row was not considered a very good financial risk.

Now Doc of the Western Biological Laboratory had no right to practice medicine. It was not his fault that everyone in the Row came to him for medical advice. Before he knew it he found himself running from shanty to shanty taking temperatures, giving physics, borrowing and delivering blankets and even taking food from house to house where mothers looked at him with inflamed eyes from their beds, and thanked him and put the full responsibility for their children's recovery on him.

— From *Cannery Row* by John Steinbeck,
copyright 1945 by John Steinbeck.
Renewed ©1973 by Elaine Steinbeck,
John Steinbeck IV, and Thom Steinbeck.
Used by permission of Viking Penguin,
a division of Penguin Group (USA) Inc.

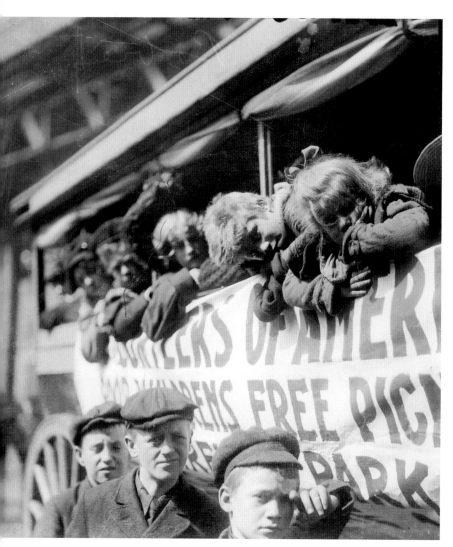

Children on their way to a Volunteers
of America poor children's free picnic
in Chicago, IL, on June 26, 1902.

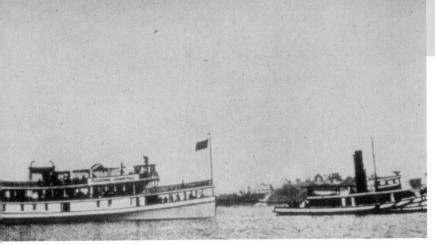

The Boston, MA, Floating Hospital (known as "Clifford"), a boat based in Boston Harbor that brought children and their mothers on a day voyage of ocean breezes and salt air, circa 1903.

A group of children and nurses waiting to board a floating hospital in New York, NY, sometime between 1909 and 1916.

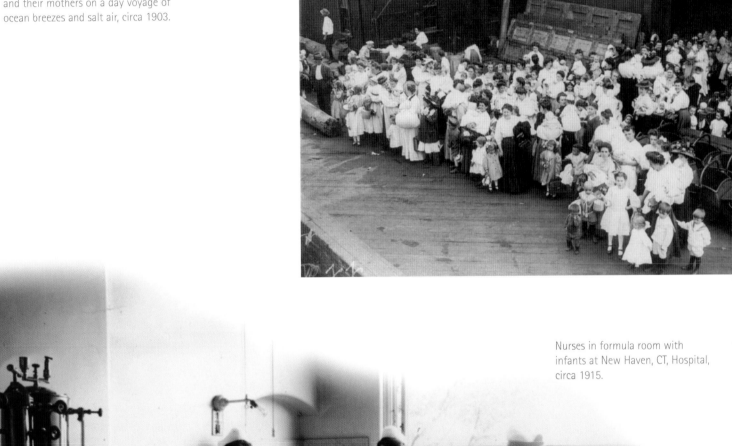

Nurses in formula room with infants at New Haven, CT, Hospital, circa 1915.

THE BEGINNINGS OF AMERICAN PEDIATRICS

The first 2 centuries in America were perilous times for children. Great epidemics of infectious diseases swept through the country killing literally thousands of infants and children. Smallpox was particularly feared, and epidemics occurred with regularity. In 1721 an epidemic in Boston, MA, led to the first significant advance in American medicine when the Reverend Cotton Mather persuaded a physician, Zabdiel Boylston, to employ variolization (inoculation of pus from a small pox lesion) in an attempt to curb the spread of the disease. This procedure was not widely accepted by either the medical or theological communities, and it was not until 80 years later when Benjamin Waterhouse, MD, professor of medicine at the Harvard Medical School, introduced vaccination using cowpox material obtained from Edward Jenner, that more effective prevention became possible.

During 1735 to 1740 in New England, a huge epidemic of the "throat distemper," or diphtheria, occurred that killed more than 5,000 people, of a total population of about 200,000 people. Eighty percent of these deaths occurred in children younger than 10 years old. One of the great tragedies of the epidemic was the death of multiple children in the same family.

As Ernest Caulfield, MD, an important American pediatric historian, wrote:

"In addition to diphtheria, dysentery, measles, and scarlet fever, smallpox, influenza, and tuberculosis should certainly be included in the list of common diseases of colonial children. A surprisingly large proportion of them had worms. Deaths from falls, burns, and poisonings were frequent. It seems a little surprising that any of them survived."

The infant death rate during these times has been estimated to be as high as 300 per 1,000 births. The high rate of death was accompanied by a high birth rate, the average family having about 9 children. Reverend Mather had 14 children, only 1 of whom survived him. Only 1 of President Thomas Jefferson's 6 children survived him.

Although the medical care of children in the English colonies in the 17th and 18th centuries was largely provided by parents, midwives, and nurses, a few colonial leaders who were concerned with children's diseases can be identified. John Winthrop, Jr, governor of Connecticut in the mid-17th century, conducted an extensive, if unusual, pediatric practice through the colonial mails. Winthrop's correspondence described a wide range of pediatric problems such as rashes, jaundice, seizures, and diarrhea.

In one of the letters to Winthrop requesting his medical advice, there even is a clear description of child abuse.

Colonial physicians, who were usually uneducated, poorly trained practitioners, wielded a variety of mostly ineffective remedies and anecdotal treatments, but some of them were careful

1650
Governor John Winthrop, Jr, of Connecticut practiced pediatrics and dispensed medications through the colonial mails. (New Haven, CT, and Hartford, CT)

1721
Reverend Cotton Mather and physician Zabdiel Boylston introduced variolization to abort a smallpox outbreak. (Boston, MA)

Gravestones of Mrs Martha Gott and her 5 children, who died of "throat distemper" (diphtheria)—Nathaniel, died October 29; Rebekah, died November 14; Martha, died November 15; John, died November 29; and Josiah, died December 5, 1737, Wenham, MA.

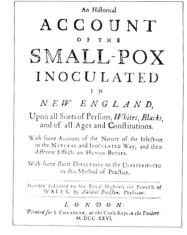

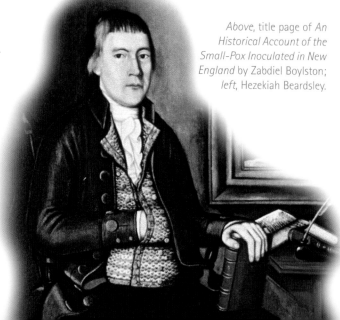

Above, title page of *An Historical Account of the Small-Pox Inoculated in New England* by Zabdiel Boylston; *left,* Hezekiah Beardsley.

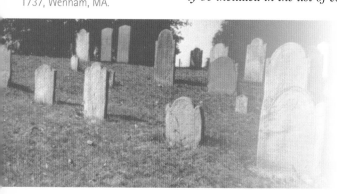

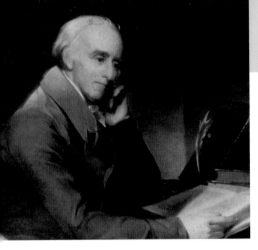

Benjamin Rush, MD.

1735–1740
New England diphtheria epidemic killed 5,000 people, mostly children.

1765
Founding of the Medical College of the College of Philadelpia (now University of Pennsylvania), the first American medical school. (Philadelphia, PA)

1788
Hezekiah Beardsley described a patient with hypertrophic pyloric stenosis of infancy. His paper was rediscovered and republished by William Osler, MD, in 1903. (New Haven, CT)

observers. Hezekiah Beardsley, a Connecticut physician and pharmacist, described the clinical course and autopsy findings of a child with a "schirrhus" of the pylorus, writing in the *Cases and Observations* publication by the Medical Society of New Haven County, CT, in 1788. In 1903, this early report was rediscovered by William Osler, MD, who said that Beardsley had first described the disease of hypertrophic pyloric stenosis "clearly and accurately."

Although universities and colleges were founded early in the American colonial period, they emphasized classical and theological curricula. Training in secular subjects such as medicine came much later with the establishment of colleges of medicine. The first American medical schools were the Medical College of the College of Philadelphia (now University of Pennsylvania) in Philadelphia, PA, established in 1765; the School of Medicine of King's College (now Columbia University), founded in New York, NY, in 1768, which became the College of Physicians and Surgeons in 1813; and Harvard Medical School, established in Boston in 1783. Teaching about children and their diseases was done sporadically, if at all, at the early medical schools and then by professors of physic (medicine) or midwifery (obstetrics).

At the University of Pennsylvania, Benjamin Rush, MD, a preeminent American patriot physician and a signer of the Declaration of Independence, was professor of medicine between 1789 and 1813. Dr Rush's medical lectures included a section on "Diseases Peculiar to Children." He published articles describing children's diseases such as spasmodic asthma, diseases of the mind, and diphtheria. Dr Rush also coined the term *cholera infantum* to describe the lethal summer diarrhea that killed thousands of American children well into the middle of the 20th century.

In 1825 William Potts Dewees, MD, professor of midwifery at the University of Pennsylvania, published his *Treatise on the Physical and Medical Treatment of Children*. This book (which had 8 subsequent editions) was divided into 2 parts: a section on the care of the pregnant woman and the newborn, and a section on the care of older infants and children.

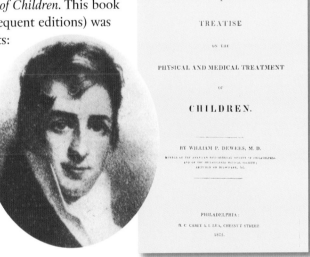

William Potts Dewees, MD, and the title page of his *Treatise on the Physical and Medical Treatment of Children*.

> "The European practice is generally too slow and too mild for children's diseases in this country. Diseases here are more violent, owing probably to the greater vicissitudes of the weather."

ELI IVES, MD, IN THE INTRODUCTION TO HIS COURSE ON DISEASES OF CHILDREN, 1820

1789
Benjamin Rush, MD, gave lectures on the diseases of children at the University of Pennsylvania School of Medicine and coined the term *cholera infantum* for summer diarrheal disease. (Philadelphia, PA)

1800
Benjamin Waterhouse, MD, introduced vaccination for smallpox using the cowpox vaccine of Edward Jenner, discovered a few years earlier in England. Dr Waterhouse's 5-year-old son was the first person in the American states to be vaccinated. (Boston, MA)

Eli Ives, MD, and the frontispiece of one of his lectures on the diseases of children.

The first formal medical school course and the first faculty appointment in the diseases of children in the United States were at the Medical Institution of Yale College in New Haven, CT. Between 1813 and 1852, Eli Ives, MD, who was appointed as professor of the diseases of children, presented a series of lectures on the topic.

His motivation for teaching this subject was because

> *"Diseases and remedies of the infantile state (are) a subject that has received little attention from Enlightened Physicians. The difficulty of acquiring a knowledge of disease in infants results from their inability to communicate their sensations by language."*

Dr Ives' lectures, recorded by hand in his students' notebooks, consisted of discourses on a wide range of subjects ranging from angina to worms. Dr Ives ascribed many illnesses to offending substances in the intestines. Teething was the cause of many infantile diseases and lancing of the gums was considered essential. Dr Ives' therapeutic sheet anchors were calomel (mercury) and ipecac, but he mainly emphasized a wide variety of herbal remedies. Dr Ives rarely employed bloodletting or leeches or other "heroic remedies."

As the 19th century progressed, there was increasing skepticism about the effectiveness of medical remedies, leading Oliver Wendell Holmes, MD, to quip in 1860:

> *"I firmly believe that if the whole materia medica, as now used, could be sunk to the bottom of the sea, it would be all the better for mankind and all the worse for the fishes."*

The first medical institutions for the care of children were foundling homes for the shelter of abandoned infants. Infants committed to these institutions had a virtually 100% mortality from infections as indicated by remarks by Job Lewis Smith, MD, to the American Pediatric Society (APS) in 1889.

> *"The steamboat every morning brought foundlings to the [Randall's] Island and every afternoon removed an equal number for burial in Potters' Field."*

The 12-bed Children's Hospital of Philadelphia, which opened in 1855, was dedicated to the treatment of poor children. The 20-bed Children's Hospital Boston opened in 1869. These were the first American hospitals to offer treatment of children's diseases and accidents exclusively.

The need to separate sick children from adult patients was increasingly recognized, especially by nonphysicians, as illustrated by an 1886 report by the Lady Visitors (women's auxiliary) to the directors of the New Haven Hospital:

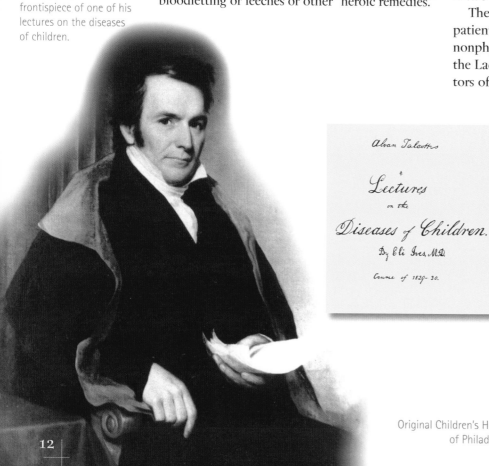

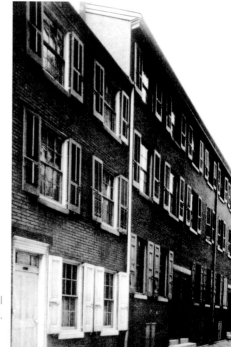

Original Children's Hospital of Philadelphia.

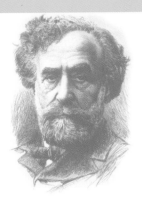

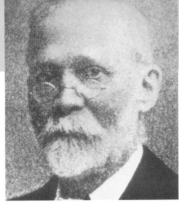

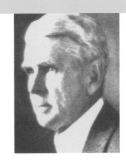

Three pediatric pioneers. *Left to right,* Abraham Jacobi, MD; Job Lewis Smith, MD; and L. Emmett Holt, Sr, MD.

1813
Eli Ives, MD, was appointed professor of the diseases of children and conducted the first formal courses in pediatrics in the United States at the Medical Institution of Yale College. (New Haven, CT)

1825
William Potts Dewees, MD, published the first American pediatric textbook *(Treatise on the Physical and Medical Treatment of Children).* (Philadelphia, PA)

"The Lady Visitors must urgently call attention to the great need of a separate Children's Ward. At present, children and nervous women patients are in the same ward to the detriment of both. Patients with nervous complaints should not be subject to noise; nor should poor children, whose lives are dull enough at best, be deprived of the small amount of pleasure and fun that is available."

By the end of the 19th century, there were more than 2 dozen children's hospitals around the country, and many more children's wards and nurseries within general hospitals.

Pediatric progress was evident in New York, where Abraham Jacobi, MD, and Dr Job Lewis Smith were contemporaries in the latter part of the 19th century. Dr Jacobi received his medical training in Germany. After graduation, he was imprisoned for 2 years as a suspected communist revolutionary. He emigrated to New York in 1853 and devoted most of his professional life to caring for children and treating their diseases.

In 1860, Dr Jacobi established a children's clinic at the New York Homeopathic Medical College (now New York Medical College), and held an appointment as professor of infantile pathology and therapeutics. He was instrumental in the founding in 1880 of the Section on Diseases of Children of the American Medical Association (AMA), the first national pediatric association. He effectively championed causes that promoted the welfare of children. His drive and enthusiasm were instrumental in establishing pediatrics as a separate discipline in the United States, and he has been rightly designated *"the father of American pediatrics."*

Dr Smith, who entered practice in Manhattan, NY, at about the same time as Jacobi, also played a major role in American pediatrics. Dr Smith worked primarily at the Bellevue Hospital

Medical College, where he was appointed clinical professor of diseases of children in 1876. One of Dr Smith's signal accomplishments was the founding of the APS. In 1888, 43 physicians who were interested and involved in pediatrics were the founders. The 43 founding members were mostly from the northeastern United States, but there were 2 members from Chicago, IL; 2 from Canada; and 1 each from St Louis, MO; Cincinnati, OH; and Ann Arbor, MI. For nearly 50 years, the APS was the preeminent pediatric organization in the United States. The presentations and discussions that took place at the APS annual meetings, as recorded in the annual *Transactions of the American Pediatric Society,* documented progress and advances of the specialty.

L. Emmett Holt, Sr, MD, of New York, can be largely credited with establishing a scientific basis for modern pediatrics in the United States. Following his graduation from the College of Physicians and Surgeons in 1878, Dr Holt entered private practice in midtown Manhattan. He became the medical director of a failing New York Hospital, which he redesigned as the modern Babies Hospital in 1910. In addition to outpatient facilities and 70 inpatient beds, the hospital had a dedicated research laboratory. Dr Holt also played a major role in the founding of the Rockefeller Institute for Medical Research and, with Rockefeller scientists, published a score of papers dealing with the chemical analysis of milk and milk proteins, salt and water balance, and absorption of nutrients and electrolytes in diarrheal diseases.

One of Dr Holt's greatest accomplishments was the authorship of a classic pediatric textbook, *The Diseases of Infancy and Childhood.* First published in 1897, it had 11 subsequent editions during Dr Holt's lifetime. It became the standard

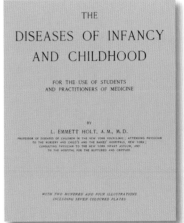

Title page of first edition of *The Diseases of Infancy and Childhood* by L. Emmett Holt, Sr, MD (1897).

1854
The founding of the Children's Hospital of Philadelphia.

1860
Abraham Jacobi, MD, was appointed professor of infantile pathology and therapeutics at the New York Medical College.

1869
Founding of Children's Hospital Boston.

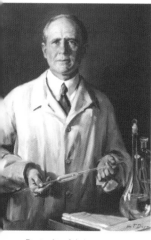

Portrait of John Howland, MD.

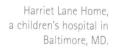

Harriet Lane Home, a children's hospital in Baltimore, MD.

American pediatric textbook and was considered the equal of Dr Osler's monumental *Textbook of Internal Medicine*. This textbook has continued since 1897, and is published today as *Rudolph's Pediatrics*. Dr Holt also authored an enormously popular and influential manual for parents entitled, *The Care and Feeding of Children*. Dr Holt was mentor and teacher of a number of physicians who became pediatric leaders, including John Howland, MD.

Dr Howland, one of the greatest figures in American pediatrics, became a full-time professor of pediatrics at the Johns Hopkins University School of Medicine and the Harriet Lane Home, its affiliated children's hospital. In the years between 1912 and 1926, he built and directed the first modern, full-time, scientifically based department of pediatrics. Howland trained a large group of men and women who became leaders of American pediatrics for the next quarter of a century, including Edwards A. Park, MD; Grover F. Powers, MD; James L. Gamble, MD; Kenneth D. Blackfan, MD; Benjamin Kramer, MD; and many others.

By the end of the 19th century, there were 119 American medical schools (excluding the many proprietary diploma mills). About half of these had designated chairmen of pediatrics, although most of these were also private practitioners. The APS was in its second decade and had 60 active members who met annually in the spring to report their research studies. The APS conducted national studies of scurvy and the effects of antitoxin in diphtheria. There were 4 active pediatric journals as well as several definitive pediatric textbooks. There were more than 2 dozen

children's hospitals, widely scattered in cities across the United States.

The terms *pediatry* or *pediology* were often used to describe the specialty and children's physicians were called *pediatrists* or *pediologists*, but, toward the end of the 19th century, the designations *pediatrics* and *pediatrician* became nearly universally used. Thus, by the turn of the 20th century, pediatrics had an accepted name as well as a significant body of clinical and scientific knowledge, plus a cadre of bright, motivated, and committed practitioners, investigators, and teachers. These provided a solid base for launching the century of progress to follow, which was given further impetus by progressive societal and political changes occurring at the dawn of the 20th century.

INFANT FEEDING AND NUTRITION

"Nutrition," wrote Dr Holt in his classic textbook, *The Diseases of Infancy and Childhood*, in 1897, "in its broadest sense is the most important branch of pediatrics." The first generation of pediatric specialists had little to offer their ailing patients in the way of effective drugs or therapies. One can argue that it was expertise in infant feeding that first gave credibility to pediatricians in the eyes of mothers. The story of the pediatrician as "baby feeder" thus constitutes one of the most important concepts leading to modern pediatrics.

Feeding and nutrition were especially important issues in the late 19th century, when an estimated 10% to 15% of babies in large urban areas never lived to see their first birthday. Of the many social and environmental factors contributing to this appalling loss of life, early pediatric leaders, such as Drs Jacobi, Smith, and Holt, singled out gastroenteritis as the number one killer of infancy.

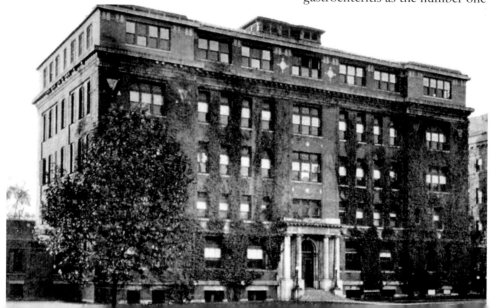

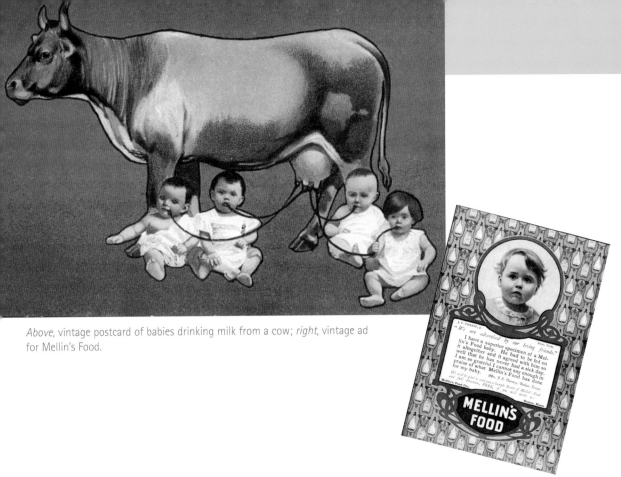

Above, vintage postcard of babies drinking milk from a cow; *right*, vintage ad for Mellin's Food.

1876
Job Lewis Smith, MD, was appointed clinical professor of the diseases of children at Bellevue Hospital Medical College. (New York, NY)

1880
The founding of the American Medical Association Section on Diseases of Children (later to become known as the Section on Pediatrics) by Abraham Jacobi, MD.

Every summer in New York and other eastern cities, epidemic diarrhea swept through the sweltering heat of the tenement districts. Countless infants died of dehydration. Those who survived were frequently left weakened and vulnerable to later illness, initiating a vicious cycle of malnutrition and recurrent infection all too often culminating in death.

Though many environmental factors likely contributed to this phenomenon, Dr Jacobi and his pediatric colleagues increasingly pointed to the role of contaminated or impure milk. Breastfeeding rates had declined over the course of the 19th century. Many mothers of the urban poor, compelled to work outside the home, weaned their infants at an ever-younger age out of sheer necessity. Middle- and upper-class women increasingly chose not to breastfeed as well. The late 1800s witnessed the rise of a great deal of pseudoscientific speculation that the conditions of city life were somehow unfavorable to the constitutions of women and their capacity to nurse. Finally, wet nurses were expensive and often came from a social class difficult to accommodate into a "respectable" middle-class household.

Instead, mothers increasingly turned to modifications of cow's milk becoming available on the market by the late 1800s. Many of these early infant formulas built on the scientific foundations laid by the great German chemist Justus von Liebig, who showed that milk could be characterized according to its proportions of carbohydrate, fat, and protein. The discovery spawned the rise of a fledgling infant formula industry that directly advertised its products to mothers. These early "infant foods" typically consisted of powdered supplements promising to bring the chemical constituents of cow milk in line with that of breast milk. The role of vitamins was unappreciated. These products, unfortunately, had to be mixed with commercially available cow milk that was, itself, highly suspect. Prior to later regulation, commercial dairy farming and processing standards in the 1800s left much to be desired. Reports abounded of milk contaminated by open sores on the cows and excrement, allowed to spoil in open cans exposed to flies, and adulterated with molasses or other additives to mask the taste. Though reformers recognized that other environmental factors such as contaminated water contributed to infant diarrhea, it was the shortcomings of modified cow milk that occupied their attention.

All pediatricians agreed in proclaiming "pure milk" to be the solution, but disagreed vehemently over what this meant. For Dr Jacobi, the answer was simple—some form of sterilized milk. During the 1880s, the bacteriological revolution, led by Louis Pasteur and Robert Koch, MD, was in full swing. Boiling milk to eliminate pathogens, however, changed its color and taste, making it objectionable for both doctor and baby. A better solution gradually emerged in the form of what became known as pasteurization—briefly heating the milk to a set temperature (eventually defined as 140°F). This had originally been devised by Louis Pasteur as a way to prevent the souring of wine, and Pasteur was credited for saving the French wine industry. Before it was recognized as a way to prevent milk-born infections, pasteurization was used commercially to extend the "shelf life" of liquid milk. Dr Jacobi championed this approach, initially hoping that it could be accomplished at home with inexpensive equipment. The difficulties of implementing this scheme led to a second approach—the provision of pasteurized and modified infant milk free of charge in so-called "milk stations." New York merchant and philanthropist Nathan Straus opened the first of these in 1893. Within 10 years, Straus's milk stations were dispensing nearly 2 million bottles annually, and his approach was becoming a central strategy of infant mortality reformers in other cities.

For years, many leading pediatricians were ambivalent about pasteurization. The role played by microbes in diarrhea remained unclear until well into the 20th century. Though today it is suspected that enteropathogenic *Escherichia coli* accounted for much of the summer gastroenteritis phenomenon, contemporary investigators lacked the tools to distinguish pathogenic from normal gut flora, much less identify viruses. To many physicians it seemed more likely that bacteria played a secondary role. The oppressive heat and poor ventilation of summer, it was argued, generated a chemical degeneration of milk that predisposed infants to indigestion and secondary infection. By this reasoning, milk had to be more than bacteriologically pure; it had to be chemically sound. Pediatricians focused their energy on improving the quality of artificial milk to match breast milk.

The greatest proponent of *scientifically based* artificial feeding was Harvard's first professor of pediatrics, Thomas Morgan Rotch, MD. Feeding babies was too important, from Dr Rotch's view, to be left to commercial interests or to mothers. It was not enough to imitate the basic chemical composition of breast milk; the components of artificial milk had to be modified on an *individual basis*, to the needs of the particular infant. For this purpose, Dr Rotch devised an elaborate set of calculations that became known as the "percentage system," which won wide adherence

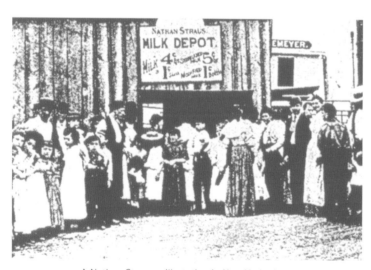

A Nathan Straus milk station in New York, circa 1893.

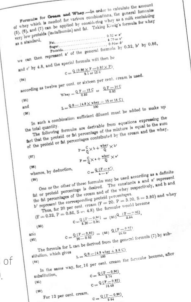

Infant formula calculations of
Thomas Morgan Rotch, MD.

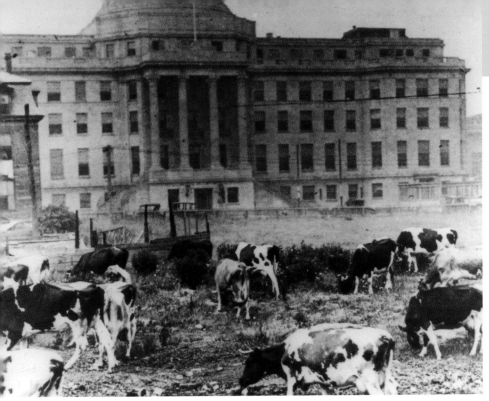

The fourth Children's Hospital Boston in 1914; the cows grazing nearby provided certified milk for Thomas Morgan Rotch, MD.

1894
Charles W. Townsend, MD, described "hemorrhagic disease of the newborn." (Boston, MA)

1896
The American Pediatric Society published results on the use of antitoxin for the treatment of diphtheria—the first national American pediatric investigation.

1897
L. Emmett Holt, Sr, MD, published his classic textbook, *The Diseases of Infancy and Childhood.* (New York, NY)

among his fellow pediatricians at the turn of the century. Just as the surgeon wielded his scalpel and the eye specialist an ophthalmoscope, the pediatric specialist carried a slide rule, working out minute calculations using complex algebraic calculations to prescribe a highly specific milk "formula" tailored to the infant in question. The system proved so complicated that Dr Rotch encouraged the development of commercial milk laboratories in Boston that could function as the equivalent of pharmacies for pediatricians' milk prescriptions.

"Percentage feeding" was enormously popular in the United States during its heyday at the turn of the last century, and, though short-lived, had a number of important consequences for the specialty's future. For one, it helped fix the pediatrician in the public's mind as a "baby feeder"—a role that has remained central to general pediatrics today.

Regrettably, by associating artificial feeding with "science," Dr Rotch's system further undercut the value of breastfeeding in the eyes of many pediatricians and at least some mothers. In the short term, the emphasis on calculating the chemical balance of infant milk so precisely initially led most pediatricians to oppose pasteurization as well, since it could be easily shown that heating disrupted milk's chemical composition. Pediatricians recognized that pure milk had to be free of contamination, but favored voluntary milk certification over pasteurization. This solution, adopted in a number of cities, set up boards of pediatricians charged to "certify" a particular model dairy farm as providing milk of the highest quality, allowing the dairy to charge a considerably higher price. Though acknowledged by all sides as the ideal solution to the milk question, the great expense and limited availability of

"A pair of substantial mammary glands has the advantage over the two hemispheres of the most learned professor's brain in the art of compounding a nutritious fluid for infants."

OLIVER WENDELL HOLMES, MD

1898
Joseph B. DeLee, MD, established the first premature infant incubator station in the United States. (Chicago, IL)

1908
The Chicago Board of Health mandated pasteurization of milk.

S. Josephine Baker, MD, developed an effective approach to combat infant mortality via preventive education. (New York, NY)

1909
The first White House Conference on the Care of Dependent Children was convened by President Theodore Roosevelt. (Washington, DC)

certified milk limited its application and diverted attention from the vast majority of infants.

Dr Jacobi, always sensitive to the constraints of the poor, continued to advocate simple modifications of pasteurized milk over Dr Rotch's system. Jacobi once characteristically quipped, *"You cannot feed babies with mathematics, you must feed them with brains."*

By 1910 most pediatricians were inclined to agree. The system to some extent collapsed under the weight of its own complexity. Newer pediatric science, while continuing to recognize that Dr Rotch's basic goal of imitating breast milk was sound, suggested that he had gone too far in manipulating formula so precisely on a changing day-to-day basis. Dr Rotch's successor at Harvard (and later second president of the American Academy of Pediatrics [AAP]), John L. Morse, MD, conducted important studies that marked a shift from calculating percentages to determining the caloric content of milk. These principles, as well as others elaborating the key components of breast milk and cow milk, laid the groundwork for much more fruitful collaboration between pediatricians and public health workers that would soon have dramatic results.

First among these accomplishments was the rise of commercial pasteurization. By 1908, when Chicago became the first American city to mandate pasteurization, refinements in the process itself had made it less objectionable to pediatricians. At the same time, the limitations of the milk station approach had become increasingly evident. Though the milk depots dispensed literally millions of bottles, they still reached only a fraction of the poor. Obtaining fresh milk on a daily basis was simply not practical for many mothers. Moreover, gastroenteritis rates failed to decline even after a decade of intensive milk station work. As it became evident that pasteurization had to be applied on a broad scale, the twin strategies of milk stations and milk certification gave way to mandatory commercial milk pasteurization in the second decade of the century. Pasteurization joined other public health strategies, notably improved water quality and maternal education efforts supporting breastfeeding. Mortality from gastroenteritis fell sharply in eastern cities and, by 1920, New York's once devastating summer diarrhea epidemics had largely vanished.

Sterilizing milk for children at Northwestern University, IL, settlement houses in 1903.

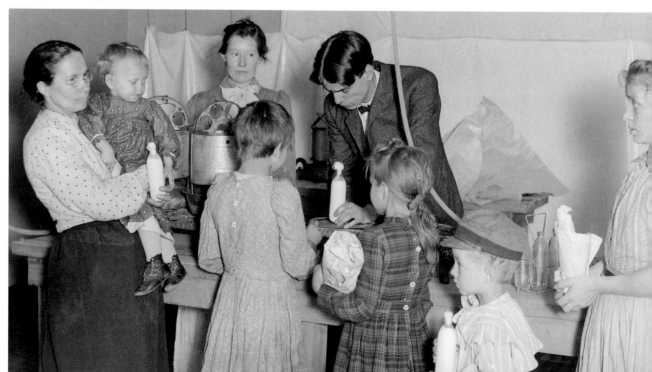

Scurvy and Rickets

In the mid-1940s, we began to see a number of cases of scurvy, despite their mothers insisting that they were getting their "orange juice" every day. It turns out that some mothers were using orange soda pop instead of orange juice because it was much cheaper—a 12-oz portion of orange soda was only 5 cents and lasted 3 or 4 days. Education of mothers eliminated the problem.

The prevention of rickets had some mishaps as well. It had been proven in the 1930s that cod liver oil prevented rickets, but in the 1940s, new concentrated vitamin D preparations such as oleum percomorph were introduced. Babies were liberated from having to take the thick, horrendous tasting, awful smelling teaspoonful a day of cod liver oil. Then we began to see a number of infants with hypervitaminosis D who presented with severe headaches and hair loss. We discovered that mothers were giving their infants teaspoonfuls of the new concentrates instead of 0.6 cc. It took several years to reeducate mothers about the conversion.

— *David Annunziato, MD*

1912
John Howland, MD, was appointed as professor of pediatrics at the Johns Hopkins University School of Medicine and the Harriet Lane Home for Invalid Children. (Baltimore, MD)

The US Children's Bureau was established by Congress. (Washington, DC)

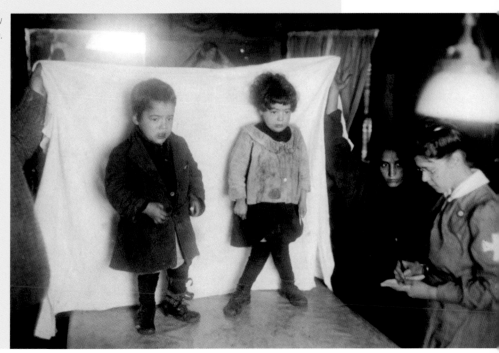

Children with rickets visiting a New Haven, CT, nurse clinic, circa 1920.

Sir William Osler on Infant Feeding

"According to exhaustive research by the Pediatric Society there is no single question before this nation today of greater importance than how to return to natural methods in the nurture of infants. You can easily tell a man who was bottle fed by feeling the tip of his nose. In all sucklings, because of the physical effects of breast pressure on the nose, the two cartilages are kept separate and do not join. In the bottle fed baby, where there is no pressure on the tip of the nose, the cartilages rapidly unite and in the adult present to the finger a single sharp outline, entirely different from the split, bifed condition of the breast fed infant. Research by the Pediatric Society on the future of bottle fed babies clearly shows that all kinds of intellectual obliquity, moral perversion, and special crankiness in adults result from the early warp given to the mind by this gross and unworthy deception during the most plastic period of a baby's life."

— *Tongue-in-cheek remarks by Sir William Osler at a "Festival" honoring Abraham Jacobi on his 70th birthday, New York, May 5, 1900. (Adapted from Cushing H.* The Life of Sir William Osler. *Oxford, England: Clarendon Press; 1925.)*

19

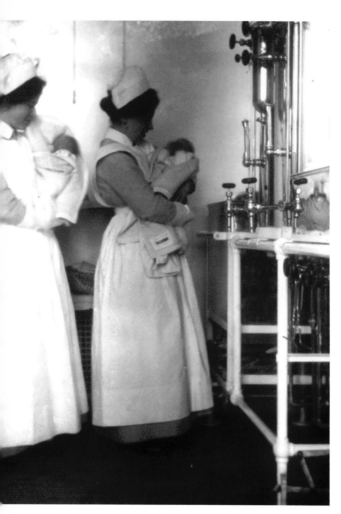

Nurses holding infants in a formula room.

The recognition of vitamins constituted the next success story. Pediatricians had long asserted that proprietary infant foods, and later pasteurized milk, contributed to scurvy and rickets. Yet the real causes for these common afflictions remained uncertain. Scurvy continued to be regarded as essentially a disease of seamen long after the famous shipboard experiments of James Lind, MD, in the mid-1700s demonstrated the role of lime juice in its prevention. Pediatricians finally recognized the condition in infants in the late 1800s, but tended to blame it on artificial or sterilized milk per se. Gradually Henry Koplik, MD, and others began to discard this theory in favor of hypothesizing a missing factor, later to be designated vitamin C. Ascorbic acid was isolated in 1928 and shown to cure scurvy 5 years later.

Perhaps the most notable contribution of American pediatrics to infant feeding in the early 20th century was its role in the identification of vitamin D. Rickets was a condition that had actually become more common during the course of industrialization, and by the 1880s had become one of the most common afflictions of children. Theories over its causation tended to be polarized between those emphasizing the roles of nutrition versus fresh air and sunshine. Cod liver oil had been used as a folk remedy since the late 1700s, but was dismissed as empirical by most investigators in the early 20th century. The search for the nature of the "anti-rachitic factor" became one of the driving forces behind the team of clinicians and biochemist assembled by the first chairman of pediatrics at the Johns Hopkins University School of Medicine, Dr John Howland. There, biochemist Elmer Verner McCollum scored a major breakthrough by showing that cod liver oil contained a factor that protected laboratory rats from rickets even when fed a diet with an unfavorable balance of calcium and phosphorous. After the essential factor was designated vitamin D, an Iowa pediatrician, Philip C. Jeans, MD, convinced the AMA Council on Foods and Nutrition in the 1930s to recommend that milk be routinely fortified. The incidence of nutritional rickets declined dramatically over the course of the 20th century.

Aided by the discovery of vitamins and many other advances in nutritional research, confidence in bottle-feeding continued to rise throughout the first half of the 20th century. Interestingly, artificial formula itself became simpler. Studies in the 1920s seemed to show that infants grew as well with simple standardized formulas or even evaporated milk as with breast milk or complex formulas. The problem of iron deficiency was not anticipated until much later. The percentage method was relegated to an amusing anecdote that many pediatricians recalled from training, its most tangible legacy being the fact that infant milk in the United States continues to this day to be called "formula." The profession also as a whole became much more comfortable with manufactured infant formula so long as it was not

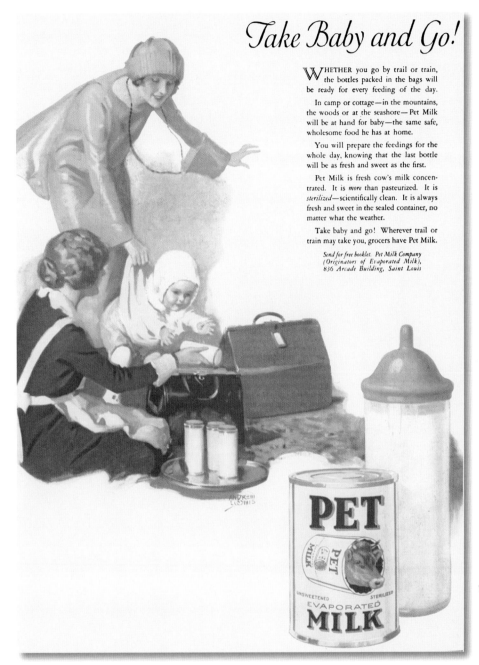

Take Baby and Go!

WHETHER you go by trail or train, the bottles packed in the bags will be ready for every feeding of the day.

In camp or cottage—in the mountains, the woods or at the seashore—Pet Milk will be at hand for baby—the same safe, wholesome food he has at home.

You will prepare the feedings for the whole day, knowing that the last bottle will be as fresh and sweet as the first.

Pet Milk is fresh cow's milk concentrated. It is *more* than pasteurized. It is *sterilized*—scientifically clean. It is always fresh and sweet in the sealed container, no matter what the weather.

Take baby and go! Wherever trail or train may take you, grocers have Pet Milk.

Send for free booklet. Pet Milk Company (Originators of Evaporated Milk), 836 Arcade Building, Saint Louis

PET MILK

UNSWEETENED   STERILIZED
EVAPORATED
MILK

Vintage Pet Milk advertisement.

advertised to the public (a move enforced by the AMA "seal of approval" in the 1930s). There would be troubling consequences of this relationship to be sure, and the AAP, in the late 20th century, would dramatically shift its efforts back to the advocacy of breastfeeding.

But in the 1920s, physicians and mothers alike saw the rise of artificial feeding as one of the greatest gifts bestowed by modern science to children. Infant mortality from gastroenteritis had indeed fallen dramatically at the same time as the rise of bottle-feeding. For many mothers, the bottle had become a symbol of science, and

the pediatrician had attained a new level of prestige as an expert in nutrition. Still, the increasing reliance on artificial feeding cannot fully explain how the pediatrician became a trusted adviser on many issues going far beyond formula. The many facets of raising children, ranging from moral guidance to toilet training, had long been the purview of women. It would be women who would play a central role in the invention of well-child care as a central task of pediatrics by the 1930s, for historical reasons closely linked to first blossoming of social feminism in the Progressive Era.

A Brief History of Infant Feeders

1922
Elmer Verner McCollum;
Edwards A. Park, MD;
Benjamin Kramer, MD;
and John Howland, MD,
described blood
chemistries in rickets and
the benefit of sunlight
and cod liver oil.
(Baltimore, MD)

Julius H. Hess, MD, pub-
lished *Premature and
Congenitally Diseased
Infants*, the first
American textbook on
prematurity. (Chicago, IL)

1928
Alexander Fleming
serendipitously discov-
ered penicillin. (London,
England)

1930
Founding of the
American Academy of
Pediatrics. (Detroit, MI)

Over the centuries, it was recognized that breastfed babies survived, while artificially fed infants survived poorly. Indeed, breastfeeding remains the gold standard of infant feeding today and producers of artificial milk have strived to emulate nature's product. Figures 1 and 2 show examples of early feeding devices from more than 2,000 years ago. Their primary use may have been in weaning from the breast and rarely for initial feeding of newborns.

During the middle ages, there were few significant changes except increased use of feeders provided by nature, such as animal horns and gourds. Infants in those years had the advantage of large extended families in close proximity allowing for wet nursing if the biologic mother was not available. Factors such as

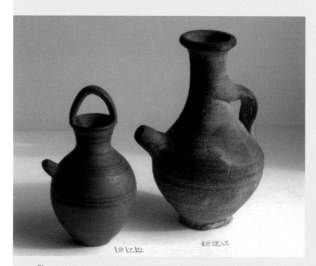

Figure 1

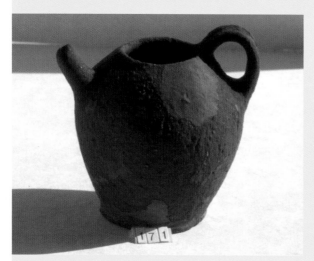

Figure 2

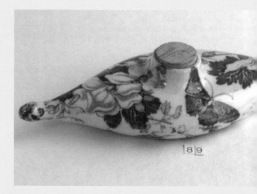

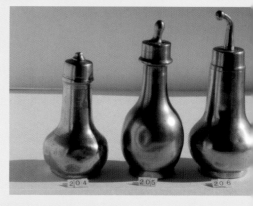

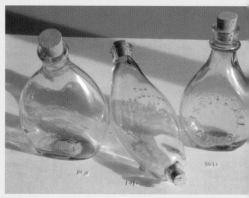

Top to bottom, figures 3, 4, and 5

the Renaissance, the Industrial Revolution, and migration for religious reasons broke the bond of the close extended family, necessitating the use of nonfamily wet nursing. Solicitations for wet nurses were one of the common advertisements in colonial newspapers, usually resulting in unsatisfactory results for the family. Thus began the need for other feeders and, in the late 1600s and 1700s, a profusion of bottles were marketed, including ceramic, metal, and glass types (Figures 3, 4, and 5). Glass-blown products were preferred; blowing glass into molds allowed for a large variety of feeders, including the Windship feeder (Figure 6). This was the first US patented feeder. It was mammary shaped and meant to be worn under the clothing, the nipple protruding through, fooling the infant into pseudo-nursing!

Elijah Pratt patented the first rubber nipple in 1845, after which the long-tube feeder became popular. This was finally outlawed by the city of Buffalo, NY, in 1897, being labeled the "murder bottle" (Figure 7)! (The rubber tubing developed small cracks allowing a haven for bacteria).

Sterilizers became popular as did bottles that would fit into them. William Decker, MD, of Kingston, NY, introduced the Hygeia feeder (Figure 8) that allowed ease of cleaning. Although the nipples were also improving, they were often dislodged by the infant's sucking action, until the clamped-on nipple was developed in 1937. Glass feeders were totally phased out by the mid-1970s in favor of plastics.

During the mid-1900s, breastfeeding incidence dropped to a low of 20%. The urgings of pediatricians, certified lactation consultants, and La Leche League deserve credit for the resurgence in nursing. Will the 1900s be remembered as the century where the majority of infants were fed milk from other species in a plethora of oddly shaped bottles?!

— *Darroll J. Erickson, MD*

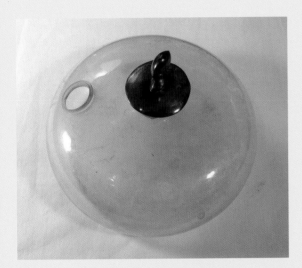

Figure 6

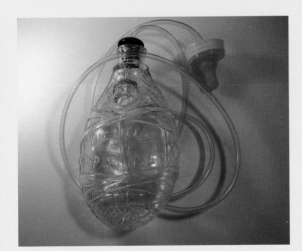

Figure 7

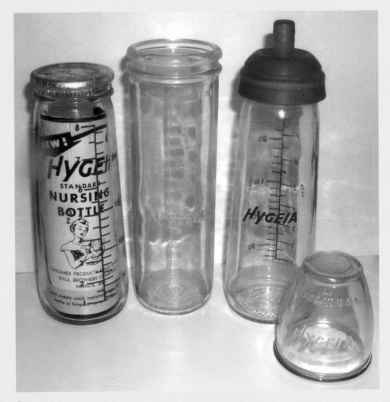

Figure 8

THE RISE OF PREVENTIVE PEDIATRICS

In 1900 the entire American pediatric profession could have been seated in a single, large conference room. Though ranging in interest and temperament, its members were united by Dr Holt's enthusiasm for the potential of science to transform the medical care of children. Days consisted of long hours attending largely indigent hospital patients in the morning, seeing private patients in the home or office in the afternoon, and writing case reports in the evening or any other time that could be found. Few effective drugs were available (a notable exception was diphtheria antitoxin). The pediatrician's chief therapeutic tool was his knowledge of infant feeding. The APS remained an exclusively male organization with a membership almost completely limited to eastern cities.

Not Just Formula Changes Anymore

I was advised by my academic teachers that pediatric practice was changing formulas and assuring patients that their child would "grow out of it." During my first week as the town's pediatrician, I was confronted with 2 retinoblastomas, one previously undiagnosed diabetic in a coma, and a preemie weighing 18 oz. Where were those formula changes?

— *Milton Arnold, MD*

By the time the AAP was founded in 1930, the profession had changed profoundly. Pediatricians could now be found in virtually every state, and in both rural and urban areas. Though hospital-based consultants continued to remain vigorous, most pediatricians were now community practitioners seeing most patients in the home or office. Most remarkably, the supervision of well infants and children had become a central feature of office pediatrics.

The rise of primary care pediatrics was not inevitable. British pediatricians, for example, continue to function chiefly as consultants. The reason why American pediatricians followed a different path reflects their own distinctive historical situation—namely, the reaction of physicians to the great child and infant welfare movements that swept the United States during the early 20th century.

It is not easy to pinpoint why such an outpouring of enthusiasm for improving the status of children erupted in the early 1900s. Child welfare reform was one facet of the broader Progressive reform movement that overtook the United States between the 1890s and the First World War. Confronted by what had previously seemed to be intractable social ills, Progressive reformers took great interest in childhood as the period of life during which outside intervention, especially education, would most likely have lasting influence. Middle-class women, often college-educated and yet with few career opportunities outside of teaching and nursing, became heavily involved in these campaigns. Women's clubs met to discuss the latest articles on child-rearing or social issues such as child labor and maternal health. Some women went so far as to move into the inner city and attempt to live life among the poor in urban "settlements," most famously the Jane Addams Hull-House

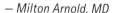

Jane Addams of Hull-House, Chicago, IL, circa 1913.

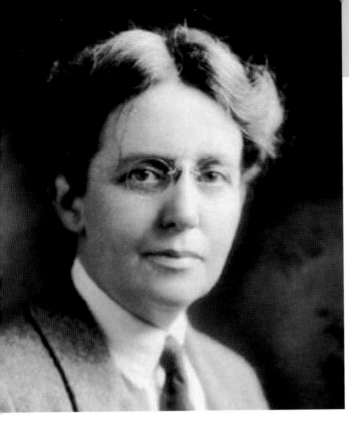

S. Josephine Baker, MD.

in Chicago. From the settlements would emerge some of the most influential child welfare leaders, such as Julia C. Lathrop, first director of the US Children's Bureau, and Lillian Wald, the American pioneer of visiting home nursing.

As the APS increasingly restricted its focus to the biomedical problems of childhood, these infant welfare reformers became the driving force for change. By 1910, summer deaths from gastroenteritis had hardly declined despite millions of bottles of pure milk being dispensed annually by the milk stations. Many reformers lost patience with this approach, pointing out that dispensing a bottle of clean milk was hardly likely to do much good if provided to the baby in a crowded and filthy tenement. The antidote, many believed, was already at hand in the form of the established principles of child health and hygiene. For the next 10 years, between 1910 and 1920, reformers enthusiastically embraced maternal education as the panacea for infant mortality. Milk stations

were transformed into infant welfare stations, staffed with nurses and voluntary physicians who could provide scientific advice to low-income mothers. Notably, and in marked contrast to most pediatricians of the era, these clinics encouraged breastfeeding.

Just how persuasive the new approach appeared to contemporaries is captured in the experience of New York, whose Bureau of Child Hygiene became a model for many other cities to follow. The division's director, S. Josephine Baker, MD, was a graduate of Women's Medical College of the New York Infirmary who, it can be argued, practiced pediatrics outside of the APS by working in a health department rather than a children's hospital. Assigned to the city's notorious Hell's Kitchen district just in time for the annual devastation from summer diarrhea, Dr Baker conducted a novel experiment. Instead of relying on milk stations, she sent the city's school nurses into the district to educate mothers on

Assigned to the city's notorious Hell's Kitchen district just in time for the annual devastation from summer diarrhea, Dr [S. Josephine] Baker conducted a novel experiment.... The infant mortality rate decreased by more than 1,200 deaths that summer, a success that soon won Dr Baker the directorship of the city's newly created Bureau of Child Hygiene.

breastfeeding, cleanliness, and infant care. The infant mortality rate decreased by more than 1,200 deaths that summer, a success that soon won Dr Baker the directorship of the city's newly created Bureau of Child Hygiene.

Dr Baker used the bureau to develop a 2-tiered approach to combat infant mortality via preventive education. She expanded the school nurses' duties into visiting home nursing, making each nurse responsible for meeting and educating all new mothers in a particular district during the entire summer. If breastfeeding was not possible or the infant was ill, mother and baby were referred to the second level of the system—examination by a volunteer physician at an infant welfare station. Visiting nurses held well-baby clinics and made home visits. As the system was expanded between 1908 and 1914, New York's infant mortality rate fell sharply from 144.4 to 94.6 per

1,000, the lowest of any major city in the United States or Europe. By the end of the decade, summer diarrhea epidemics had become a memory of the past. Though other factors, such as commercial pasteurization and improved sanitation, likely contributed, contemporaries saw Dr Baker's accomplishment as a vindication of the maternal education strategy.

"Baby-saving work" reached a crescendo at the time of the First World War (1914–1919), at which time a blast of patriotic energy infused the movement. Women's voluntary associations collaborated with churches and municipal governments to call for the reduction of infant mortality with an intensity approaching a religious revival. Many cities launched "baby week" campaigns promoting child health. Parades featured mothers marching like war heroes. A wide variety of exhibits, displays, and literature offered educational

Infants waiting to be examined at a 1913 "better babies contest."

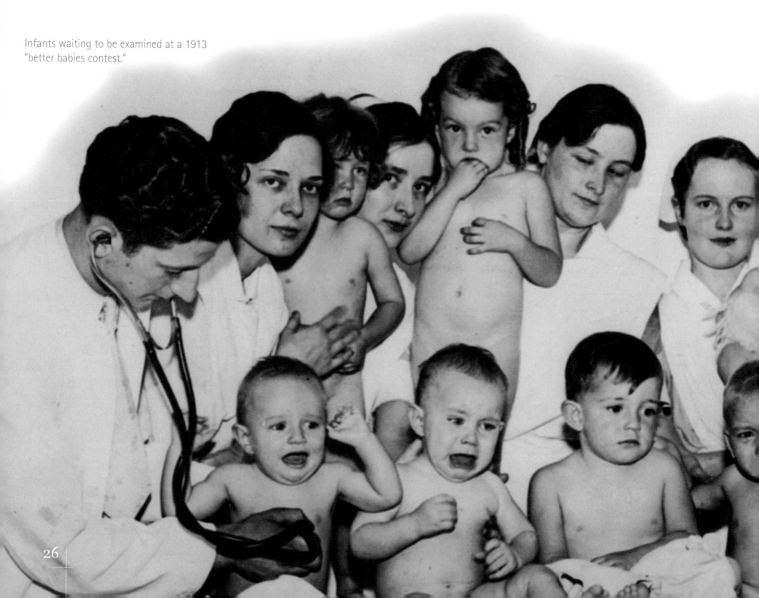

advice. Especially popular were "better baby contests," competitions in which plump infants were rated by judges using scorecards. Many reform leaders, it might be noted, frowned upon these contests, noting that blonde and blue-eyed babies tended to win disproportionately. All of these various enticements were intended to attract mothers to the central attraction, the chance to have a baby examined in a formal health consultation. Cities typically retained some combination of infant welfare stations and visiting nurse programs after the excitement had settled. Infant mortality rates dropped substantially around the country during the second decade of the century in concert with these changes, further energizing reformers.

Federal leadership was almost nonexistent prior to 1920, with one notable exception, the Children's Bureau. Established in 1912 as a result

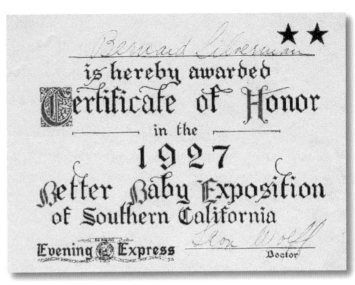

"Certificate of Honor" from a 1927 California better baby exposition.

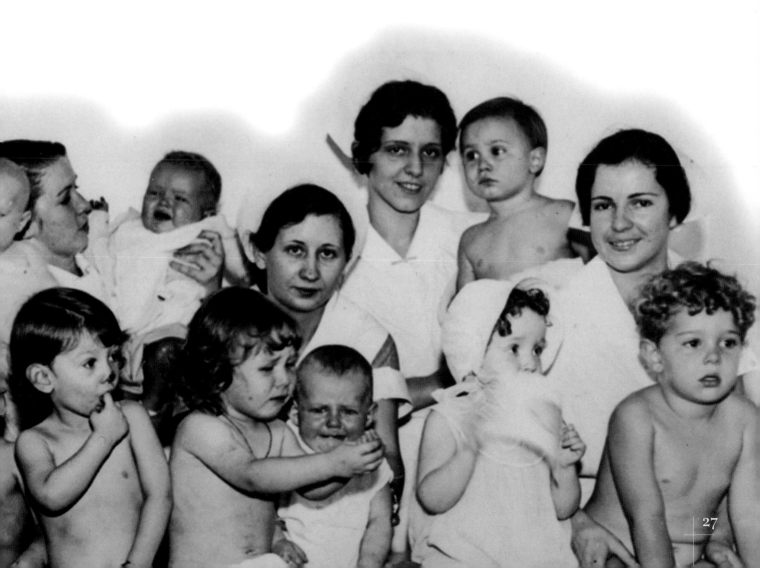

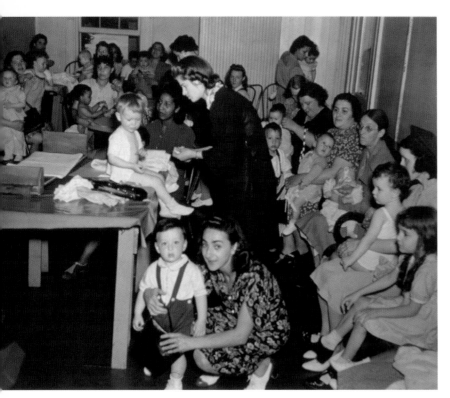

New Haven, CT, well-baby visiting nurse clinic, 1930.

letters requesting child health advice, to which bureau members often responded either with a personal reply or by contacting a local women's association to assist the writer.

All of these efforts reached a climax in 1921 with the passage of the Sheppard-Towner Maternity and Infancy Protection Act. Though relatively modest by today's standards, Sheppard-Towner marked the first major involvement of the federal government on behalf of children. Its passage was a direct consequence of the passage of the 19th amendment, providing women's suffrage the previous year. Women had long argued that infant welfare issues would be neglected until mothers could vote and, immediately following the amendment's passage, did in fact deluge Congress with a sea of letters advocating a federal law aimed at improving maternal and child health. Caught in an unprecedented political situation and fearful that women might truly vote in a block, Congress passed the legislation.

In its final form, the resulting Sheppard-Towner Act provided just over $1 million annually in matching funds for states to set up programs promoting infant health such as visiting nurses and preventive health clinics. Staffed by volunteer or (less often) by health department doctors, these clinics were free but referred problems requiring therapy to local physicians. They popularized child preventive health in rural areas, notably in the south and west. The Sheppard-Towner clinics also examined preschool children as well as infants. The response from mothers appears to have been overwhelmingly enthusiastic.

Nonetheless, as discussed in the next chapter, Sheppard-Towner quickly set off a political battle that would have direct consequences for pediatricians. The AMA condemned the act as "state medicine" and intrusion of government

of a recommendation from the first White House Conference on the Care of Dependent Children in 1909, the Children's Bureau consisted of a small staff composed entirely of women, led by the politically astute Julia Lathrop, a graduate of Hull-House with close ties to numerous women's associations around the country. The bureau relied on these organizations to conduct surveys of infant mortality and child health conditions around the country. It published a highly popular guide to childrearing, *Infant Care,* that popularized feeding schedules and early toilet training for the generation preceding Benjamin M. Spock, MD (of "Dr Spock" fame). Many mothers wrote

*Thus, the stage was set for the creation
of a new pediatric organization to represent
the new pediatrician.*

into private practice. Its opposition must be understood in the context of the more conservative political climate of the 1920s. Progressivism had expended much of its energy in the "War to End All Wars," and the success of the Soviet Bolshevik Revolution had incited a wave of anti-communist fear around the country. The AMA and a coalition of state medical societies joined a variety of unlikely allies, notably the Daughters of the American Revolution, to undercut support for Sheppard-Towner. Sustained opposition led to the act's expiration in 1929.

Even in defeat, Sheppard-Towner triumphed on one level. Physicians, particularly specialists in pediatrics and obstetrics, recognized the market demand for preventive health care. During the 1920s, a new generation of pediatrician emerged. One reason the infant welfare clinics had little trouble finding volunteer physicians, before and after Sheppard-Towner, was that these clinics provided experience in child health supervision that could not be obtained in hospitals. Physicians in these clinics learned to incorporate standardized medical records and growth charts into their own practice, and to offer well visits by appointment. In doing so they greatly expanded the scope of pediatrics. Between 1914 and 1934 the number of pediatricians in the country expanded more than tenfold. By the early 1930s most surveys indicated that well-child supervision accounted for roughly 40% of all office visits, not far from the proportion today.

The American pediatric profession had thus expanded dramatically by 1930 to a broad base of primary care physicians and a narrower contingent of hospital-based specialists. Thus, the stage was set for the creation of a new pediatric organization to represent the new pediatrician.

Reflections on Life and Death and Pediatrics

Having completed 50 years as a practicing pediatrician, my recollections are dominated by what lays out as a drama of life and death. Pediatrics is unique in that it allows us to pursue all of the ends of medicine—the diagnostic, the therapeutic, the preventive, and the perfective. As primary care, it certainly has its share of the tedious and the mundane. Life and death experiences in pediatrics, however, are remembered with a crystalline clarity—because they are never anything less than momentous. The first time I undertook the resuscitation of a premature newborn infant in the Hospital Lying-in Nursery at the University of Chicago, I felt a surge of emotion that I was not prepared for, even as a resident. Who could ever turn away from such need?

By the time I chose pediatrics as a career, I had already spent time as a corpsman in World War II and as a Marine battalion surgeon in the Korean War. I would have thought that I was prepared for the end of life events including those that were sudden, unexpected, and sanguinary. Nothing, however, truly prepares a physician for the death of a child. Standing at the bedside of a recently lost young life, it is almost impossible to convince yourself of the reality that "I am innocent." Did I prepare adequately for this moment of our joint jeopardy? Was this calamity really inevitable? Could this vibrant, blooming, captivating, pulsating luminescence really be snuffed out so seemingly effortlessly?

Yet, so much in our profession truly warms the soul. To gaze into those new eyes of a newborn. To spend an afternoon gazing down on those uniformly beautiful faces of infants and children. There is the incredible power of recuperation that turns a febrile, fearful, obtunded school-aged child into a smiling, grateful follow-up visit.

— *Eugene F. Diamond, MD*

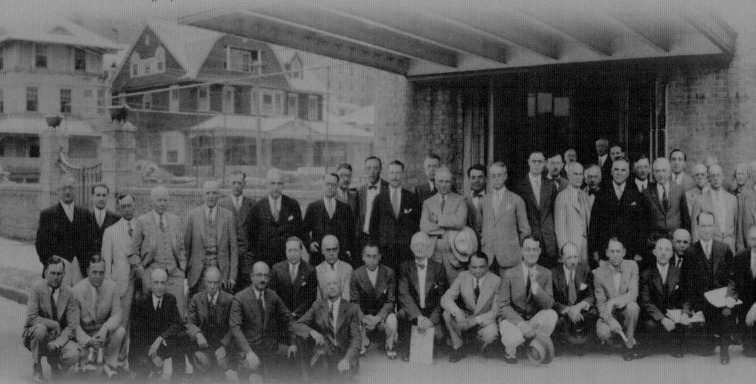

Panoramic shot of attendees (including at least 3 women) at the first Annual Meeting of the American Academy of Pediatrics in Atlantic City, NJ, 1931.

The actual origin of the
American Academy of Pediatrics can be traced to a
fateful gathering on July 19, 1929....
It was not long after the first course of dinner
that the subject of a new national pediatric society
was raised. It was immediately evident that many
pediatricians had been thinking the same way....

Chapter 2
The Birth of the American Academy of Pediatrics

1922 to 1935

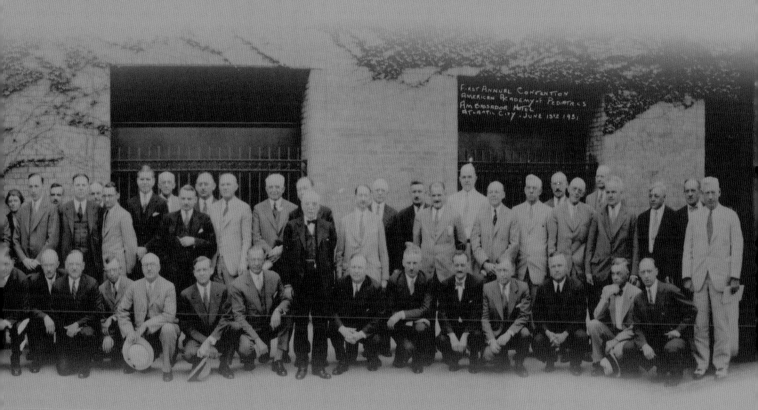

First Annual Convention
American Academy of Pediatrics
Ambassador Hotel
Atlantic City - June 13th 1931

1922
The American Medical
Association (AMA)
Section on Diseases of
Children was rebuked
by the AMA House of
Delegates for its public
statement in support of
the Sheppard-Towner Act.
(St Louis, MO)

1929
The formation of a new,
national pediatric society
was discussed in meet-
ings in Portland, OR,
and Chicago, IL.

LOOKING FOR A VOICE

The founding of the American Academy of Pediatrics (AAP) in 1930 was made nearly inevitable by several factors and issues surfacing in the 1920s in the United States. One of these was the increasing numbers of American physicians who were restricting their practices to the care of children. In 1929, the American Medical Association (AMA) American Medical Directory listed about 1,330 men in the United States who claimed to practice pediatrics exclusively, and an additional 2,150 who stated that they mainly practiced pediatrics.

At this time, there were only a few local or state pediatric societies. There were at least 2 regional organizations—the Central States Pediatric Society, which met regularly and included nearly all the practicing pediatricians (about 300 members) in the area between the Rocky and Appalachian mountains, Canada, and the Gulf; and the North Pacific Pediatric Society, which first met in 1919, and continues to meet. However, there were only 2 national pediatric organizations—the Section on Diseases of Children of the AMA and the American Pediatric Society (APS), neither of which were believed, by many, to serve the needs of the increasing numbers of practicing pediatricians across the nation for an effective vehicle for education and expressing their views on national issues. The APS had a constitutional limit of 100 in its active membership. Most APS members were involved in academics, teaching, and research. In addition, there was strong sentiment within the APS that the society should not become involved in social or political activities.

In 1909, Thomas Morgan Rotch, MD, gave his APS presidential address entitled, "The Position and Work of the American Pediatric Society Toward Public Questions." Dr Rotch proposed active involvement of the APS in social and public health issues that affected children. His presentation evoked a long and heated discussion by APS members, most of whom believed that the society should

not be smeared with the pitch of politics, however praiseworthy the objectives.

Isaac A. Abt, MD, of Chicago, IL (an eminent American pediatrician who had edited a comprehensive textbook of pediatrics, and, ironically,

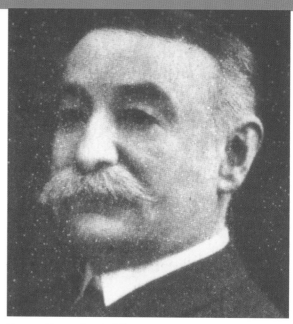

Thomas Morgan Rotch, MD.

became the first president of the AAP in 1930), stated the thoughts of most APS members:

"I should feel sorry to see a large part of the work of this Society devoted to subjects of this kind, which though of sociological interest, are not so much along the line of work of most of us. I believe we can do our best along the lines of research. We have a duty to the public, but that should not be the most important side of our work."

In his concluding comments to the society, Dr Rotch stated prophetically:

"I supposed that the Society would wish to lend its influence to broad questions of the time connected to Pediatrics. If it does not so wish, these questions can be discussed elsewhere."

The Section on Diseases of Children of the AMA had been formally established back in 1880, largely by initiatives of Abraham Jacobi, MD. At the first meeting of the section, Dr Jacobi gave an address entitled, "The Claims of Pediatric Medicine," in which he outlined the rationale for pediatrics as a medical specialty. The section had annual scientific meetings in conjunction with the AMA, which many practicing pediatricians felt were too brief and superficial to meet their need for continuing education. Some pediatricians were unhappy by their perception of a lack of attention and appreciation by the AMA to pediatric issues. They were also uncomfortable with the subordinate role of the section to AMA policy, without much opportunity for independent action.

This latter concern was brought to a climax in 1922 when Congress was considering the Sheppard-Towner Act, which was a modest program to authorize the Children's Bureau to provide grants to the states for maternal-child health initiatives, including prenatal clinics, infant welfare stations, and child hygiene divisions. This act was discussed at the 1922 spring meeting of the Section on Diseases of Children in St Louis, MO, and by a unanimous resolution, the section supported the act. The action of the section was prominently featured in the St Louis newspapers. On the same day at a meeting across town, the House of Delegates of the AMA passed a separate resolution condemning the Sheppard-Towner Act

as government intrusion into private medical practice and an attempt to introduce socialized medicine. When the House of Delegates learned, through the newspapers, of the section's action, anger erupted. As Marshall Carleton Pease, MD, commented in his 1952 history of the AAP:

> *"A Committee of wrath was sent by the House of Delegates to reprimand the Pediatric Section but they were met with unrepentance and jeers."*

The House of Delegates then promptly passed a ruling that no section of the AMA could independently adopt a resolution or, in any way as a group, indicate approval or disapproval of matters concerning AMA policies. Further, it directed that sections of the AMA should confine their activities solely to social gatherings and presentations of a scientific program and they were not permitted to have any input into AMA policy.

Dr Pease summarized the predicament of pediatricians at that time:

> *"The status of being an unwanted child in the family of medicine was not a happy one for the average clinical pediatrician. He longed for a worthy place in the group of specialists where his opinions would have the weight they deserved on the basis of his unique knowledge of children. Legislation on matters of public health often began with the mother and child, but pediatricians were not only not consulted, but worse, were often ignored. The only 'out' seemed to be to form a unified national pediatric society, which by its integrity and its open-mindedness to new approaches in all fields of child health, could win the respect that was its due."*

1930
Founding of the American Academy of Pediatrics. (Detroit, MI)

1931
Founding of the Society for Pediatric Research (began as the Eastern Society for Pediatric Research in 1929 before going national in 1931).

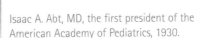

Isaac A. Abt, MD, the first president of the American Academy of Pediatrics, 1930.

1932
Louis K. Diamond, MD; Kenneth D. Blackfan, MD; and James M. Baty, MD, unified hydrops fetalis, icterus gravis, and anemia of the newborn as manifestations of erythroblastosis fetalis. (Boston, MA)

Publication of the *Journal of Pediatrics* as the official organ of the American Academy of Pediatrics. (St Louis, MO)

These issues and sentiments were widely discussed and debated by many pediatricians, including those attending meetings of the Central States Pediatric Society, but no real action was taken for 7 years—7 years of discontent and discussion, but very little action.

It is of some interest that, in 1929, Congress allowed the Sheppard-Towner Act to expire. In 1934, Martha Eliot, MD, participated in drafting Title V of the Social Security Act, which revived the maternal and child health measures that the Sheppard-Towner Act had encouraged during the 1920s (see Chapter 3 for more about these efforts in the 1930s).

THE FORMATION OF THE AMERICAN ACADEMY OF PEDIATRICS

The actual origin of the AAP can be traced to a fateful gathering on July 19, 1929 during the AMA Section on Diseases of Children meeting in Portland, OR. James W. Rosenfeld, MD, invited all of the section attendees, about 35 pediatricians from around the country, to an elegant dinner at his home. William P. Lucas, MD, of San Francisco, CA, described some of what transpired at that dinner in a 1941 letter to AAP historian Ernest Caulfield, MD. Dr Lucas was seated at the same table with Dr Abt; C. Anderson Aldrich, MD, of

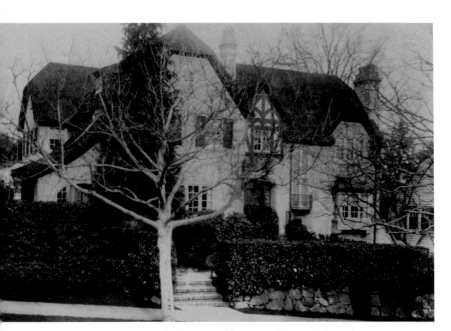

The Portland, OR, home of James W. Rosenfeld, MD, the site of the fateful dinner gathering on July 19, 1929, that launched the formation of the American Academy of Pediatrics.

Chicago; and Joseph Bilderback, MD, of Portland. It was not long after the first course of dinner that the subject of a new national pediatric society was raised. It was immediately evident that many pediatricians had been thinking the same way. They believed that such a new pediatric society should include most of the practicing pediatricians of the nation as members, and be a unified group of practitioners and academicians to further the field of pediatrics and advance the medical care and social needs of children.

The discussion ultimately included all 35 of the group, most of whom supported the forming of a new society. Issues such as qualifications for possible charter members, the role of the new society in national child health and welfare programs, and the initial steps necessary for establishing the new society were discussed. It was suggested by Dr Abt that the name of the new society could be the American Academy of Pediatrics. It was also unanimously recommended that Clifford G. Grulee, MD, of Chicago should be asked to serve as the first executive secretary. Drs Abt and Aldrich agreed to meet with Dr Grulee, on their return to Chicago, to discuss this matter and to ask him to serve as secretary-treasurer of the projected society.

Lest it be thought that this watershed meeting was strictly business, Dr Pease wrote:

> *"The food seems to have been of a quality that causes nostalgia after twenty years."*

In addition, despite the fact that this was during the height of Prohibition, Dr Lucas commented:

> *"Our discussions had little levity although Bacchus flowed freely his libations (good scotch) well into the wee hours of the night."*

The choice of Dr Grulee to spearhead the initiative was apparently unanimous. At the time, Dr Grulee was 50 years old. After he graduated cum laude from the Northwestern Medical School in 1903, his major academic appointments were at Rush Medical College, where he served as clinical professor of pediatrics and chairman of pediatrics between 1919 and 1941. He was elected president of the Section on Diseases of Children of the AMA in 1925, and served as editor in chief of the AMA *American Journal of Diseases of Children (AJDC)* from 1923 to 1955. Dr Grulee lived and practiced in Evanston, IL, for 37 years. He was

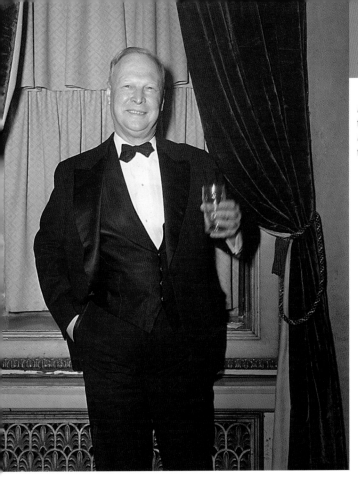

1933

Gerhard Domagk, MD, discovered Prontosil— the first sulfonamide. (Germany)

Founding of the American Board of Pediatrics.

involved in practically all activities that had to do with pediatrics and children in the Chicago area and was well-known and highly regarded both regionally and nationally.

When Drs Abt and Aldrich met with Dr Grulee in his office in Evanston, they found that he had already been contemplating the formation of a new pediatric society and, in fact, had already drafted a letter that he was going to send to pediatricians in key locations around the nation calling for the formation of such a society. Despite the sketchiness of the planning thus far, he readily agreed to be secretary-treasurer and, from then on, took the lead. In all written accounts of the early days of the AAP, Dr Grulee's role is described as being absolutely essential for the success of the project. He, along with Drs Abt and Lucas, were the key figures in the founding of the AAP, but, as Dr Lucas wrote later:

> *"With no budget and no money in sight, Dr Grulee, with his vision and imagination, his dynamic force, threw himself into the organization, and the result is the work that Dr Grulee did and we were simply accessories to it."*

In December 1929, Drs Abt, Aldrich, and Grulee met to draw up a detailed plan of organization. They drafted an outline of the purposes of the new society, which was mailed to pediatricians around the country in February 1930. Most of the recipients of the letter were receptive to the possibility of joining a new and expanded association devoted to children. The Central States Pediatric Society endorsed the new organization, as did the APS. In fact, 52 of the founders

> *"This is a memorable day in the history of American pediatrics. The founding of the Academy will have a far-reaching significance in developing the scope and field of pediatrics and, I hope, a beneficent influence on the life and health of those patients whom the pediatricians will reach."*

ISAAC A. ABT, MD, FROM THE FIRST PRESIDENTIAL ADDRESS OF THE AMERICAN ACADEMY OF PEDIATRICS ON JUNE 12, 1931

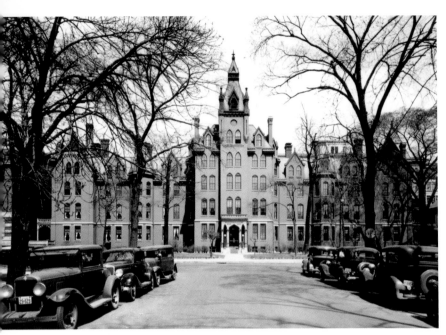

Harper Hospital in Detroit, MI, site of the founding meeting of the American Academy of Pediatrics on June 23 and 24, 1930.

of the AAP, its first 8 presidents, and its first secretary-treasurer were members of the APS.

An organizational meeting for the new society was held in the library of Harper Hospital in Detroit, MI, on June 23 and 24, 1930, with a group of 35 pediatricians in attendance. The actual founding meeting took place on June 23. At that meeting, committees were established to lay the groundwork for the new society: to draft a constitution; develop a name for the new organization; establish rules for membership; establish procedures for running the central office; and more. The committees reported the next day, a constitution and bylaws were adopted, and the new organization was formally named the American Academy of Pediatrics. Additional committees were appointed, including a Committee on Medical Education and a Committee on Relation to the White House Conference and Publications.

A list of approximately 400 pediatricians was compiled and these pediatricians were invited to become charter members. Most of those invited were personally or by reputation known to the 35 pediatricians who attended the organizational meeting and compiled the mailing list. Officers for 1930–1931 were elected. The first president was Dr Abt and the initial vice president was

John L. Morse, MD, who was a respected and admired pediatrician from Boston, MA.

An Executive Board was appointed, consisting of the chairmen of 4 regions into which the country was divided: Region I, the East, consisted of New England, New York, Pennsylvania, Maryland, the District of Columbia, and Delaware; Region II, the South, consisted of the states south of Virginia, West Virginia, Kentucky, Arkansas, and Oklahoma, including Texas; Region III, the Midwest, included the states between Ohio and the Rocky Mountains; and Region IV, the West, included the states between the Rocky Mountains and the West Coast.

The AAP was officially incorporated in July 1930 in Dr Grulee's home state of Illinois and the central office was established in Evanston. The officers and Executive Board met again in February and April 1931. At the February meeting, a formal statement of the purposes of the AAP was issued.

1. *To create reciprocal and friendly relations with all professional and lay organizations that are interested in the health and protection of children.*

2. *To foster and encourage pediatric investigation, both clinically and in the laboratory, by individuals and groups.*

At the time of the first AAP Annual Meeting in Atlantic City, NJ, held on June 12 and 13, 1931, there were 304 enrolled members of the AAP. There were members in many of the states, making the AAP, from the beginning, a national organization. Ninety-three members, including

Right, Isaac A. Abt, MD, and John L. Morse, MD, the first American Academy of Pediatrics president and vice president, respectively.

at least 3 women, attended the Atlantic City meeting, which was highlighted by the presidential address of Dr Abt, in which he stated:

"It is our desire to build an association so that every qualified pediatrician could seek membership. It will be necessary for the Academy to interest itself in undergraduate and postgraduate instruction and to exert a regulatory influence over hospitals. As an organization we should assist and lead in public health measures, in social reform, and in hospital and educational administration as they affect the welfare of children."

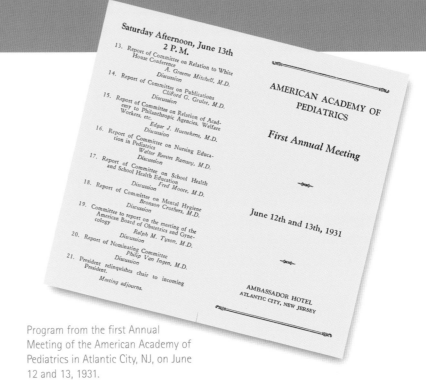

Program from the first Annual Meeting of the American Academy of Pediatrics in Atlantic City, NJ, on June 12 and 13, 1931.

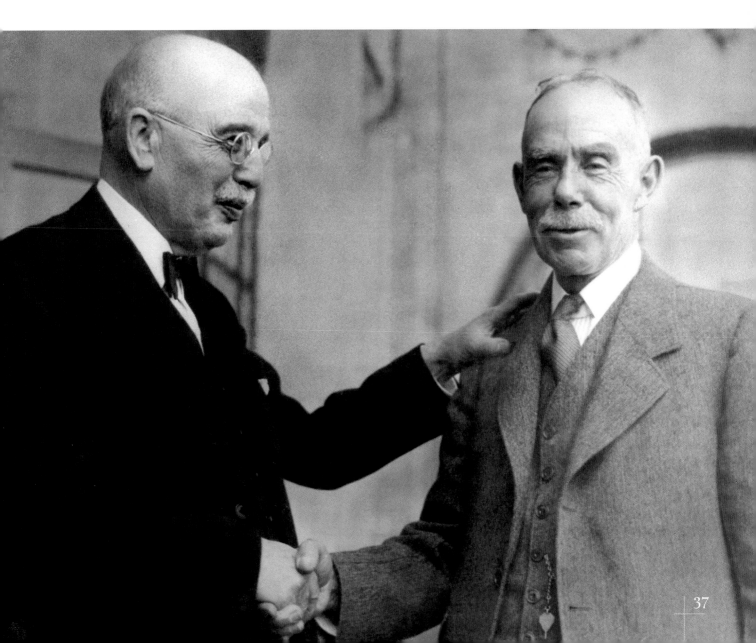

THE ORGANIZATION GETS RIGHT TO WORK

The first few years of the AAP were marked by a number of significant accomplishments. Among the most important were the establishment of the *Journal of Pediatrics* and the formation of the American Board of Pediatrics (ABP).

During a discussion at the 1931 Annual Meeting, sentiment for establishment of a new journal became apparent, as evidenced by a dialogue between Borden Veeder, MD, and Dr Grulee:

> Dr Veeder: *"I think that there is a strong possibility of the development of another pediatric journal, which might be the official journal of the Academy."*

> Dr Grulee: *"It seems to me that the time is rapidly approaching when we must have more pediatric journals in this country. No one realizes more than I do the pressure on a pediatric journal [Dr Grulee was editor of the AJDC]. The only question is one of money."*

In November 1931, Dr Grulee was authorized to negotiate a contract with the C. V. Mosby Company of St Louis, which included the following provisions:

1. *The AAP would underwrite 400 subscriptions at $5.00 apiece.*

2. *The $5.00 would be included in the annual AAP dues.*

3. *The Editors and Editorial Board members would be appointed by the AAP.*

4. *The policies, articles and review of advertising would be the responsibility of the AAP.*

5. *The* Journal of Pediatrics, *as the new journal was to be named, would be the official publication of the AAP and the* Journal *would publish Executive Board Proceedings, reports, Round Table and Seminar abstracts, and special sections, such as News, Book Reviews, and Social Aspects of Medicine.*

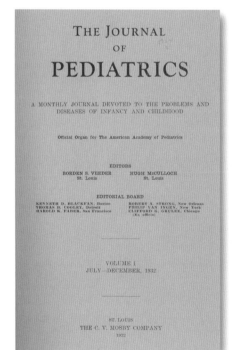

Title page of the *Journal of Pediatrics*, Volume 1, Number 1, July 1932.

It was specified that the C. V. Mosby Company would own the journal, assume complete financial control, including debts and profits, and be responsible for publication and distribution and the solicitation of advertising. It was remarkable that both the AAP and Mosby were willing to take the risk of launching a new journal at the height of the Great Depression. The Executive Board appointed Dr Veeder and Hugh McCulloch, MD, both of whom lived in St Louis, as coeditors, and a strong editorial board. The first issue of the *Journal of Pediatrics* was published in July 1932, only 2 years after the AAP was founded.

In 1934, the AMA directory listed approximatly 1,734 American physicians who were self-identified as pediatric practitioners. Any physicians in the United States could designate themselves as a pediatrician. Some of these physicians had significant pediatric training experience, some of them had taken short courses of pediatric training (frequently in Europe), and many had no formal training at all.

The original founders and leaders of the AAP were very cognizant that, if the AAP was to gain professional stature and public recognition, it would be essential to develop high standards for membership. It was felt that this should include a description of necessary training to be called a pediatrician and that there was a need to create a mechanism for assessing clinical competence.

A committee chaired by Dr Veeder was appointed to study and define the necessary credentials to become an AAP member. The committee decided that formation of an American Board of Pediatrics would be the best way to address the problems of defining training and competence. To avoid the appearance of being self-serving, the committee recommended that the ABP should be created by the 3 national pediatric organizations then in existence: the AAP, the APS, and the AMA Section on Diseases of Children. All 3 societies endorsed the concept and, in early 1933, each nominated 3 members for the first ABP Board. The ABP charter was registered in Delaware on December 9, 1933. The charter set 3 objectives for the board:

1. *To review accreditation of training programs*

2. *To develop credentials for those to be certified*

3. *To examine applicants for certification*

The first meeting of the ABP Board was held on January 18, 1934, in St Louis. Dr Veeder was elected president; Henry F. Helmholz, MD, was elected vice president; and Dr Aldrich was elected secretary. A list of physicians who might be certified by the board was constructed, which included many members of the AAP and APS. These were assigned into 3 groups. Group I consisted of physicians who had limited their practices to pediatrics for more than 10 years. These physicians could be certified *on record (grandfathered)* without an examination. Group II consisted of physicians who had limited their practices to pediatrics for 6 to 10 years. These physicians, mostly academicians, were required to have at least 1 year of hospital training and an additional year in a pediatric center, and continue to work in a pediatric institution or center. An examination was required. Group III consisted of recent graduates of medical school. Physicians in this group were required to have had at least 2 years of formal pediatric training followed by 2 or 3 years of pediatric practice. Certification required an examination. These criteria were widely circulated and were printed in the extant pediatric journals, and applications were solicited.

By the second meeting of the board in June 1934, 195 Group I applications had been received and 162 of these were certified on record. At the same time, an oral examination was administered to physicians from groups II and III. The oral examination consisted of 4 twenty-minute sessions with 4 different examiners consisting of case presentations, interpretation of x-ray films, slides of pathological specimens, and questions on growth and development. (Supplementary true-false written examinations were not instituted until 1939.) Seven candidates from Group II and 3 candidates from Group III successfully passed. Over the next few years, additional Group I physicians were grandfathered, ultimately reaching a total of 504 physicians, and, in 1938, on-record certification ended. Most of the Group II physicians had also been processed. At that time, there were only about 300 two-year pediatric residency positions available in the United States, so it was estimated that only about 150 recent residency program graduates would need to be examined each year.

There was not unanimous appreciation of the board. Some academic leaders in the Northeast, particularly at the medical schools of Harvard,

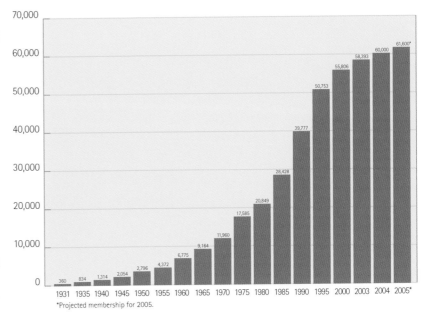

American Academy of Pediatrics Membership (1931–2005)

*Projected membership for 2005.

Yale, and Johns Hopkins, believed that their training program credentials were higher than those required by the ABP. For several years, they resisted recommending certification for their faculties. However, once the ABP was established and functioning, certification by the ABP was made the principal requirement for membership in the AAP. The AAP began to rapidly grow and become increasingly important on the national political scene. Ultimately, even some of the recalcitrant northeastern pediatric academicians realized that AAP membership (and its requirement for ABP certification) was increasingly desirable for academicians and urged their faculties to take the examination.

Thus, in a very short span of years, the AAP was conceived, created, and expanded into a national institution that was involved in all aspects of pediatric education and practice and in a broad range of child health issues. It was conducting a well-attended national Annual Meeting. At least 10 committees were established to provide guidance for the Executive Board in a wide number of areas. However, a number of controversies and confrontations would develop about the involvement of government agencies in activities that affected pediatric practice.

Young boy near Cincinnati, OH,
circa 1940.

*Having been the offspring of the idealistic
child-saving crusades of the Progressive Era,
the American Academy of Pediatrics was to face
the greatest crisis of its existence as it reached
adolescence during the 1940s....*

Chapter 3
Pediatrics in Transition

1935 to 1950

1936
Philip C. Jeans, MD, persuaded the American Medical Association Council on Foods and Nutrition to recommend fortification of milk with vitamin D.

1938
Charles C. Chapple, MD, introduced the forerunner of the Isolette infant incubator. (Philadelphia, PA)

Robert E. Gross, MD, surgically ligated a patent ductus arteriosus. (Boston, MA)

Dorothy H. Anderson, MD, described pathological features of cystic fibrosis. (New York, NY)

RISING CONFLICT: THE 1930s

Having been the offspring of the idealistic child-saving crusades of the Progressive Era, the American Academy of Pediatrics (AAP) was to face the greatest crisis of its existence as it reached adolescence during the 1940s. Ironically, the chief point of contention was the relationship between the pediatric profession and the federal Children's Bureau. In 1922, the Section on Diseases of Children of the American Medical Association (AMA) sided with the Children's Bureau against the AMA House of Delegates by refusing to condemn the Sheppard-Towner Act. This action triggered a growing schism with the AMA that eventually led to the founding of the AAP. But many pediatricians had deeply ambivalent feelings about federal involvement in children's health, fearful that it would eventually impose limits on their freedom to practice medicine.

Physicians' fears of government intrusion into health care became acute during the Great Depression. At its worst point in 1933, 1 in 4 workers was unemployed. Malnourished and poorly clothed children became a common sight, especially among those fleeing from the devastated farmlands of the dust bowl. An estimated 1 to 2 million mothers,

Two Depression-era scenes from a New Mexico highway, 1936. *Above left*, members of an impoverished family who left their home in Iowa in 1932 because of the father's ill health (tuberculosis); *above right*, mother feeding sick child (tuberculosis).

fathers, and children wandered the countryside seeking food and shelter. Even the most basic medical care was impossible for many to afford. As federal powers expanded under the New Deal, advocates of government-sponsored health insurance gained more influence than ever before.

Primary care doctors, in turn, struggled to make their own ends meet. Working long hours that routinely extended into nights and weekends, physicians often failed to collect fees, and competed intensely for the few patients who could pay. Such frustration eventually boiled over into an aggressive campaign, orchestrated by the AMA, opposing compulsory health insurance. Though physicians desperately needed income, they feared that government intervention would fundamentally challenge their freedom to practice.

The AAP leadership attempted to walk a tightrope with respect to its position toward the roles of the private and public sectors in providing child health care throughout the 1930s. The passage of Title V of the Social Security Act in 1935 revived many of the federal matching grant programs that were lost with the expiration of the Sheppard-Towner Act, and greatly increased the power and funding of the Children's Bureau. Its new medical adviser, Martha Eliot, MD, was a member of the AAP. The AAP also appointed a Committee on Legislation in 1935, led by the articulate and formidable Joseph S. Wall, MD, charged to analyze the most important national health insurance proposal of the time, the Wagner National Health Bill. The Committee on Legislation approved the bill "in principle" in 1939, but recommended its revision with greater input from the medical community and the use of a means test to determine eligibility for coverage. At a time when the AMA and private insurers were leading an intense drive to warn the public of the dangers of national health insurance, this was a moderate stance. Peace between the AAP conservatives and liberals was maintained for the time being.

Allan Butler and the Wagner-Murray-Dingell Bill

In the early 1940s, the United States was considering entering World War II as a full participant. Some pediatric giants were studying how to lessen the infant and child mortality from diarrhea. James L. Gamble, MD, had published his first edition of *Gamblegrams;* Alexis F. Hartmann, MD, showed the value of correcting acidosis; Allan M. Butler, MD, documented the essentiality of potassium in intravenous fluids; and Daniel C. Darrow, MD, researched the balance of electrolytes in intravenous fluids.

Simultaneously, the US Congress was engaged in attempting to document the possible benefit of the federal government supporting a form of universal medical insurance, which was vigorously opposed by the American Medical Association (AMA). The Wagner-Murray-Dingell Bill was drafted by several members of Congress and was supported by some members of academia.

The AMA claimed that this bill was the first step to Communism and would ruin the private practice of medicine. By chance, the president of the AMA was a Harvard faculty member, Roger I. Lee, MD. In contrast, Dr Butler, a star pediatrician and also a member of the Harvard faculty, was an outspoken supporter of the bill.

As consideration of the bill dragged on, the AMA decided to take its argument to Congress. The AMA prepared its president to challenge Dr Butler. Dr Butler invited me and other Harvard medical students assigned to pediatrics to come to Washington, DC, to hear the discussion. Dr Lee gave a very detailed list of objections to the Wagner Bill, after which Dr Butler, in very measured words said, "Roger, have you ever read the Wagner Bill?" A very chagrined Dr Lee very quietly responded, "No, I have not." The debate ended and the bill passed. On the ride back to Boston, MA, Dr Butler was obviously very happy, and then told us, "I'm very glad that no one asked me if I had read the bill, because I hadn't."

— Lewis A. Barness, MD

1939
The American Academy of Pediatrics held its first "independent" Annual Meeting (not held in conjunction with another medical conference). (Cincinnati, OH)

1940
Karl Landsteiner, MD, and Alexander Wiener, MD, discovered the Rh (Rhesus) factor.

Four babies standing in a crib at Saint Vincent's Asylum, Chicago, IL, 1929.

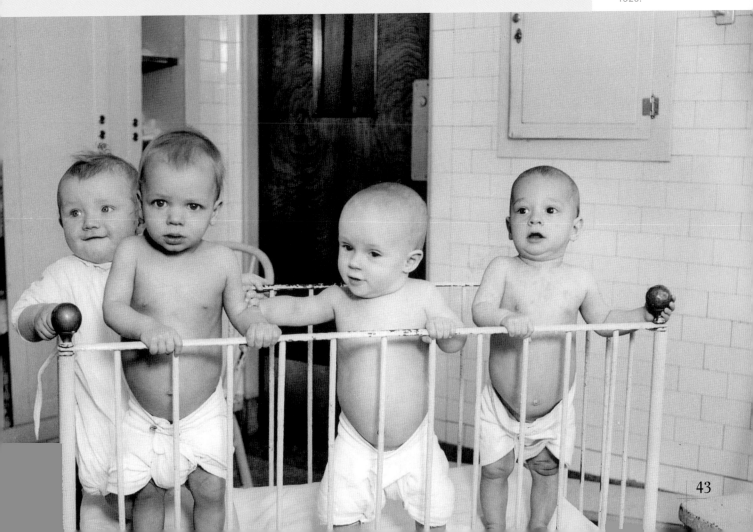

43

1941
The United States entered World War II.

1943
Congress enacted the Emergency Maternity and Infant Care Act.

Ethel C. Dunham, MD, and the Children's Bureau published *Standards and Recommendations for the Hospital Care of Newborn Infants, Full Term and Premature.* (Washington, DC)

Selman A. Waksman discovered streptomycin. (New Jersey)

Alfred Blalock, MD, and Helen B. Taussig, MD, described a palliative surgical treatment of tetralogy of Fallot (the first operation was performed in 1944). (Baltimore, MD)

CRISIS AND RESOLUTION: THE 1940s

In 1941, the United States entered World War II. With the introduction of the draft, large numbers of young men were inducted into the armed services as the nation mobilized for war. Young women were marrying these servicemen and frequently following them to training camps around the country. Their pregnancies often occurred in places that were far from home and family support, and access to obstetrical and pediatric care was often marginal at best, even for those who could afford them—and most could not.

The situation of these young families became so acute that requests for governmental assistance were ultimately forwarded to the Children's Bureau. Dr Eliot, who was now associate chief of the bureau, moved to create a national program, the Emergency Maternity and Infant Care Act (EMIC), to meet what was considered to be a wartime emergency. Originally, the EMIC was meant to assist only those families that could not pay, but a means test was never set up and all families, regardless of financial status, were soon covered. The program expanded rapidly and soon became very unpopular among many members of

the medical community. A 1949 AAP report recited a litany of complaints, including predelivery solicitation of service wives by the EMIC, excessive paper work, inadequate compensation of physicians, denial of the right of physicians to charge supplemental fees for those who could afford to pay, and the imposition of "arbitrary" administrative rules for establishing minimum levels for quality and competence of care provided. It was evident that the long-time cooperation between the AAP and the Children's Bureau was severely strained.

Most obstetricians and pediatricians had participated in EMIC expecting that the program would be terminated at the end of the war. In 1945, however, Senator Claude E. Pepper introduced legislation that would have extended the provisions of EMIC into peacetime. Some of the AAP leadership believed that they had been "blindsided" and that the Maternal and Child Welfare Bill (also referred to as the "Pepper Bill") had been essentially written by the Children's Bureau, a charge that Dr Eliot denied vigorously. Nevertheless, the AAP president and Executive Board seriously considered withdrawing AAP support from the Children's Bureau. The possibility

Posters from the Works Progress Administration (WPA) Federal Art Project, 1936 to 1938.

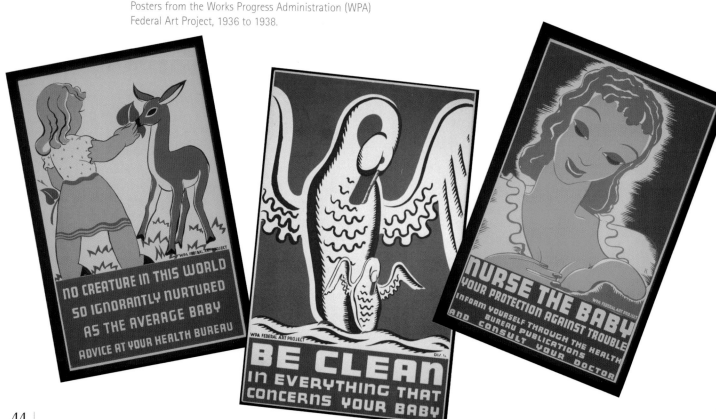

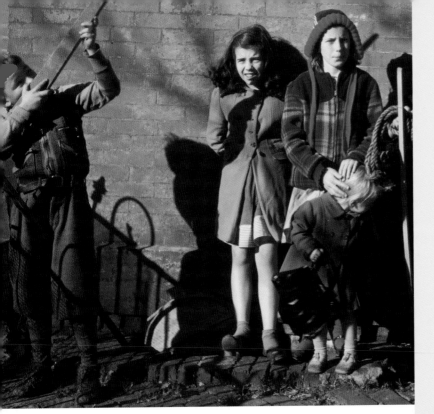

Group of children in Washington, DC, circa 1940.

Two girls sitting on porch steps in Colorado in the 1930s.

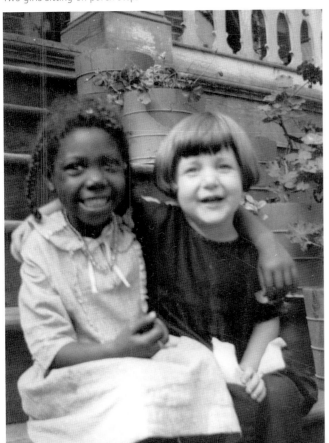

Grover Powers' Plea for Cooperation

In 1944, Grover F. Powers, MD, professor of pediatrics at Yale University School of Medicine and mentor to Martha Eliot, MD, at Yale and the Children's Bureau, wrote an impassioned letter to the editor of the *Journal of Pediatrics,* in response to the fears of many in the American Academy of Pediatrics that the federal Emergency Maternity and Infant Care Act might serve as an opening wedge for "socialized medicine." Dr Powers' letter is excerpted here:

"No one should be satisfied with the distribution of medical care in the United States and no one knows the complete solution of the various problems involved.... Only if we are alert to new concepts and procedures and eager for experimentation in medical practice as in the laboratory will we be able to give effective counsel and guidance. In the Emergency Maternity and Infant Care program, through fortuitous circumstances, we have been presented with an experimental study of a segment of the medical care problem, well defined and clearly limited. Shall we discard valid experimental data thrown in our laps, so to speak, by the exigencies of war or shall we welcome the opportunity to salvage something constructive from the holocaust! And would it not be ungrateful, short-sighted, and unscien-

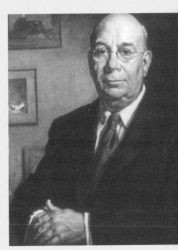

Grover F. Powers, MD.

tific, contrary to our own high purposes and, above all, against the best interests of America's children to cease collaboration with our experienced Children's Bureau friends—tried and true crusaders in our common cause of maternal and child welfare—because of blind fears which the Emergency Maternity and Infant Care program may have on the course of pediatric practice....

American pediatrics has a glorious reputation of scientific achievement, an enviable reputation for unselfish public service, and eager appreciation of the fact that 'new occasions teach new duties'! Let us by no overt act place a 'blot on the 'scutcheon' of our heritage!"

Martha Eliot, MD: Persistent Pioneer

1946
Louis K. Diamond, MD, described exchange transfusion through the umbilical vein as a treatment for erythroblastosis fetalis. (Boston, MA)

Benjamin M. Spock, MD, published *The Common Sense Book of Baby and Child Care.* (New York, NY)

1948
Publication of *Pediatrics* as the official journal of the American Academy of Pediatrics.

John F. Enders; Frederick C. Robbins, MD; and Thomas H. Weller, MD, successfully grew polio virus in tissue culture. (Boston, MA)

When Martha Eliot applied to medical school, Harvard was closed to women, but she applied as a matter of principle before she entered Johns Hopkins. When she graduated in 1918, she faced the pervasive discrimination against women in postgraduate training. Regardless of women's ability, for much of the 20th century they were routinely denied internships, appointments, and promotions. Dr Eliot wanted to do a pediatric internship at Johns Hopkins but was rejected by John Howland, MD, who rarely considered women—even the most talented of them—for training. After serving as an intern at Bellevue, the wartime [World War I] shortage of male doctors enabled her to obtain a medical internship at the new Peter Bent Brigham Hospital and then a pediatric residency at the St Louis Children's Hospital. After completing her residency, she opened an office in Boston, but entered this practice with "little enthusiasm and much dissatisfaction." To her great relief she received a letter from Edwards Park, MD, who had just become the first chairman of the new Department of Pediatrics at Yale. Park remembered Eliot from her student days at Johns Hopkins and invited her to join him in New Haven where she stayed for 14 years. In 1939, she took a full-time position with the Children's Bureau, and served as bureau chief between 1951 and 1956. At the age of 66 she "retired" from the bureau and went to Harvard as professor of maternal and child health. She also was chair of the Massachusetts State Commission on Children and Youth until her 80th birthday. Martha Eliot left a brilliant legacy of achievements in child health initiatives and advocacy for children which were recognized by the Lasker Prize in 1948 and the John Howland Award of the American Pediatric Society in 1967.

— *Marion Hunt, PhD* (Adapted from Hunt M. Extraordinarily interesting and happy years. Martha M. Eliot and pediatrics at Yale, 1921–1935. *Yale J Biol Med.* 1995;68:159–170. Used with permission.)

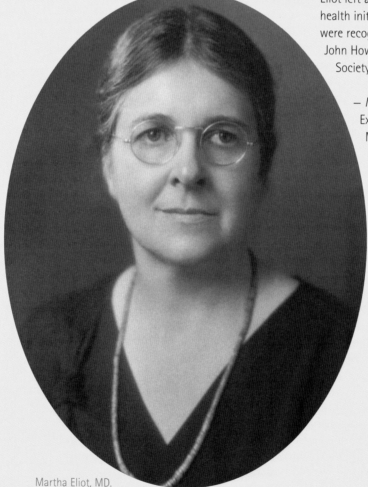

Martha Eliot, MD.

Right, homesteader and his children eating barbecue at the New Mexico Fair, 1940.

of a complete rift between the AAP and the Children's Bureau, respectively the most important organization representing the private pediatrician and the key government agency supporting child health, was viewed by many pediatricians as a potential disaster that would be detrimental to the welfare of the nation's children.

It was at this crucial point in 1945 that a possible way to resolve the controversy was suggested. It is difficult to determine who actually conceived the solution. One scenario described initiatives between Dr Eliot and Henry Helmholz, MD. Dr Helmholz, who was on the Medical Advisory Board of the Children's Bureau, had been AAP president in 1938–1939. Dr Eliot told Dr Helmholz that she believed that if the AAP membership knew how great the deficiencies in the state of the nation's children and their health needs were, that they would continue to support the bureau. She proposed an ambitious joint national study of health services for children to provide hard data on the availability and distribution of physicians and medical services for children. Dr Helmholz presented the idea to the AAP

Executive Board, which embraced the idea in principle but was frightened by its price tag. The venerable secretary-treasurer of the AAP, Clifford G. Grulee, MD, broke the deadlock after 2 days of behind-the-scenes fund-raising, and the AAP thus embarked on its most ambitious collaborative project with the federal government to date. Many American pediatricians participated in the endeavor. The AAP leadership created a new committee, the Committee for the Study of Child Health Services, to oversee the program, and appointed John Hubbard, MD, as the director of the study.

Beginning in October 1945 and continuing for the next 2 years, an enormous amount of data was amassed. In 1949, the Commonwealth Fund published the final report and a supplement on methodology. Containing 270 pages and 100 figures or tables, the report provided, for the first time, a complete and comprehensive national picture of the numbers and distribution of child health personnel and the venues in which they worked. Data were also provided describing the availability of pediatric hospitals and facilities, and the personnel and curricula of the 70 US medical schools and the hospitals providing pediatric training.

1949
Linus Pauling and Harvey A. Itano, MD, described sickle cell anemia as a "molecular disease" caused by an abnormal hemoglobin.

The last case of smallpox in the United States was reported.

The American Academy of Pediatrics and the Children's Bureau published a national survey, "Child Health Services and Pediatric Education."

William L. Bradford, MD; Elizabeth Day; and Frederick Martin, MD, showed that infants respond to a triple vaccine, diphtheria-tetanus-pertussis (DTP). (Rochester, NY)

Ogden C. Bruton, MD, described agammaglobu-linemia. (Washington, DC)

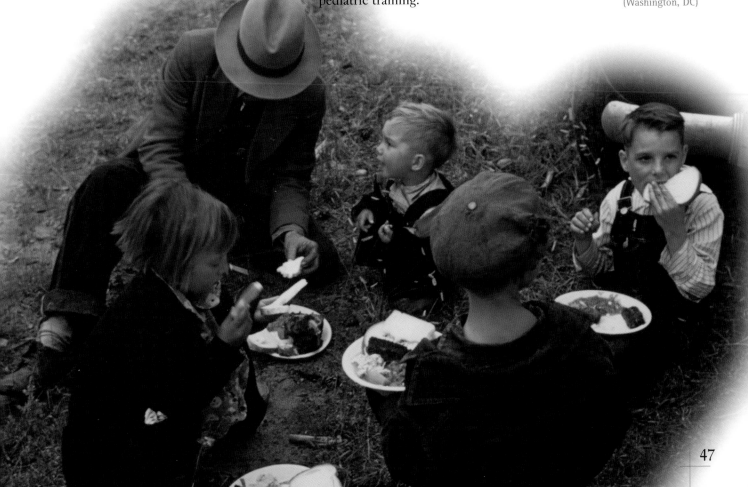

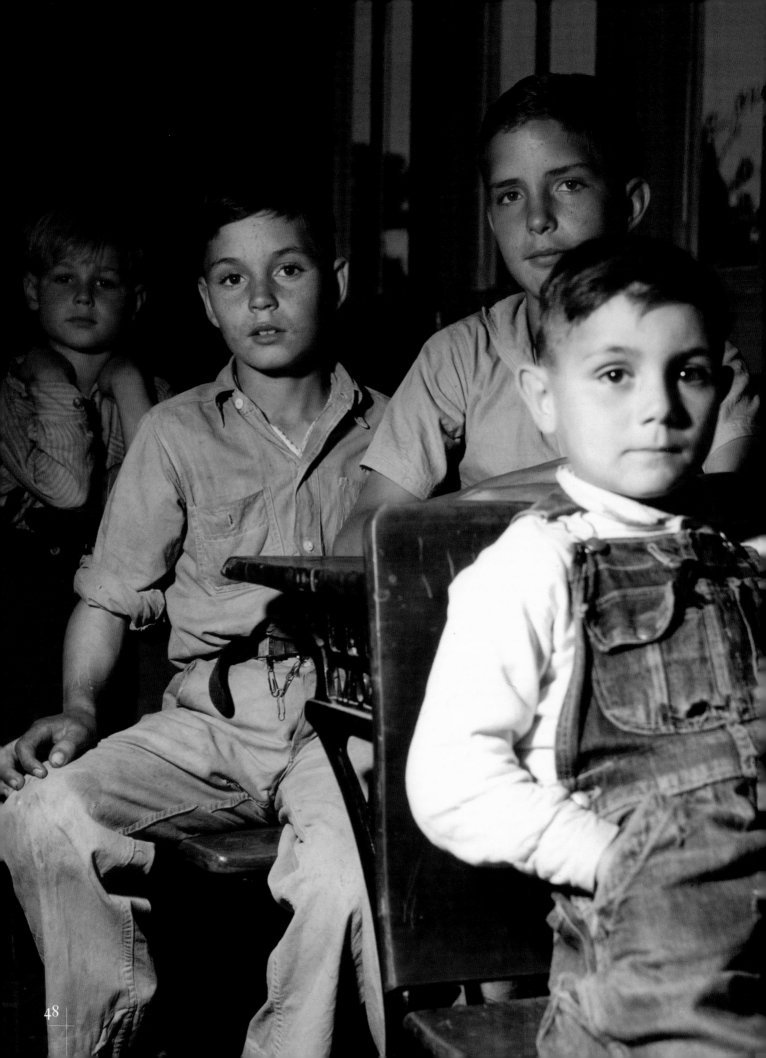

Since the appointed task of the study committee was to conduct the study and report its results rather than to make specific recommendations, the committee was disbanded following the report's publication. Because the AAP was committed to interpreting its results and making recommendations to address deficiencies, the oversight and implementation of the study was transferred in 1947 to a newly appointed Committee for the Improvement of Child Health (ICH). Perhaps not surprisingly, this committee itself soon became the focus of controversy as it set off to propose a series of new legislative activities at the federal and state levels, as well as to make recommendations about pediatric education in the medical schools. The committee's reports were accepted reluctantly by the Executive Board, and it was evident that fear of increasing government control was still a concern. Perhaps even more worrisome was the fear that the committee might be too independent and try to preempt some of the power and decision making of the Executive Board.

In early 1948, in a report to the Executive Board the ICH described a financial "emergency" in American medical schools concerning pediatric education and recommended seeking direct federal aid to the medical schools to address this. The Executive Board accepted the committee recommendation and mailed it as a fait accompli to the membership-at-large. A "storm of protest" (as described by Marshall Carleton Pease, MD) then ensued. Some members feared that federal aid to medical schools would inevitably lead to federal interference in pediatric education and teaching policies and that this might ultimately lead to interference in practice. Further, there were complaints that the committee members who made the recommendation were primarily academicians who did not understand private practice. It is unclear exactly how many of the members expressed these kinds of concerns, but those who did were very vocal! At the same time, the AMA sharply rebuked the AAP for its recommendation, but also announced an alternative effort to obtain funds from private sources to support medical education. The issue was discussed at the 1948 Annual Meeting where it was voted to hold in abeyance any action to seek federal aid for medical education—without prejudice to justification of federal aid or its need. Shortly after this, the ICH was dissolved and the activities in this area were incorporated back into the AAP and the direct purview of the Executive Board and the controversy subsided.

By 1950, the war was over, the nation was prosperous, and enormous progress was occurring in medical science. The "difficult decade" that divided the AAP and could have fragmented American pediatrics had been survived. Pediatrics and the AAP were ready to embark on the *golden age of pediatrics* of the next 3 decades.

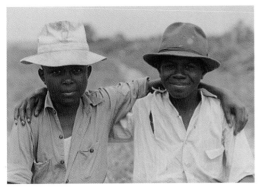 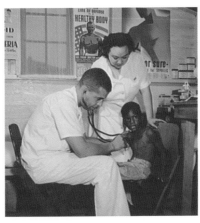 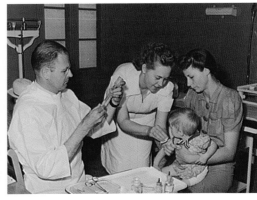

Left, schoolchildren in rural Texas, 1943. *Above left to right*, children of migrant workers at a Farm Security Administration (FSA) agricultural workers' camp, Bridgeton, NJ, 1942; doctor, nurse, and patient at FSA agricultural workers' camp clinic, Bridgeton, NJ, 1942; doctor preparing shot in FSA agricultural workers' camp clinic, Caldwell, ID, 1941.

GROWTH AND ACCOMPLISHMENTS OF
THE AMERICAN ACADEMY OF PEDIATRICS:
1935 TO 1950

Despite political conflict, AAP growth continued during these years, increasing membership from 834 in 1935 to 2,796 in 1950. The members were increasingly dispersed through all of the states. An unequal geographic distribution of members in the original 4 regions became evident and a disproportional representation of membership on the Executive Board had occurred. For example, in 1945, the Eastern Seaboard, with nearly half of the AAP membership, had only 2 of 13 votes on the Executive Board. To address this inequity, the country was redivided in 1949 into 8 geographic districts (I–VIII) plus District IX, which included Mexico and Latin America. In 1948, a major effort to democratize the AAP was made by encouraging the formation of state chapters that would

elect, by ballot, the district chairmen and alternate district chairmen.

The Annual Meetings were juxtaposed with the meetings of the AMA until 1939, when it was decided to have them independent of other medical groups. This enabled the attraction of commercial exhibits, which became a significant source of revenue. Regional (or areal) meetings were held from the early days of the AAP—some of which rivaled the Annual Meeting in attendance. Eventually, it was decided to have a national Spring Meeting, and the regional meetings were discontinued. The educational content of the national meetings was extensive and broad and included innovations such as roundtables on specific topics.

In 1949, the AAP Section on Surgery was created as a forum for the increasing number of surgeons who were restricting their practice to children. The AAP recognized pediatric surgery

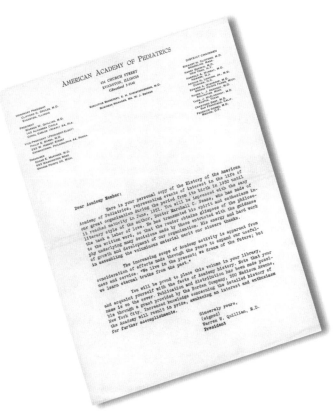

Marshall Carleton Pease, MD, wrote a fascinating history of the early years of the American Academy of Pediatrics (AAP), published in 1951. Pictured is the letter that was sent out to AAP members at the time, announcing the book with the inspiring quote, "We live in the present; we dream of the future; but we learn eternal truths from the past."

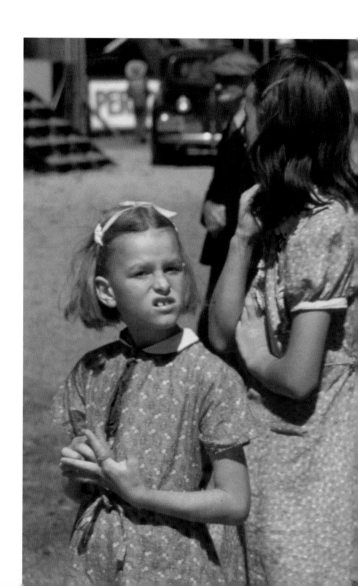

long before the specialty was accepted by surgical groups. Other sections that were formed at the same time were the Section on Allergy and Immunology and the Section on Mental Growth and Development.

The *Journal of Pediatrics* remained the official organ of the AAP until 1947. By this time, the journal had become highly successful and profitable for the Mosby Company. There was pressure to renegotiate the 1931 contract, but Mosby was unwilling to open its books for review. Instead, it offered the AAP a small share of the profits, which the AAP rejected, and, instead, a new journal, owned by the AAP, was created. The new journal was named *Pediatrics*. A contract was negotiated for publication by the Thomas Publishing Company. The editors and editorial board of the new journal were appointed by the AAP, most of whom had previously served on the *Journal of Pediatrics*. *Pediatrics* rapidly became a scientific and financial success.

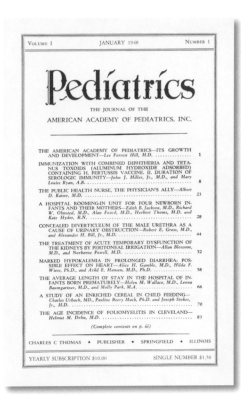

The first issue of *Pediatrics*, Volume 1, Number 1, January 1948.

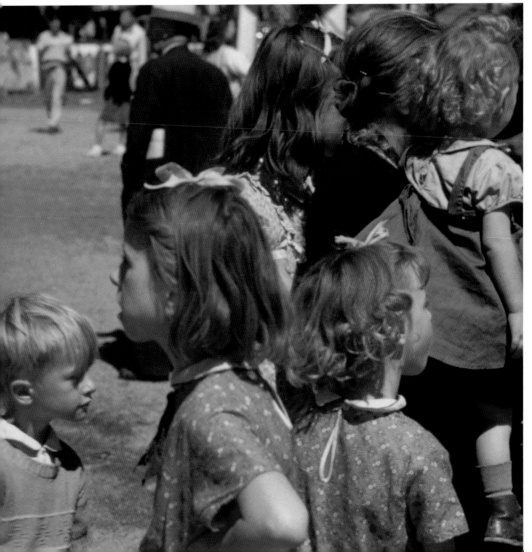

Family at Vermont state fair, Rutland, VT, 1941.

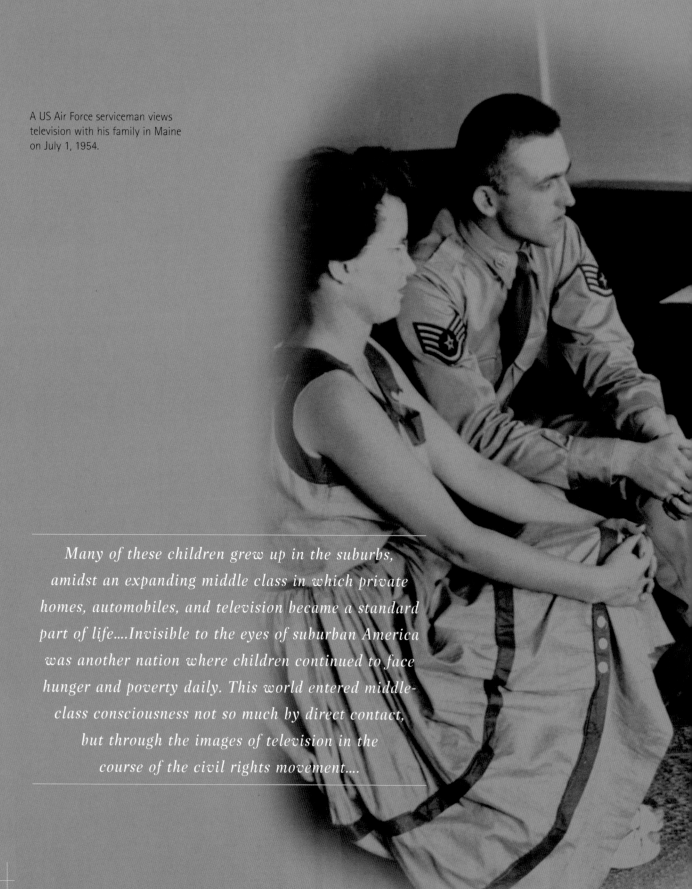

A US Air Force serviceman views television with his family in Maine on July 1, 1954.

Many of these children grew up in the suburbs, amidst an expanding middle class in which private homes, automobiles, and television became a standard part of life....Invisible to the eyes of suburban America was another nation where children continued to face hunger and poverty daily. This world entered middle-class consciousness not so much by direct contact, but through the images of television in the course of the civil rights movement....

Chapter 4
An Expanded Agenda for Children

1950 to 1980

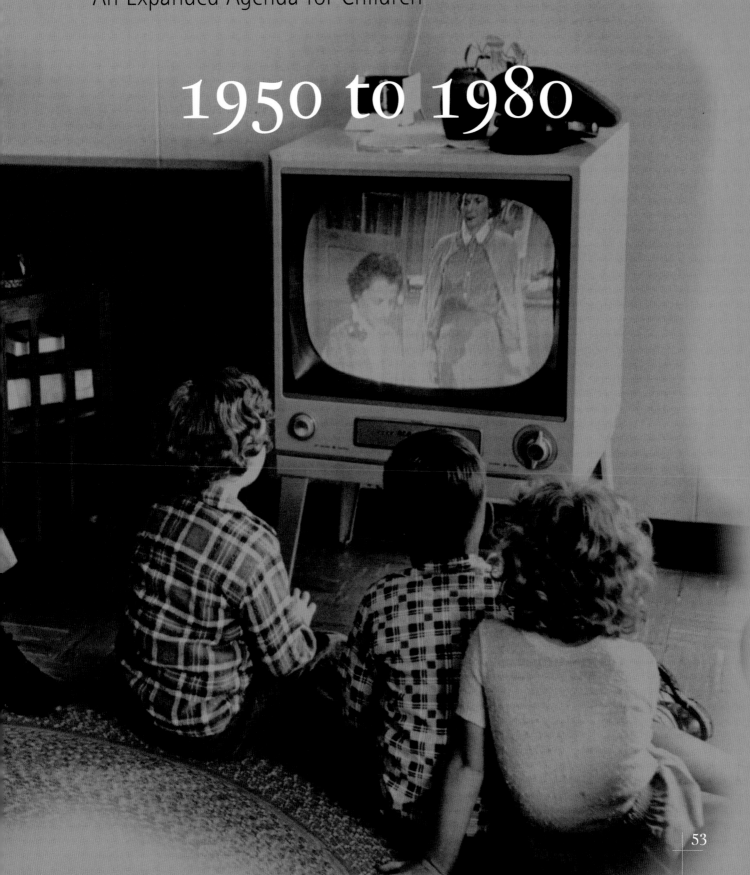

1950
Floyd W. Denny, MD, and
Charles H. Rammelkamp,
Jr, MD, reported the
effectiveness of penicillin
therapy of beta-hemolytic
streptococcal pharyngitis
in preventing acute
rheumatic fever.
(Minneapolis, MN)

1954
Surgeons Joseph E.
Murray, MD, and J.
Hartwell Harrison, MD,
and nephrologist John P.
Merrill, MD, performed a
kidney transplant
between identical twins.
(Boston, MA)

THE BABY BOOM GENERATION

The end of the Second World War brought unprecedented prosperity to the United States. Fertility rates, after having fallen to historical lows in the depression, now rebounded dramatically with an average of 4 million babies born annually between 1946 and 1964. Many of these children grew up in the suburbs, amidst an expanding middle class in which private homes, automobiles, and television became a standard part of life. Popular magazines and television idealized the nuclear family. Many women who had entered the workplace during the war now returned to full-time responsibilities in the home. Child rearing itself became more relaxed. Child advice books prior to the war had emphasized strict feeding schedules, early toilet training, and a fear of "overindulging" babies. Now mothers turned to the reassuring tone of *The Common Sense Book of Baby and Child Care*, by Benjamin M. Spock, MD, encouraged by its opening words—*"You know more than you think you do"*—to rely on maternal instinct to raise children.

Dr Spock's writing, drawing upon psychoanalytic theory, affirmed a positive and loving relationship between mother and infant as of paramount importance. Office pediatricians increasingly faced questions on preventive and emotional health.

Of course, many did not share in this new prosperity. Invisible to the eyes of suburban America was another nation where children continued to face hunger and poverty daily. This world

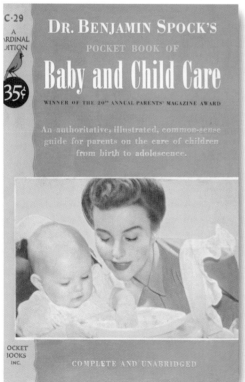
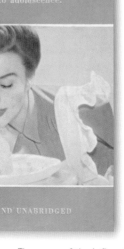

The cover of the influential child-rearing book, *Baby and Child Care*, by Benjamin M. Spock, MD—"Dr Spock."

entered middle-class consciousness not so much by direct contact, but through the images of television in the course of the civil rights movement. Children played a central role in this story. While politicians, lawyers, and activists jousted in the aftermath of the *Brown v Board of Education* decision, first-grade African American schoolchildren walked to school each morning past jeering mobs of white demonstrators held back by police officers. In 1963, the use of fire hoses and police dogs against women and children joining Martin Luther King, Jr's, Birmingham demonstrations raised widespread national indignation and marked a turning point for the civil rights movement.

The resilience of children under such circumstances (documented eloquently in the influential *Children of Crisis* series by child psychiatrist, Robert Coles, MD) astonished many observers and attracted great sympathy. The administration of President John F. Kennedy began to draw attention to the problem of what was sometimes called the "forgotten America," encompassing the segregated south as well as Appalachia and, increasingly, the inner city. The Aid to Dependent Children (ADC) program was refashioned and expanded as Aid to Families and Dependent Children (AFDC) in 1962, and was later joined by Medicaid, food stamps, and many other programs addressing poverty. President Lyndon B. Johnson continued these efforts to launch a "war on poverty" that would have a major impact on children's lives.

These same years witnessed a resurgence of social activism among pediatricians not seen on such a scale since the child welfare crusades of the early 20th century. Julius B. Richmond, MD, was instrumental in the creation of Head Start, one of the most innovative and successful initiatives of the war against poverty. University of Colorado pediatrician C. Henry Kempe, MD,

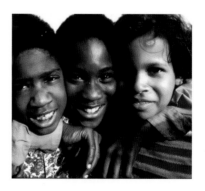

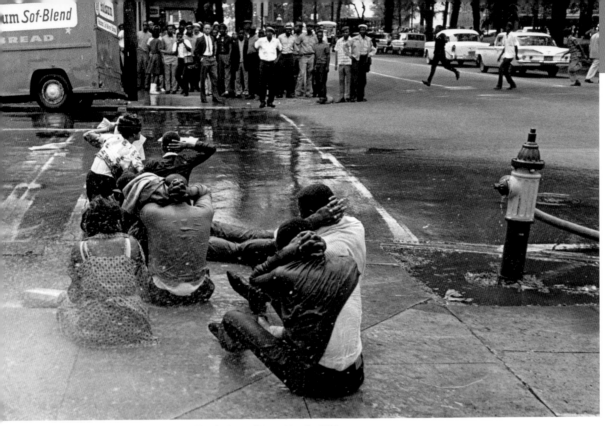

Demonstrators at a civil rights rally in Birmingham, AL, on May 3, 1963.

1955
The Salk polio vaccine is vindicated by the largest field trials in history. The subsequent decline of polio is widely regarded as the greatest triumph of postwar medicine.

1959
Jerome Lejeune, MD, described trisomy of chromosome 21 in Down syndrome. (Paris, France)

Mary Ellen Avery, MD, and Jere Mead, MD, described a deficiency of pulmonary surfactant in respiratory distress syndrome. (Boston, MA)

joined by many members of the American Academy of Pediatrics (AAP), spearheaded a movement to report and prevent child abuse. Dr Spock attracted considerable controversy as a third-party candidate for US president in 1972, running principally against the Vietnam War. Indeed, conservatives derided college antiwar activists as products of his "permissive" child-rearing philosophy.

The legacy of the 1960s for children was complex. The advances made on behalf of minority civil rights were countered by white flight, urban renewal, and the economic collapse of many inner cities. These trends became particularly acute as the civil rights movement radicalized and inner-city riots swept the nation with the 1968 assassination of Martin Luther King, Jr. Though federal investment in the AFDC and other programs did indeed lower the percentage of Americans living below the poverty line, a conservative backlash emerged by the late 1960s. Influential observers such as Daniel Patrick Moynihan (assistant secretary of labor in the Johnson administration) characterized the roots of these problems in the "tangle of pathology" that was the legacy of slavery on the black family. In truth, later historical research has shown that 2-parent families remained the norm among African Americans until jobs vanished from the inner city in the 1950s. Nonetheless, few could dispute that guns, violence, drug use, and homicide became prominent features of life for all too many urban children and adolescents.

Though the civil rights movement focused attention on African Americans, observers recognized that many groups of children struggled for their share of the country's prosperity. Rural areas such as Appalachia contended with

"I affirm that a child who occupies a bed in a children's ward, whether he is a millionaire, belongs to the middle class, or is a pauper, no matter what his race, color, or creed, receives as a rule the best possible medical attention and the most devoted care from the physician in attendance."

ISAAC A. ABT, MD, FROM THE FIRST PRESIDENTIAL ADDRESS OF THE AMERICAN ACADEMY OF PEDIATRICS ON JUNE 12, 1931

1960
A report describing the first successful testing of the first live measles vaccine by John F. Enders and Samuel L. Katz, MD, was published. (Boston, MA)

The first neonatal intensive care unit (NICU), designed by Louis Gluck, MD, was opened. (New Haven, CT)

The American Board of Pediatrics established its first subspecialty certification for pediatric cardiology.

unemployment and poverty as rural economies declined. Native American families on reservations struggled to preserve their cultural identity as well as improve their financial situation. A rising tide of new immigrants, notably Asians and Hispanics, further diversified the country and created new challenges for pediatric providers.

The 1960s and 1970s also witnessed a revolution of the middle-class family. Women were increasingly free to enter the workplace. Many did so out of choice, others out of economic necessity amidst the sluggish economy of the 1970s. Most parents, however, continued to place great value upon the emotional nurture of their young children. Family life was often characterized by more warmth and communication, and less rigid separation of parental roles. Yet it frequently became more volatile as well. Divorce rates, which had been creeping upward slowly for most of the century, rose sharply in the early

1970s. At the same time, society as a whole remained ambivalent about federal support for child care, which conservatives characterized as undermining the traditional family. All of these factors raised new hurdles for children and adolescents to overcome, raising challenges not only for their parents but their pediatricians as well.

Against this background, in 1975, pediatric leader Robert J. Haggerty, MD, and his colleagues coined the term *new morbidity* to assert the necessity for pediatrics to expand its agenda to encompass psychosocial as well as more traditionally medical diseases. In embracing this calling, many pediatricians recognized that their efforts to advocate for children necessarily carried them beyond the confines of the office visit. The AAP itself reaffirmed its own origins as an organization dedicated to the welfare of children, and escalated its advocacy efforts to an unprecedented level.

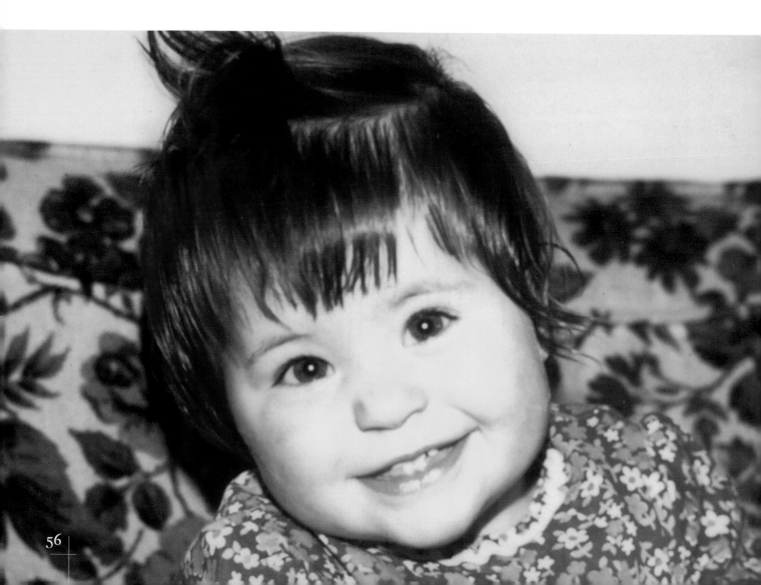

The 1960s were a time of increasing size and an ever-widening involvement of the AAP in national issues and legislation through the work of its committees. Several initiatives begun in the 1950s (and earlier) were expanded in the 1960s, including the continued establishment of early Poison Control Centers (PCCs) through the work of the Committee on Accident Prevention, as well as the publication and circulation of definitive manuals by the Committee on Fetus and Newborn (*Resuscitation of the Newborn Infant* and *Standards and Recommendations for Hospital Care of Newborn Infants, Full-Term and Premature*). The Committee on Infectious Diseases continued to publish new editions of its popular *Report of the Committee on Infectious Diseases* (the *Red Book*) that was first published in 1938. The Committee on Nutrition issued a number of reports addressing a wide range of pediatric nutritional issues, including a recommendation that infant formulas should be fortified with iron.

In 1961, the AAP strongly supported the establishment of the National Institute of Child Health and Human Development (NICHD), which, through its grant programs, supported a wide range of research endeavors, many of which were conducted by the faculties of medical school departments of pediatrics. Grants from the NICHD facilitated the growth of pediatric departments and expansion of their general pediatric and subspecialty faculties.

In the mid-1960s, the AAP had to face another internal controversy that again threatened to split its membership. Although the AAP had many activities involved with health legislation and socioeconomic issues, some members from California who believed that these issues were not being adequately addressed founded an organization called the California Federation of Pediatric Societies. This group went national in 1966 and began to solicit membership of pediatricians in what they now called the Federation of Pediatric Societies. This raised the distinct possibility of a new national pediatric society that would pre-empt functions of the AAP.

The AAP leadership responded to this challenge by emphasizing its belief that the AAP could best influence the quality of child health

1961–1963
The licensure and introduction of the live attenuated polio vaccine, developed by Albert B. Sabin, MD, occurred, following trials in the Soviet Union.

1962
An article describing the "battered-child syndrome" was published by C. Henry Kempe, MD. (Denver, CO)

The creation of the National Institute of Child Health and Human Development was authorized by Congress, with Robert A. Aldrich, MD, as its first director. (Bethesda, MD)

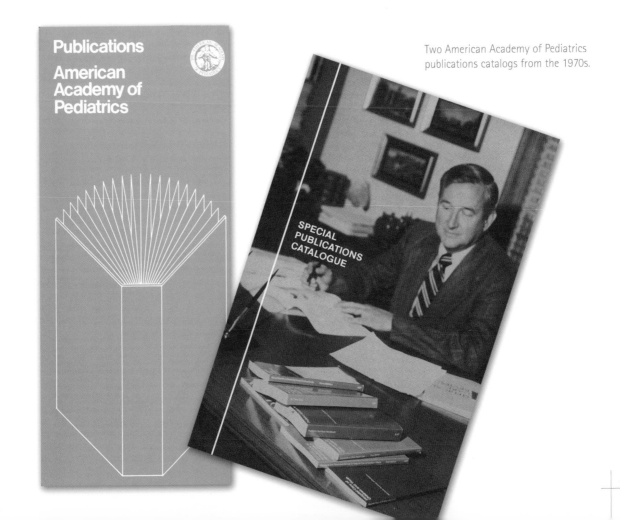

Two American Academy of Pediatrics publications catalogs from the 1970s.

services by continuing to concentrate on education and science rather than becoming an organization primarily concerned with the business and economic aspects of pediatric practice, although it listed a wide range of AAP activities in this arena. In mid-1966, the federation proposed an amendment to the AAP constitution that called for establishment of a Socio-Economic Council, separate and independent from the AAP Executive Board, that could speak for the Fellows of the AAP in legislative and socioeconomic matters. Clearly, passage of such an amendment would have created 2 national pediatric societies and split the AAP into 2 groups. As a result of many discussions between the 2 groups, the amendment was withdrawn, and the AAP was not divided. However, a consequence of this episode was greater emphasis by the AAP on issues that related to pediatric practice.

In 1968, the AAP became an important force in the medical consultation aspects of the Head Start program, as described later in this chapter. The AAP continued to be involved in directing the medical aspects of Head Start until the contract with the Department of Health,

Education, and Welfare was terminated in 1976. During those 8 years, more than 700 AAP members served as medical consultants to Head Start in 50 states.

In addition to the educational activities (lectures, workshops and seminars) at the Annual and Spring meetings, the AAP offered the membership programs for continuing education and self-assessment, including the Self-evaluation and Education Program (SEEP) in 1970 (which had been approved in 1968) and the Professional Assessment for Continuing Education (PACE) program in 1974. In 1978, the Pediatric Review and Education Program (PREP) was introduced by the AAP and the American Board of Pediatrics (ABP). PREP was, at least in part, a response to increasing discussion about pediatric board recertification, and, especially, concerns whether recertification would be voluntary and whether a cognitive examination would be required. PREP initially had 2 components. One was an educational program provided through a new journal, *Pediatrics in Review* (*PIR*), which published review articles of important pediatric subjects, as well as other articles on recent advances in pediatrics. PREP also contained a self-assessment exercise based on the published articles. A voluntary, proctored recertification examination was offered annually. However, only a few hundred pediatricians took the examination each year.

Despite the voluntary nature of the recertification examination, controversy continued. Each year at the Chapter Presidents' Forum, recertification was heavily debated, with most participants opposing any recertification. When Dr Haggerty, who was AAP vice president in 1983, spoke in favor of recertification, he recalls being accosted by an irate member who grabbed his tie and said, "If you mention recertification again, I'll personally see that you are impeached!" In 1987, the ABP introduced time-limited certification. After 1988, those certified by the ABP were required to take a proctored, cognitive recertification examination every 6 years, but those certified prior to 1988 were essentially "grandfathered" and exempted from reexamination. With this compromise, the recertification controversy abated.

From 1976 to 1978, the AAP spearheaded a Task Force on Pediatric Education, which conducted an exhaustive survey of pediatric practice and education. The task force was made up of 16 members from 10 different pediatric

Materials from the Self-evaluation and Education Program (SEEP), 1970.

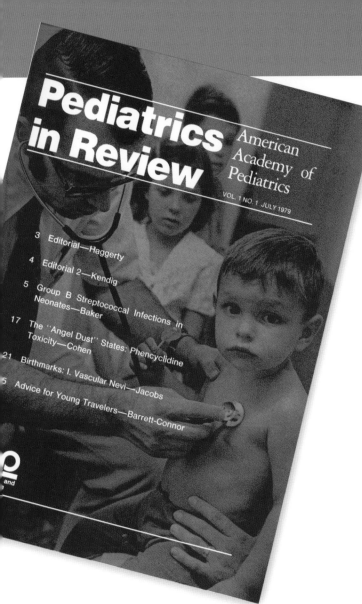

Pediatrics in Review

American Academy of Pediatrics

VOL. 1 NO. 1 JULY 1979

3 Editorial—Haggerty

4 Editorial 2—Kendig

5 Group B Streptococcal Infections in Neonates—Baker

17 The "Angel Dust" States: Phencyclidine Toxicity—Cohen

21 Birthmarks: I. Vascular Nevi—Jacobs

5 Advice for Young Travelers—Barrett-Connor

Left, the first issue of *Pediatrics in Review*, Volume 1, Number 1, July 1979; *below*, *The Future of Pediatric Education (FOPE)* report, 1978.

AUG 2 1 1978

The Future of Pediatric Education

A Report

by

The Task Force on Pediatric Education

1968
Robert Good, MD, performed a successful bone marrow transplantation for severe combined immunodeficiency syndrome. (Minneapolis, MN)

1970–1980
Robert J. Haggerty, MD, and Morris Green, MD, described a "new morbidity" of pediatric practice. (Rochester, NY, and Indianapolis, IN)

organizations, and included AAP Fellows in private practice. The task force conducted 2 studies: a survey of a large number of mothers from all over the country and walks of life, and a study of 7,000 recent graduates of pediatric residency programs around the country. In 1978, the task force published a report, *The Future of Pediatric Education (FOPE)*, that made a number of recommendations concerning the content of medical school pediatric curricula as well as the duration, structure, and content of pediatric residency. They called for 36 months of pediatric residency during which increased emphasis would be given to ambulatory experience including biosocial and developmental problems as well as counseling.

During the 1960s, socioeconomic and legislative activities of the AAP were greatly expanded. To assist with these efforts, the AAP established its Department of Government Liaison in Washington, DC, in 1970. The role of this office was to foster communication between the AAP,

federal agencies, and Congress on issues affecting child health and to facilitate early AAP participation in discussions of proposed legislation. The Washington office also published a useful *Legislative Handbook* to instruct AAP members on how to more effectively influence the legislative process.

Continuing Medical Education: "Pediatrics Is Not Static"

The need for continuing medical education (CME), which the AAP so skillfully provides in a diversity of venues, became obvious early in my career. It permitted practitioners to interact and learn from colleagues via seminars, hands-on workshops, and publications (both hard copy and, ultimately, online). Our faculties are carefully vetted for their knowledge, abilities in engaging the registrants, and skills in preparation of audiovisual materials. Pediatrics is not static. We must maintain what we've learned and be willing to modify and update our skills. We also have an obligation to educate ourselves, patients, parents, and colleagues.

— *Milton Arnold, MD*

The Early Years of the American Academy of Pediatrics Washington, DC, Office

Since July 1970, the American Academy of Pediatrics (AAP) has had an established office in Washington, DC, to help lead and facilitate active participation by its members in the legislative and regulatory processes. Our challenge was, and still is, to move forward constructively, by understanding emerging trends or needed changes and finding ways to address them.

I began work at the AAP in November 1973, when President Richard Nixon called national health insurance his top domestic priority. In June 1974, Donald W. Schiff, MD, who later served as AAP president, asked the Congress to "mark the 1970s as the decade for children." Increased funding for numerous programs from the Department of Health, Education, and Welfare was requested at annual appropriations hearings, with emphasis on Title V of the Social Security Act, the National Institute of Child Health and Human Development, and immunizations. We enjoyed many victories in spite of tight budgets, and child health programs began to grow.

The biggest challenge at the time was actually modifying the National Health Planning and Resources Development Act of 1974 to include children's needs and then delivering the 50 state plans within an 8-month time frame. To hold down the mounting national medical bill of $100 billion, this law was intended to make sure that costly health services and facilities were developed only where and when they were needed. Through the leadership of AAP president John MacQueen, MD, handbooks and sample plans were provided to AAP chapters to accomplish this task. Lessons learned by AAP members at the local level proved invaluable in building our strong chapters as we know them today.

— *Jackie Noyes, MA* (Ms Noyes is an associate executive director of the AAP, based in the AAP Washington, DC, office.)

The accomplishments of the AAP pediatricians advocating and providing health care for children during the span of 1950 to 1980 are numerous and profound. The following accounts, necessarily highly selective, can only give a flavor of the many efforts taken by the membership of the AAP and its allies on behalf of children.

Poison Control Centers and Aspirin Poisoning

In 1950, the AAP created the Accident Prevention Committee (APC) to explore methods to combat childhood injuries. World War II had led to the marketing of many potentially toxic household chemicals and drugs. A 1952 study by the APC estimated that 51% of childhood injuries resulted from unintentional poisoning. There was an obvious need for reliable information on ingredients and toxicity of household products that would facilitate decisions on appropriate management in childhood poisonings. The APC study contributed to the opening of the first Poison Control Center in Chicago, IL, by Edward Press, MD, a pediatrician who recognized the need for timely and accessible product information, toxicity data, and management recommendations. Although it was originally only an informational resource for health care providers, the Chicago center's success stimulated a national proliferation of centers that offered direct information on management and poison prevention to both the public and professionals.

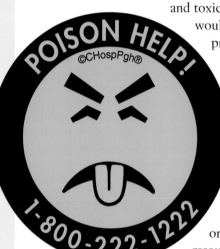

"Mr Yuk" poison control sticker from the Children's Hospital of Pittsburgh, PA.

The early PCCs usually were located in hospital emergency rooms, and response time to calls was highly variable. It was often difficult to find product information, and the advice given all too often was to "bring them in," leading to frequent and often unnecessary gastric lavage or syrup of ipecac. (The era of gastric emptying by syrup of ipecac has come to an end. The November 2003 issue of *Pediatrics* contained an AAP policy statement, "Poison Treatment in the Home," that recommended the removal of ipecac from the home.)

Since there were no published resources, each PCC had to laboriously collect its own product information. In 1955, Robert H. Dreisbach, MD, authored *Handbook of Poisoning*, followed in 1957 by a huge data-based book, *Clinical Toxicology of Commercial Products*, by Marion N. Gleason, MD; Robert E. Goesslin, MD; and Harold C. Hodge, MD. In 1963, *Poisoning*, by Jay M. Arena, MD, was published.

In 1957, at the suggestion of the AAP, the Surgeon General established the National Clearinghouse of Poison Control Centers, which developed an index card system containing product information that was distributed to PCCs. It ultimately consisted of 16,000 cards, which required considerable hand shuffling and searching. When this proved too cumbersome, the data were made available on microfiche. In the 1980s, the growing database became accessible on a computerized, frequently updated source marketed commercially as Poisindex.

The American Association of Poison Control Centers (AAPCC) was founded in 1958, and its first president was Robert Grayson, MD. Its charge was to foster cooperation between centers, to establish standards, and to develop educational programs for professionals and the public. In 1978, the AAPCC established criteria for the development of regional poison control centers including uniform standards and resources as well as the availability of trained poison information specialists. By 2003, there were 64 regional centers in the United States, 80% of which were certified. A national toll-free hotline was established to give advice to pediatricians and parents, as well as instructions on how to contact the nearest regional or local PCC.

For many years, salicylate (aspirin) overdosage, often accidental, was among the most important causes of poisoning in children, especially children younger than 5 years old. In the 1960s, when salicylates were widely used for a variety of ailments, it was estimated that there were more than 10,000 cases of severe salicylate intoxication each year in the United States, leading to 140 deaths from aspirin poisoning in 1963. But improvement in these statistics was seen in the 1970s. Data from the National Clearinghouse of PCCs showed a drop in salicylate poisoning from 21.7% of total poisonings in children younger than 5 years old in 1968 to only 3.4% in 1977. This improvement was attributed to the introduction of safety packaging in 1970 and the use of 81-mg "Baby Aspirin" tablets. At the same time, there was increased use of acetaminophen instead of aspirin, in large part because of the recognized association between salicylates and Reye syndrome.

— *Howard Mofenson, MD; Joseph Greensher, MD; and Robert Grayson, MD*

1972
Congress enacted the Special Supplemental Nutrition Program for Women, Infants, and Children (WIC).

The United States ended requirement for routine smallpox immunization.

1975
Robert H. Bartlett, MD, performed the first successful neonatal extracorporeal membrane oxygenation (ECMO) at the University of California at Irvine.

Reflections on Childhood Poisoning

In the early 1950s, the toddler daughter of an otolaryngologist in Birmingham, AL, "investigated" the highly alkaline dishwater detergent under the sink. She gasped, stopped breathing, and the father had to do an emergency tracheotomy on his own daughter. I wrote a furious letter to the president of the company, pointing out that the detergent's caustic nature was not revealed, and that there were no precautions on the box, other than not to use it as a shampoo. I got a response from the company (though from a much lesser luminary than the president) stating that the detergent, in legal terms, was not a caustic and, besides, if too many warnings were displayed on the box, nobody would buy it. The letter also noted dispassionately, "Probably choking on flour would be just as bad."

In 1970, the Poison Prevention Packaging Act mandated protection of dangerous medications from marauding children. St. Joseph aspirin featured the first "child-proof" cap, which was a *surmountable* challenge for my youngest child, who had a merry old time eating St. Joseph aspirin and scoffing at science and the industrial engineers.

— *S. Donald Palmer, MD*

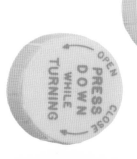

Left, boy playing with medicine bottle; *right*, child safety cap from the early 1960s.

1979
Thomas E. Cone, Jr, MD, published the *History of American Pediatrics.* (Boston, MA)

Godfrey N. Hounsfield and Allan M. Cormack received the Nobel Prize for their development of computer-assisted tomography.

The Beginning of Head Start

In 1965, the AAP played a very important role in bringing comprehensive child development programs to many poor children and their families throughout the United States. As the first national director of Head Start, I feel it's a story that the AAP membership should know. The 1960s were heady days of social ferment. After the assassination of President Kennedy in 1963 and the concomitant civil rights resolution, the nation was ready for a "war on poverty," made possible by the passage of the Economic Opportunity Act of 1964. President Johnson appointed Mr Sargent Shriver, the first director of the Peace Corps, to lead the antipoverty effort. Shriver had learned much about child development and mental retardation as executive director of the Joseph P. Kennedy, Jr, Foundation, and his thoughts immediately turned toward interrupting the transmission of poverty from one generation to another.

He appointed a 15-person advisory committee that had 4 pediatricians represented, including Robert Cooke, MD, professor of pediatrics at Johns Hopkins medical school, as chairperson. Within 3 months, the committee issued a bold report indicating the importance of improving the environments of poor, young children. Among other things, it stated, "It is clear that successful programs of this type must be comprehensive, involving activities generally associated with the fields of health, social services, and education." Mr Shriver recruited me, a professor of pediatrics, to direct what would become a very comprehensive program, and the challenge was daunting. In February 1965, we made the decision to have a nationwide, 8-week summer program starting in June of that year.

As we contemplated how to mount the health program, the role of the AAP became central. As an AAP member, I was familiar with its organizational structure and I saw the state chapters as the way to ensure high-quality services throughout the United States. We appealed to the AAP Board of Directors for help and its response was favorable and enthusiastic. This was not a simple matter because, at that time, organized medicine,

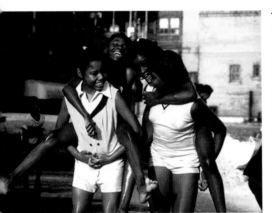

Girls playing in fire hydrant water, Chicago, IL, June 1973.

especially the American Medical Association (AMA), opposed any collaboration with government. In fact, the AMA was engaged in the most bitterly fought political campaign of the 20th century against the passage of Medicare (which, of course, it lost). The members of the AAP Board of Directors had great vision and courage!

The contractual relationship between the AAP and the Head Start program involved providing quality assurance for health programs at the local level. The state chairpersons recruited AAP members to serve as consultants for every program in the country. Many of the children received their first-ever physical examinations through the program and there were many dramatic stories of previously undetected health problems.

In our pluralistic society, the program developed unique local approaches. The ingenuity of pediatric consultants knew no bounds in getting children to appropriate services. This was especially important then, for Medicaid had just been passed, but was not yet implemented. We had no funds for treatment, so local hospitals and clinics were asked to provide these additional services. When we received occasional protests about the burden of the new requests, we had to remind communities that we didn't generate the need— only the demand—for services.

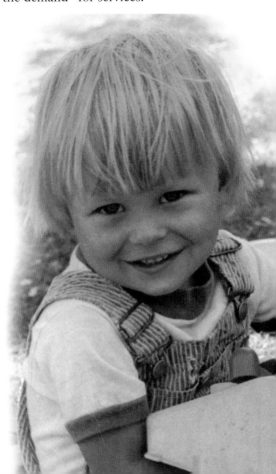

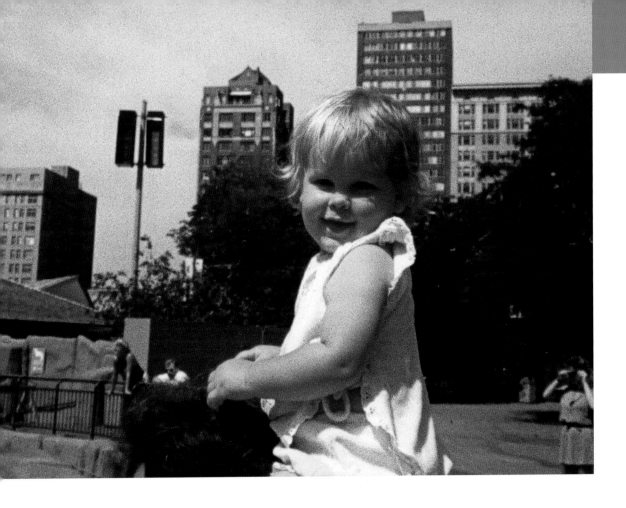

The nation owes a great debt to the leaders of the AAP and its many members who responded, under emergency circumstances, to implement one of the great successes of the social programs of the 20th century.

— *Julius B. Richmond, MD*

Behavioral Pediatrics and a Preventive Model for Pediatricians

Medical school was a disappointment for me. One of my professors, Robert Loeb, MD, at Columbia P & S [Columbia University College of Physicians and Surgeons] stood out. "No questions. Watch a patient for 15 minutes and then tell me his age, his occupation, married or not, what is he in here for, and is he getting better?" We found that in time we could do this! During medical school, I realize now that I was being diverted from the reason I went into medicine— wanting to make relationships that helped others to health. Although Dr Loeb taught me to value observation, I needed to develop my own tools for making relationships and using them to prevent illness. In pediatrics, child development is our language for reaching out to parents. I went into pediatrics because I didn't want to work with adults and I wanted to find a preventive model that could prevent illness, rather than attempting to treat it. During my internship and residency in Boston, MA, I learned the physical aspects of illness, but treating them felt, to me, like applying Band-Aids after the fact.

I began to look at children at the beginnings of their lives, a time when we thought a baby was a blank slate, and devised our Neonatal Behavioral Assessment Scale in 1956. We have learned so much from it. Newborn babies not only "see and hear," but they are responsive and can help guide parents into their new role by their responsive behavior. Studying disruptions of the attachment between working parents and their infants over the first few months of life led me to testify before Congress in favor of the Parental Leave Bill, which allowed working parents to be at home with their new infants for the first few critical months. I also supported appropriations to fund Early Intervention sites countrywide.

We have a training model at Children's Hospital Boston called "Touchpoints," which evaluates families' strengths, reaches out for vulnerable families, and embraces them with a nurturing model, using the child's behavior, temperament, and developmental progress as a basis for these relationships. Touchpoints is already successful in 52 multidisciplinary sites around this country and abroad, and will continue to grow. We are on our way to a preventive model for the new morbidity, failures in social and cognitive developments. Pediatricians should be leaders in this initiative.

— *Thomas Berry Brazelton, MD*

Practicing Political Medicine

For the past 40 years, I have been a part-time practitioner of political medicine, which I define as employing the political process to improve health. Virtually all my political activity came about as a result of patients I saw in hospital outpatient clinics and emergency rooms serving the poor.

In the fall of 1966, 6 children were admitted to our hospital with dreadful burns sustained when their clothing ignited. In October of that year, at the AAP Annual Meeting in Chicago, I saw a demonstration by scientists from the Department of Agriculture on how cotton for children's clothing could be made flame resistant. I contacted Senator Warren Magnuson, who then chaired the Senate Commerce Committee, and asked him to introduce legislation mandating that children's clothing be flame resistant. I was not nearly as persuasive as the words of burn victims and their parents during a visit the senator and his wife made to Children's Hospital (Seattle, WA). The result was the Flammable Fabrics Act Amendment of 1967. Because of heavy political and economic pressure from the cotton industry, it was 5 years before the law was implemented but, after that, the toll of flammable fabric burn injuries dropped markedly.

Pediatric wards in those days were also full of children admitted with toxic ingestions, especially aspirin ingestions. Robert Scherz, MD, a colleague at nearby Madigan Army Hospital, carried

out an elegant study showing fewer ingestions in households where aspirin was kept in child-resistant containers. I brought this work to Senator Magnuson's attention. Lo and behold, the Poison Prevention Packaging Act of 1970 was enacted and a steady drop in admissions for toxic ingestions ensued.

My interactions with Washington's senators helped in the enactment of a number of other measures, such as creation of the National Health Service Corps in 1970, the Sudden Infant Death Syndrome Act in 1974, and the Indian Health Care Improvement Act in 1976. Influencing national legislation was "heady," but, in reality, these successes probably had more to do with my getting to know 2 powerful senators, than any particular talent of mine.

— *Abraham B. Bergman, MD*

Child Passenger Safety—Speaking Up for Children

It was an otherwise ordinary evening in the early 1960s when I saw Seymour Charles, MD, a well-respected senior pediatrician, on the network evening news. I had seen him that very morning at hospital rounds, yet, now, there he was on television, marching with a large placard in a public demonstration in front of the annual auto show at the New York Coliseum. He and other members of Physicians for Automotive Safety were decrying the dangers to children of automobiles and demanding that the automobile manufacturers build safer cars and provide protection for child passengers.

That was my first experience with militant advocacy for children and the advancement of child health, but it was not my last. In the early 1960s, there were no seat belts, no child restraints, no air bags, or impact-absorbing bumpers in vehicles. There was a preoccupation with faster, bigger cars sporting deadly bullet bumpers and sharp fender fins. Children were launched like projectiles in car collisions. And no one seemed to care until Dr Charles and his Physicians for Automotive Safety taught the mighty automobile industry, and persuaded the

American Academy of Pediatrics "Make Every Ride a Safe Ride" button.

MAKE EVERY RIDE A SAFE RIDE
American Academy of Pediatrics

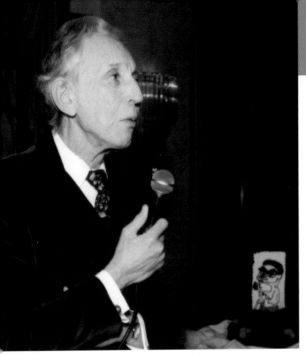

Seymour Charles, MD, speaks out for child passenger safety.

AAP and the world, that mandatory safety measures in cars were necessary.

Today, seat belts and safety restraints are a part of every vehicle, thanks to the diligent efforts of people like Dr Charles and organizations like the AAP. Dr Charles was vocal, sometimes abrasive, but always tenacious. He taught me and countless others the value of activism and advocacy in speaking up for children. Don't forget to buckle up!

— *Arthur Maron, MD*

Children With Special Health Care Needs
An entry-level position as a staff pediatrician at a state residential facility (institution) in the 1960s helped shape my future career in pediatrics, which has been devoted to children with special health care needs. My responsibilities at the residential facility included preventive and acute care for 150 residents of school age. These children, 6 to 18 years old, left their homes and families, oftentimes a considerable distance away, to be educated in the school at the facility. There were no community-based, special education school programs for children with mental retardation or other developmental disabilities in that era.

After 2 years as a staff pediatrician, I became the director of the diagnostic center at this facility. This center performed comprehensive evaluations of every child with a developmental disability in the state that was being considered for admission to any state institution. During a 90-day inpatient stay, the evaluation was complet-ed and a treatment plan developed. The child or adolescent was then placed in an appropriate institution. This proved to be a self-taught fellowship in developmental disabilities for me.

In 1965, because of the experience I gained at the state facility, I was offered the position as chief of the Handicapped Child Division in the Department of Pediatrics, and director of the Birth Defects Center at Columbus Children's Hospital. This clinical/academic role afforded me the opportunity to serve children with special needs who were living in the community with their families; quite a different perspective than my earlier one while working in a facility. Community or school programs for special education were almost nonexistent, but were created through community action. Two vignettes are illustrative:

> *An 18-month-old boy with moderate mental retardation and autistic-like behavior was seen upon referral. He lived in a semi-urban community with no training program. The mother was urged to "lead the charge" in establishing such a program, which she did. It resulted in the Starlight School being established in her community. She incidentally showed her appreciation to our program by donating a stroller and playpen to the Birth Defects Center.*

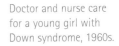

Doctor and nurse care for a young girl with Down syndrome, 1960s.

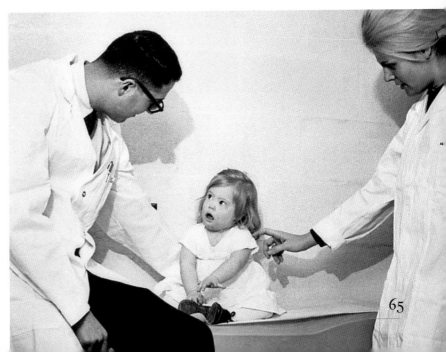

A 6-year-old boy with dual handicaps—a severe visual disability and mild mental retardation—was seen in consultation. The boy's family lived in a semirural area with no community resources to address his needs. The mother was encouraged to advocate for an appropriate community-based program for him. Imagine my surprise when, 10 years later I met the mother at a State Superintendent's Advisory Council on Special Education meeting. She has formed a strong statewide advocacy organization of parents of children with special needs.

The passage of the Education for All Handicapped Children Act in 1975 was revolutionary in mandating an appropriate education for children with special needs. Parents and professionals in this country addressed a major need through their legislative advocacy.

As my pediatric career focusing on children with special health care needs continued to unfold, there were 2 other important initiatives.

While I was a Maternal and Child (Title V) director, a statewide system of regionalized genetic services was planned and implemented and has been in place for almost 2 decades. This regional system of clinical services, professional and public education as well as research, became a national model for similar programs in other states.

Child Abuse: Not a New Phenomenon

As you might imagine, despite the relatively recent efforts to identify and combat child abuse, the problem itself is not a new one to society, as evidenced by this chilling letter from colonial times...

"My second wife pinched her step daughter Mary until she was black and blue and knocked her head against the dresser which made her nose bleed much."

— *Theophilus Eaton in a letter to Governor John Winthrop, Jr*
  New Haven, CT, 1665

Recognizing the great need to educate pediatricians in training to serve children with special health care needs, a behavioral-developmental fellowship curriculum was developed through a federal Maternal and Child Health Bureau grant. The written curriculum was disseminated across the country and has been responsible for training faculty members in behavioral-developmental pediatrics who could, in turn, prepare pediatric

residents to better serve children with special health care needs.

— *Antoinette Parisi Eaton, MD*

C. Henry Kempe, MD, and the Battered-Child Syndrome

In July 1962, University of Colorado Medical School pediatrician C. Henry Kempe, MD, published his classic paper "The Battered-Child Syndrome" in the *Journal of the American Medical Association*. Rarely has a medical article had such dramatic impact. Dr Kempe reported the results of a nationwide survey that was sent throughout the previous year to hospitals and district attorneys and had identified several hundred cases of serious physical abuse in children. Particularly among infants, many of these cases had resulted in permanent brain damage or death. Dr Kempe insisted that physicians could play a critical role in saving the lives of such children through immediate reporting and removal of the child from the environment if indicated.

Dr Kempe's article marked a wake-up call for pediatricians. Perhaps because of their valued relationships with families or perhaps because of social mores, pediatricians had not previously played a prominent role in investigating and reporting the abuse of children. For example, the well-attested presence of gonorrheal vaginitis in children early in the 20th century was widely attributed to nonsexual contact. However, pediatric radiologists had begun to question conventional wisdom about abuse as early as the 1940s. In the hands of Columbia University's John Caffey, MD, and others, an x-ray film provided an objective record that could challenge the parents' history, revealing previous and unsuspected fractures. Yet it remained common for children to be diagnosed with such obscure entities as "spontaneous subdural hematomas" and "osteogenesis imperfecta tarda." Dr Kempe, after seeing many such cases personally while supervising interns in the emergency room, played a critical role in bringing these fictions to an end.

One year before his landmark article, Dr Kempe had organized a symposium at the AAP that already begun to galvanize the pediatric profession. It was there, in fact, that at the suggestion of a colleague he coined the term *battered child*, evoking a powerful image that injected great

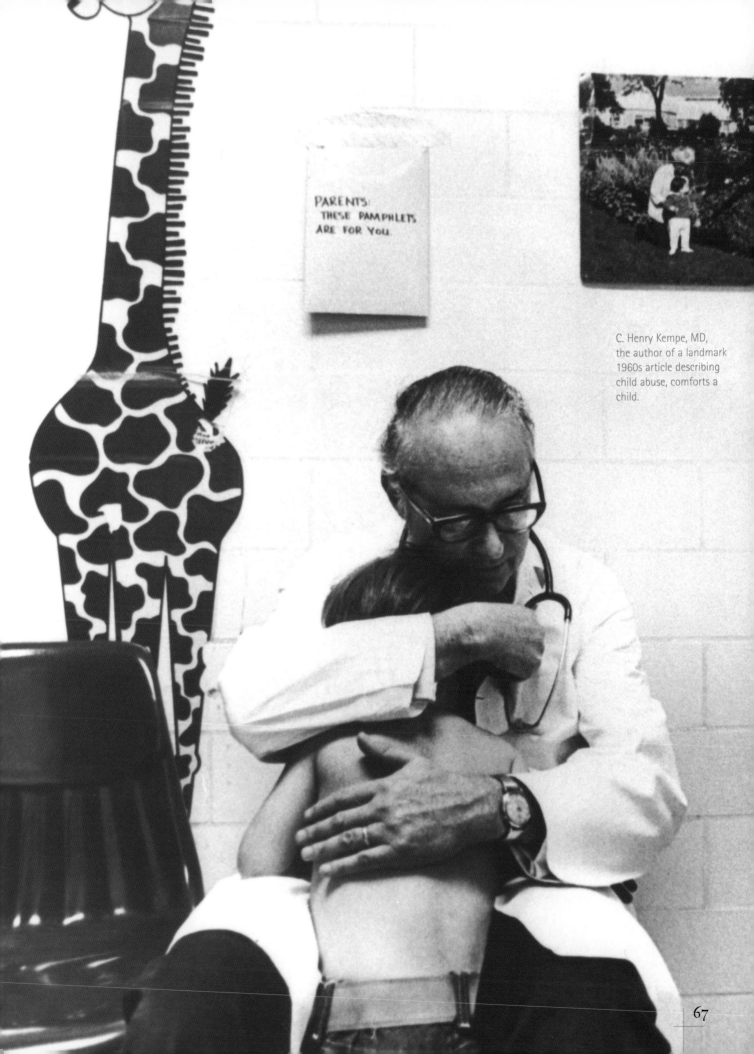

PARENTS:
THESE PAMPHLETS
ARE FOR YOU.

C. Henry Kempe, MD, the author of a landmark 1960s article describing child abuse, comforts a child.

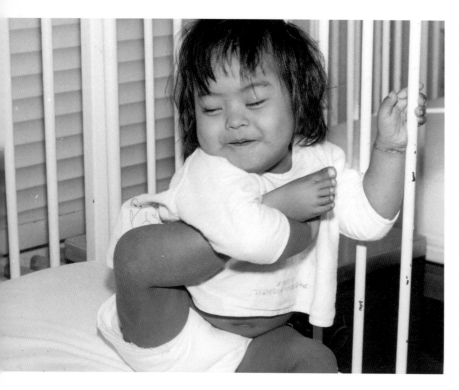

of abuse a major priority, and hospitals developed child protection teams. The definition of abuse was broadened from Dr Kempe's early focus on trauma of infants to include sexual abuse and neglect. The rapid expansion of reported cases greatly strained existing social resources. Critics charged that children were removed from the home too often and often remained in foster care for 2 years or more. In truth, fears of widespread removal of children from their homes were greatly exaggerated. In most cases, children and families were placed under home supervision. According to figures from the National Center on Child Abuse and Neglect in 1978, only about 1 in 5 abused children were placed in foster care.

Since that time, the AAP has stood at the forefront of efforts to protect children from physical and sexual abuse. It has promoted professional education, defined standards for child protection teams, and collaborated with other agencies on behalf of children. The "discovery" of child abuse provides one of the most vivid examples of the revitalization during the 1960s and 1970s of the social reform agenda so prominent in early 20th-century pediatrics.

— *Jeffrey P. Baker, MD*

Health Care for Native American Children

Into your midst has come a new life. Make its life smooth...then shall it travel beyond the four hills!
— *Omaha tribe introduction of the child to the cosmos.*

In 2005, as the AAP celebrates its 75th anniversary, the Indian Health Service (IHS), the primary federal agency coordinating the care of American Indians and Alaska Natives (AI/AN), will celebrate its 50th anniversary. The 2 organizations have changed and grown over the past 50 years and established close ties that have proved mutually beneficial.

Indian health care has not always been the responsibility of the IHS. Until 1849, the War Department was given a charge to make sure that diseases of the Indians did not affect the settlers who were taking their lands! In 1849, the Department of the Interior Bureau of Indian Affairs (BIA) took over Indian health care but, by the mid-20th century, it was clear that BIA-directed care was not working. For example, as many as 25% of Native Americans drafted into the armed services or working in defense plants

emotional power into the debate. Public response was rapid. *Time* magazine soon carried its own report, newspapers ran pieces on battered infants, and television shows such as *Dragnet* and *Ben Casey* depicted stories of battered children. Between 1963 and 1965, every state passed reporting laws designed to protect physicians from being sued for investigating and reporting instances of possible child abuse.

Resources capable of effectively responding to reports developed more slowly. Collaborating with child psychiatrists, Dr Kempe proposed that parents who beat their children recapitulated a "cycle of violence" deeply ingrained by their own violent upbringing. He developed a model program in Denver, CO, involving a team consisting of a pediatrician, psychiatrist, social worker, and lay therapist whose goal was to restore the parent's caregiving abilities. Such an approach, it was hoped, would make removal of the child from their home unnecessary in most cases.

In 1974, with broad support from American pediatricians, the AAP, and the general public, both houses of Congress easily passed the Child Abuse Prevention and Treatment Act. The act provided $85 million over 4 years to fund a National Center on Child Abuse and Neglect as well as demonstration programs around the country. Pediatric programs made the recognition during World War II had active tuberculosis. The AI/AN death rate from tuberculosis and deaths from diarrhea and dehydration were 6 times the national average. The doctors caring for the Indians on the reservations were very unhappy.

In 1955, the first IHS director of the Public Health Service, James R. Shaw, MD, noted that

> "The doctors were isolated, their pay was terrible, they had bad facilities, no books, no continuing medical education, and worst of all, they were subordinate to the local BIA superintendent."

By 1964, the IHS had addressed some of these problems by reaching out to Indian tribes and encouraging professional societies to establish alliances to promote Indian health. The AAP took this challenge and created the Committee on Indian Health (COIH). Committee members visited and inspected Indian health programs throughout the West and made recommendations to the IHS on needed improvements. Perhaps its greatest achievement, the passage by Congress of the Indian Health Care Improvement Act of 1976, came about in large part because of the strong relationships between a committee member, Abraham B. Bergman, MD, and the powerful senator from the state of Washington, Henry (Scoop) Jackson.

Lance A. Chilton, MD, who served on the Navajo Reservation at that time, remembers the fine esprit de corps that the committee members would have seen, but also the

> "remarkable amount of purulent spinal fluid that spurted out of our needles, the cutdowns we did on bone-dry infants, the pus-filled ear canals, and the rampant malnutrition, as well as the trachoma and tuberculosis."

William F. Green, MD, vividly recalls a patient who was deaf and mute with miliary tuberculosis and was brought to medical attention by newly hired community health representatives on the White River Apache reservation in 1973.

The COIH fell prey to cost- and committee-cutting at the AAP in 1982, and its functions were to be assumed by the Committee on Community Health Services (COCHS). However, COCHS's plate was too full to be able to devote much activity in Indian health services. With the help of IHS and AAP leaders, a COCHS Subcommittee on Indian Health was established.

In 1993, the AAP Board established a new Committee on Native American Child Health (CONACH). CONACH activities have expanded from dealing primarily with the IHS to relating more fully with tribally operated health systems and with urban programs as well. The relation of CONACH to the IHS remains strong. The number of Native American pediatricians has increased, and they are strongly represented on the committee.

Today, 50 years after the experiences of Dr Shaw, what is it like to be a pediatrician in the IHS? Most doctors are working in modern, well-equipped facilities such as the beautiful new hospitals in Anchorage, AK, and Shiprock, NM. Many work in tribally run programs, which are increasingly common throughout the country. The diseases of Native American children have changed as well; infectious diseases are not as prominent—tuberculosis is becoming far less common, bacterial meningitis has been nearly eradicated through immunizations (many of the vaccines were tested first on Native American children), and draining otitis is not as common as it was 50 years ago. Problems that were not present or not noticed 50 years ago have come to the fore—problems in school, the effects of violence, obesity (no longer malnutrition!), and type 2 diabetes. Tribes and the IHS can look to CONACH and the AAP as a source of

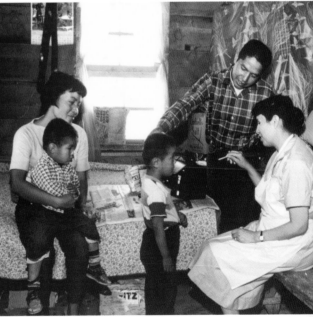

suggestions for improving the health care given to Native American children. The children themselves have strong advocates who will continue to look after their well-being beyond the 50th year of the IHS and the 75th year of the AAP.

— *Lance A. Chilton, MD, and William F. Green, MD*

A Native American doctor and nurse examining a patient.

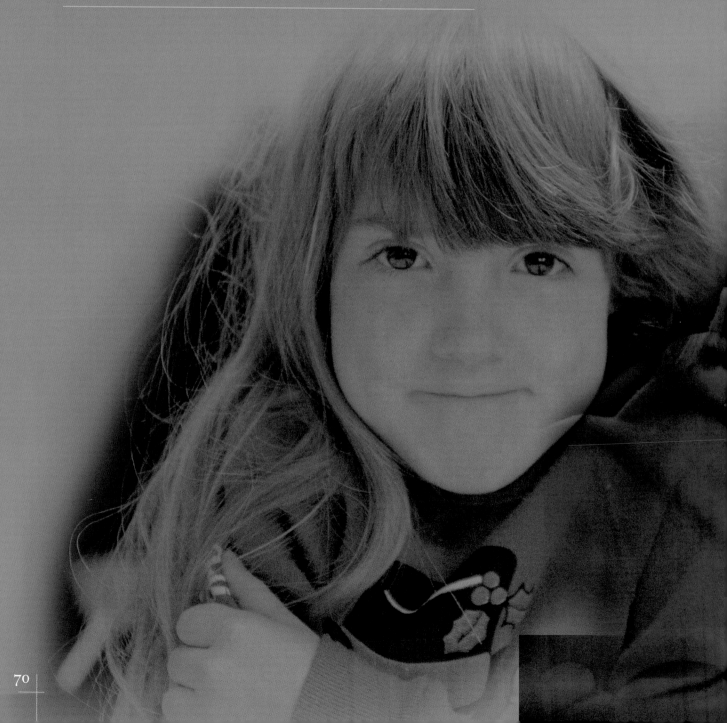

The AAP staff, approximately 350 dedicated individuals, works on behalf of children's health at offices in Elk Grove Village, IL, and Washington, DC, and the organization's membership grew to 60,000 members during the 2003–2004 fiscal year....

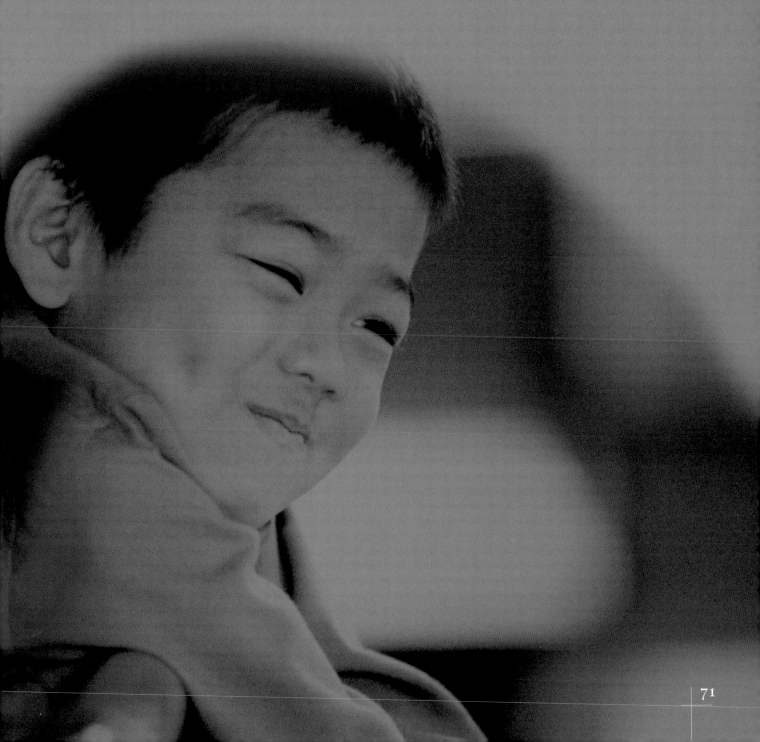

Chapter 5
Dedicated to the Health of All Children

1980 to 2005

1980
Karen M. Starko, MD, reported an association between aspirin ingestion and Reye syndrome.

1981
The human immunodeficiency virus and acquired immunodeficiency syndrome (HIV/AIDS), a syndrome that soon involved hemophiliacs and newborns of mothers infected with HIV, was described in *MMWR Morbidity and Mortality Weekly Report*.

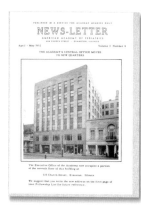

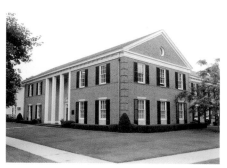

Above top, American Academy of Pediatrics (AAP) headquarters on the 7th floor of a building in Evanston, IL (image from 1952); *above bottom*, the AAP later moved its headquarters to a building at 1801 Hinman Ave in Evanston, IL (image from 1955).

ADVOCACY FOR THE HEALTH OF ALL CHILDREN—SAME PRIORITIES, NEW CHALLENGES

The winds shifted once again for the American Academy of Pediatrics (AAP) after 1980. For the previous 2 decades, it had increasingly embraced a positive relationship with government and community organizations on behalf of children. As the idealism of the 1960s diminished during the next decades, AAP members fought to preserve a voice for children in a decidedly different political climate. A variety of forces threatened to reverse the gains only recently made by disadvantaged children. Teen birth rates and deaths from violence rose, especially among inner-city youth, and poverty and teen pregnancy helped maintain high rates of premature birth. With new medical advances came new challenges, including the supervision of intensive care nursery "graduates" and children and adolescents dependent on technology such as home oxygen, feeding tubes, and even ventilators. During the 1980s, newspapers and magazines headlined desperate stories of "cocaine babies" and children with human immunodeficiency virus (HIV) that all too often conveyed a sense of hopelessness. Government cutbacks disrupted community health clinics and further threatened the health of children.

Working with child advocacy organizations and politicians from both political parties, the AAP made access to health care for all children a central priority during these years. It played a critical role in passing legislation (related in earlier chapters) providing compensation for vaccine victims and thereby protecting the nation's supply of childhood immunizations. The AAP Back to Sleep campaign during the early 1990s was followed by an unprecedented drop in deaths from sudden infant death syndrome (SIDS). Efforts to promote motor vehicle, firearm, and bicycle safety all have played a part in reducing childhood and adolescent mortality from these causes since the early 1990s; and, despite continued widespread concern, teen pregnancy rates have declined annually since peaking in 1991, most dramatically among African American girls.

Yet "new morbidities" continue to evolve, and no doubt will offer new agendas for today's and tomorrow's pediatricians. Widely available fast food and soda machines, coupled with excessive television and declining exercise, have fueled a precipitous rise in childhood obesity. The 1999 killings at Colorado's Columbine High School sent shock waves across the nation, with commentators variously blaming access to firearms, violent video games, or broken family life. Clothing designers and television advertisers seem intent on targeting children as consumers at ever younger ages, encouraging them to obsess over material adornments and body image. And beginning on September 11, 2001, pediatricians found that they had to learn to counsel children traumatized by images (and in some cases by the reality) of terrorism.

All of these challenges will consume the energy of the next generation of pediatric leaders. They will arise in a nation more diverse than ever before, requiring many pediatricians to acquire competence in Spanish and cross-cultural skills. It is hoped that the following accounts will offer inspiration about just how much can be accomplished when pediatricians and their allies work together on behalf of children.

PRESIDENTIAL HIGHLIGHTS OF THE PAST 25 YEARS

Over the past 25 years, the AAP has made great strides in advancing child health through its many advocacy, legislation, research, and education efforts. In that time, the organization's national headquarters moved from Evanston, IL, to its current location in Elk Grove Village, IL, just outside of Chicago. The AAP Washington, DC, office has become one of the most effective and admired voices for children. It would be

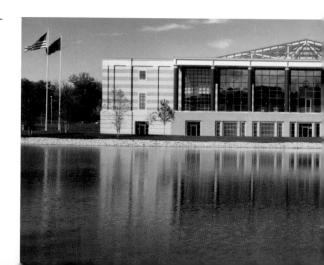

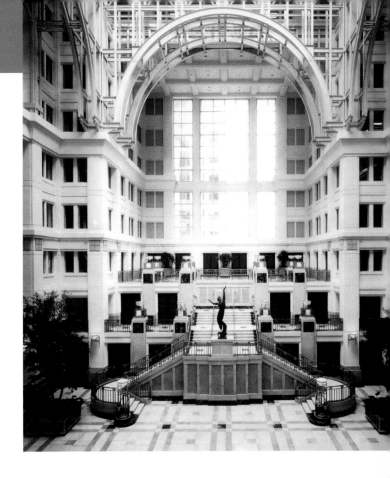

virtually impossible to comprehensively cover the many accomplishments of the past quarter century. To give an overview of what has been accomplished, James E. Strain, MD, president of the AAP in 1982–1983 and executive director from 1985–1993, was asked to poll his past-presidential colleagues and report what they believed were the accomplishments and events of special note during their presidential year.

1980–1981: R. Don Blim, MD
- M. Harry Jennison, MD, became executive director of the AAP.
- The AAP successfully advocated against the proposed consolidation of grant-in-aid programs and legislation was passed maintaining the Title V program as a separate entity administered by the Maternal and Child Health Bureau.
- The AAP launched the First Ride, Safe Ride program to promote infant passenger safety.

1981–1982: Glenn Austin, MD
- The "New Age for Pediatrics" campaign began, emphasizing the pediatrician's role in the delivery of health care to adolescents.
- A new Committee on Health Care Financing was formed, charged to develop strategies for gaining the support of labor unions for coverage of child health care.
- New guidelines on health supervision visits were published.

1982–1983: James E. Strain, MD
- The AAP was successful in a suit against the federal government that blocked the rule that regulated the care of disabled newborns.
- As a result of AAP advocacy efforts, Early and Periodic Screening, Diagnostic, and Treatment (EPSDT) rules were issued requiring

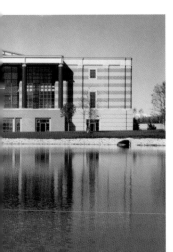

Left, the current headquarters of the American Academy of Pediatrics (AAP) in Elk Grove Village, IL, prior to new construction in 1991 and 1992. The AAP moved into this building in 1984; *above right*, the atrium of the Homer Building, Washington, DC, where the AAP Department of Federal Affairs is located on the 4th floor.

American Academy of Pediatrics Mission, Core Values, and Vision
(Effective May 2004)

Mission
The mission of the American Academy of Pediatrics is to attain optimal physical, mental, and social health and well-being for all infants, children, adolescents, and young adults. To accomplish this mission, the Academy shall support the professional needs of its members.

Core Values
We believe
- In the inherent worth of all children; they are our most enduring and vulnerable legacy.
- Children deserve optimal health and the highest quality health care.
- Pediatricians are the best qualified to provide child health care.

The American Academy of Pediatrics is the organization to advance child health and well-being.

Vision
Children have optimal health and well-being and are valued by society. Academy members practice the highest quality health care and experience professional satisfaction and personal well-being.

1985
John B. Robbins, MD;
Rachel Schneerson, MD;
David H. Smith, MD; and
Porter Warren Anderson,
Jr, MD, developed poly-
saccharide vaccine for
Haemophilus influenzae
and, later, a conjugated
polysaccharide vaccine.
(Bethesda, MD, and
Rochester, NY)

1990
Antoinette Parisi Eaton,
MD, became the first
woman to serve as presi-
dent of the American
Academy of Pediatrics.

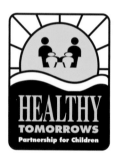

Healthy Tomorrows
Partnership for Children
logo.

states to design periodic schedules of visits in consultation with recognized medical and dental organizations.

- The "Growth for the Future" campaign to underwrite the cost of the new building in Elk Grove Village resulted in more than $3 million being pledged by AAP members. Groundbreaking took place in 1983.
- TIPP®—The Injury Prevention Program was launched. Recommendations regarding car safety seats, smoke detectors, window and stairway guards, and reduced hot water temperatures were included.

1983–1984: Paul F. Wehrle, MD

- The AAP moved its headquarters from Evanston to the new building in Elk Grove Village.
- The AAP developed the program of the International Congress of Pediatrics, which was held in Hawaii in 1986.

1984–1985: Robert J. Haggerty, MD

- The American Pediatric Society and the Society of Pediatric Research integrated their legislative efforts into the AAP Office of Governmental Liaison.
- The planning and development of the Pediatric Research in Office Settings (PROS) network occurred (and was ultimately established in January 1986).
- "Baby Doe" legislation was passed and signed by President Ronald Reagan as an amendment to the Child Abuse Prevention and Treatment Act.

1985–1986: Martin H. Smith, MD

- The National Childhood Vaccine Injury Act of 1986 was passed and signed into law.
- Model state legislation to correct the prolonged statute of limitation for children was passed in 38 states.
- A residency membership category was established.
- Dr Strain was appointed executive director.

1986–1987: William C. Montgomery, MD

- A set of guidelines supporting school-based health clinics was published.
- The AAP successfully advocated for amendments to the Education for All Handicapped

Children Act, which provided incentives to serve children with special health care needs in the 3- to 5-year age group.

1987–1988: Richard M. Narkewicz, MD

- The AAP successfully supported legislation to establish an excise tax to fund the National Childhood Vaccine Injury Act of 1986.
- The first Annual Legislative Conference to train AAP members to advocate for children in the legislative arena was held in Washington, DC.
- The AAP became a supporting member of the Pediatric Scientist Development program to support research training for pediatricians.

1988–1989: Donald W. Schiff, MD

- Access to health care for all children became the highest AAP priority.
- The Healthy Tomorrows initiative, administered jointly by the AAP and the Maternal and Child Health Bureau, was established to meet health care needs of children at the community level.

1989–1990: Birt Harvey, MD

- The AAP participated with the House Select Committee on Children, Youth, and Families in the development of a report of children's well-being throughout the world.
- The AAP successfully advocated for increased Medicaid benefits and coverage for more children.
- Legislation requiring insurance coverage for all children was promoted.

1990–1991: Antoinette Parisi Eaton, MD

- The groundbreaking occurred for a new wing of the AAP headquarters in January 1991.
- The AAP supported the Children and Pregnant Women's Health Insurance Act introduced by Representative Robert Matsui.
- The Fourth AAP Women's Leadership Conference was held at the AAP Annual Meeting in 1991 (it was the first such conference that male pediatricians were

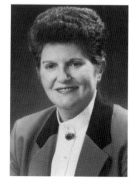

Antoinette Parisi Eaton, MD.

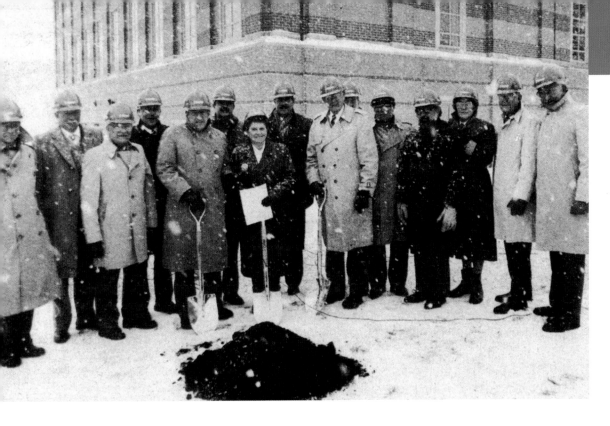

1992
The American Academy of Pediatrics advocated supine rather than prone sleeping to reduce the risk of sudden infant death syndrome (SIDS).

1994
The World Health Organization reported the elimination of poliomyelitis from the Americas.

Treatment of HIV-infected mothers with zidovudine reduced perinatal transmission to their infants.

also invited to attend). These conferences were a significant step to support women in leadership positions in the AAP.

1991–1992: Daniel W. Shea, MD
- The AAP responded to revisions of *Physicians' Current Procedural Terminology* codes, Clinical Laboratory Improvement Amendments regulations requiring certification of laboratories, new Occupational Safety and Health Administration regulations, and Vaccine Patient Information statements.

1992–1993: Howard A. Pearson, MD
- The AAP promoted a statement (that had been released in early 1992) recommending a change in sleeping position of infants from prone to supine, which has resulted in a 50% reduction in the incidence of SIDS in the United States.
- The AAP supported the Family and Medical Leave Act legislation, which resulted in regulations providing parents with unpaid leave for circumstances such as caring for newborns or sick children.
- The AAP Pediatric History Center was established
- Joe M. Sanders, Jr, MD, was appointed executive director.

1993–1994: Betty A. Lowe, MD
- The AAP supported the Health Security Act proposed by the Clinton administration.
- The AAP supported the Vaccines for Children program to provide vaccines for uninsured children.
- The AAP published a policy statement entitled, "Integrated School Health Services."
- Educational material was developed for pediatricians on how to adapt to managed care.

1994–1995: George D. Comerci, MD
- The AAP advocated incremental changes in health care coverage for children.
- The AAP successfully defended a suit brought against it by the Nestlé Food Company, alleging collusion in the constraint of trade.
- The AAP participated in the planning of the quadrennial meeting of the International Pediatric Association in Cairo, Egypt.

1995–1996: Maurice E. Keenan, MD
- A proposal to establish the Center for Child Health Research was presented (the AAP Board established the center in 1997).
- The Committee on International Child Health became a section.
- The AAP supported folic acid food enrichment regulations.

Above left, groundbreaking for the expansion of the American Academy of Pediatrics headquarters in Elk Grove Village, IL, in 1991.

1998
The Pediatric Rule, a federal regulation requiring pharmaceutical companies to test new drugs in children (as opposed to only testing in adults), was enacted. The Pediatric Rule was dismissed in 2002, but it was reestablished in 2003 as part of the Pediatric Research Equity Act. (Washington, DC)

2000
Completion of the "mapping" of the human genome.

Left, the original American Academy of Pediatrics (AAP) Della Robbia insignia, created by Jasper King in 1930; *right*, the current AAP insignia adopted in 1941 (and made official in 1955), created by Leo H. Junker. The legend of "Dedicated to the Health of All Children" was added to the official logo in 2000.

1996–1997: Robert E. Hannemann, MD
- Professional communication and education were expanded into Italy and South America.
- The AAP issued a policy statement on the physician's role in disaster preparedness, which was later expanded to include foreign as well as domestic crises.

1997–1998: Joseph R. Zanga, MD
- The AAP increased its efforts to promote pediatricians as the premier physicians for children.
- A Task Force on the Family was established to determine how the AAP should work with families.
- A multidisciplinary conference was held on the rights of children. A Constitutional Amendment on the Rights of Children was proposed.

1998–1999: Joel J. Alpert, MD
- The Task Force on Health Coverage and Access was established and developed the AAP principles regarding health insurance for all children.
- The AAP was a major participant in discussions about the use of thimerosal as a vaccine preservative.

1999–2000: Donald E. Cook, MD
- The AAP and the Pediatric Academic Societies (American Pediatric Society, Society for Pediatric Research, and Ambulatory Pediatric Association) held their first joint meeting in Boston, MA.
- The Tomorrow's Children Endowment was established to support AAP initiatives in advocacy, education, research, and community services.
- The final report of the Future of Pediatric Education II (FOPE II) Project was published.

2000–2001: Steve Berman, MD
- An International Office was created.
- The AAP developed an overall child health strategy that recognized the interrelated nature of access, quality, and cost.
- Relationships were strengthened with the Pediatric Academic Societies and the role of the Federation of Pediatric Organizations was expanded.

2001–2002: Louis Z. Cooper, MD
- Increased attention was given to Internet communication for education of members and the public.
- As a result of AAP efforts, 38 states have newborn hearing screening statutes and more than 85% of newborns are being screened.
- A Task Force on Terrorism was created.

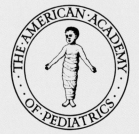
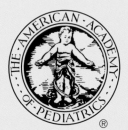

American Academy of Pediatrics

DEDICATED TO THE HEALTH OF ALL CHILDREN™

2002–2003: E. Stephen Edwards, MD

- An access retreat was held in Washington, DC, which recommended focusing on achievable goals without losing the AAP long-term vision—that families and pregnant women should be included in any national health care plan.
- A private sector advocacy initiative was created in the AAP Department of Practice and Research.
- The AAP supported legislation requiring testing of pharmaceuticals in children (passed in December 2003).

2003–2004: Carden Johnston, MD

- The Pediatric Research Equity Act was signed into law, requiring pharmaceutical companies to test new drugs and biologics to be used in children.
- The first Annual Leadership Forum was held, combining the leadership of AAP chapters, committees, and sections in one large meeting.
- Errol R. Alden, MD, was appointed executive director/CEO.

2004–2005: Carol D. Berkowitz, MD

- Dr Berkowitz will serve as the 75th AAP president during its anniversary year.

— *Compiled by James E. Strain, MD*

Joe M. Sanders, Jr, MD, and Errol R. Alden, MD, shake hands next to a statue entitled, "Together," which was dedicated to Dr Sanders for his outstanding contributions to the American Academy of Pediatrics on May 20, 2004.

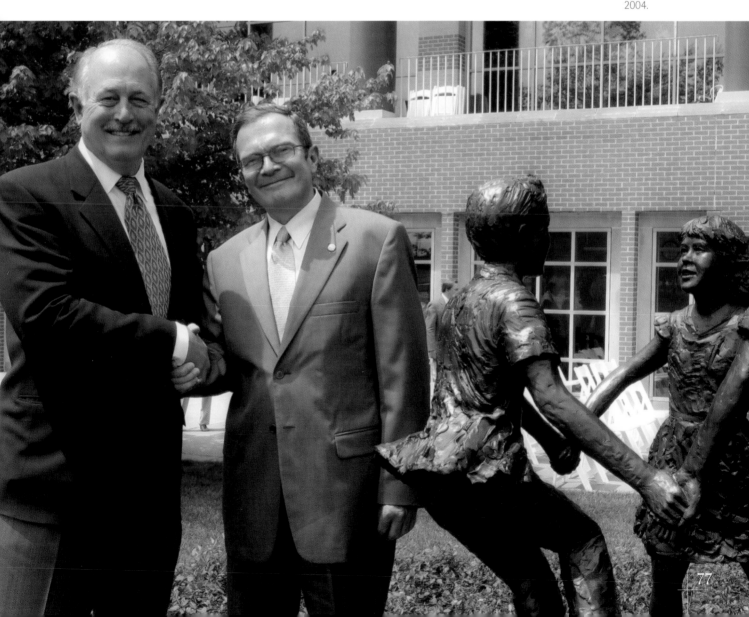

LEGISLATIVE EFFORTS—ACCESS TO HEALTH CARE

The spirit of the AAP founders in demanding quality health care for children still drives the organization's legislative agenda at the federal and state levels. Over the past 25 years, the AAP has repeatedly developed and promoted innovative solutions for the substantial numbers of children and adolescents who lack access to basic health care services. While significant progress has been made, many challenges remain.

Every year, numerous bills and regulations impacting children's health make their way through federal and state governments, and the AAP plays an active advocacy role in those efforts (though the "you win some, you lose some" mantra applies). In the 1980s, the AAP led an effort to fashion a separate Maternal and Child Health (MCH) Block Grant to plan for and deliver health services for mothers and children. Pediatrics scored a major victory with the establishment of a safety net for children through this MCH Block Grant. Soon after, the AAP spearheaded efforts to revise Early and Periodic Screening, Diagnostic, and Treatment (EPSDT) service beyond its emphasis on screening. As a result, new regulations made EPSDT a more comprehensive health program that effectively promotes the concept of a medical home for children.

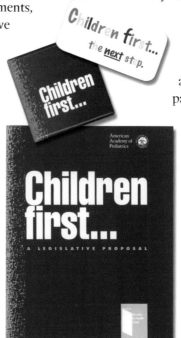

In the mid-1980s, the US Congress, left uneasy by failed health reform efforts during the term of President Jimmy Carter and drastic budget cuts by President Ronald Reagan, began to focus on Medicaid reform as a vehicle for improving children's health. Between 1984 and 1990, Congress implemented a series of reforms that fundamentally restructured children's coverage. Notably, the Child Health Assurance Program was passed in 1984 and further revisions were enacted with the Omnibus Budget Reconciliation Acts of 1989 and 1990. AAP chapters worked vigorously to urge state governments to expand eligibility for low-income children.

As a result of this legislation, Medicaid gradually became a model health insurance bill with comprehensive benefits. Yet pediatrician participation remained somewhat uneven because of administrative hassles and the common perception of "slow pay, low pay, and no pay." (In 2000, the AAP filed a legal complaint against the Health Care Financing Administration [HCFA] for failing to provide access for patient care and inappropriate professional reimbursement, and states received letters from HCFA encouraging compliance.) In the mid-1980s, the AAP moved on to the Child Health Insurance Reform Plan, which required businesses to include children's preventive care services in their employee health plans for insurance premiums to be deductible as a business expense.

Recognizing the need to build on its successes in an increasingly complex world of public policy, the first AAP Annual Legislative Conference was held in 1988 to train its members in effective legislative interaction. The public was not well informed about the deficiencies of health care for children and, to address this, strong media advocacy efforts were initiated.

In 1989, universal access to quality health care for all infants, children, adolescents, and pregnant women was designated a top priority of the AAP as it prepared to address the national problem of 37 million uninsured people, of which approximately 9 million were children. A congressional

---

An American Academy of Pediatrics President's Memories of the First "Annual" Legislative Conference in 1988

I'm not sure I knew that this would be the first annual legislative conference. We promoted it as the first legislative conference until I saw the cups that were handed out to all the people, and lo and behold, on the cup it said, "First Annual Legislative Conference" . . . another of Jackie Noyes' wonderful ideas.

— *Richard M. Narkewicz, MD*

health policy retreat, "Healthy Children: Good Policy, Good Politics," was held with key congressional staff, health agency representatives, and AAP members. It was concluded that, despite the best of efforts, the current health care system was not working for all mothers and children.

To ensure congressional commitment, the AAP drafted a joint resolution entitled "Health of America's Children," which was introduced in the Senate and was cosponsored by more than 75 members. The detailed AAP proposal, "Children First," ensured seats at key bargaining tables and before Congress, which eventually accepted many key concepts of the AAP plan.

In October 1991, Representative Robert Matsui introduced the Children and Pregnant Women's Health Insurance Act of 1991, making the AAP the first medical association to have its access objectives included in legislation. Representative Matsui and Senator Chris Dodd reintroduced the bill in the next Congress. At the time, AAP president Betty A. Lowe, MD, remarked, "We have a

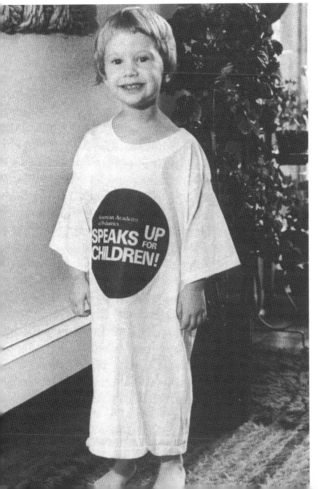

Young child wearing "American Academy of Pediatrics Speaks Up for Children!" T-shirt, circa 1980.

chance to design a system that fits the child instead of trying to fit a child into the system."

The failure of the health insurance plan proposed by President Bill Clinton led to the development of the State Children's Health Insurance Program (SCHIP), which was a block grant that allowed states discretion in eligibility, design, and implementation and encouraged participation by offering a larger match rate. The 1997 tobacco settlement made funding possible and SCHIP became a response to the growing problem of uninsured children. As an adjunct to Medicaid, it provided a chance to include more lower income children. AAP chapters provided leadership in every state to implement this new program, despite its limitations, to ensure favorable outcomes for children.

Impelled by the growing number of uninsured and underinsured children, the MediKids Health Insurance Act of 2001 was introduced in the Congress by Senator Jay Rockefeller and Representative Pete Stark and reintroduced again in the next session. As AAP president Steve Berman, MD, recounted, the bill stressed "family responsibility, affordability, quality, choice, equity, and administrative simplicity."

The AAP has established itself as a key voice in federal and state affairs relating to children's health issues, yet many challenges lie ahead in this tumultuous era of insurance reform. With that in mind, another retreat was organized by the AAP in 2003, this time bringing together policy leaders from all sides of the issue to help define new strategies. It was agreed that the AAP needs to continue to advocate for the health of all children and their families, and needs to be ready with a plan when an opportunity arises. The leadership, passion, and active participation of the AAP and its members will play a key role in determining the future of health care reform for children.

— Jackie Noyes, MA

MediKids Health Insurance Act brochure and button.

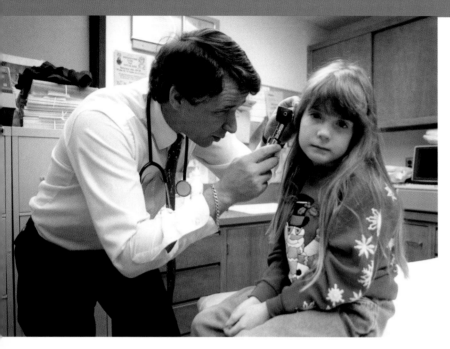

Community Access to Child Health (CATCH) at Work: Children's Clinic in Greeley, CO

Weld County is predominantly a farming community. It contains a large pocket of poverty and many physicians had stopped accepting new Medicaid patients on a regular basis. That left these families and their children with nowhere to turn for medical care except the hospital emergency room. Recognizing the need for intervention, I applied for and was awarded a CATCH planning grant, which I used to design the freestanding children's facility that ultimately became the Monfort Children's Clinic. The CATCH planning grant, along with assistance from the North Colorado Medical Center Foundation, facilitated the raising of $5.5 million in additional local funding. Since its opening in May 1995, the Monfort Children's Clinic has treated more than 10,000 area children in more than 150,000 visits. Many of the children are seeing a doctor for the first time and many have previously undiagnosed disabilities or chronic illnesses. A permanent facility has been erected where 16 full-time staff and 125 volunteers integrate dozens of services to give children health for today and hope for tomorrow.

CATCH
Community Access To Child Health

— Donald E. Cook, MD

COMMUNITY PEDIATRICS IN PERSPECTIVE

The history of modern medicine is usually told as the triumph of technologically sophisticated medical care rendered in operating rooms and hospital wards. There has always been a vocal minority of physicians, however, urging their colleagues to remember that patients are people who live together in communities, and that physicians have a responsibility to that community. Since pediatrics emerged as a distinct medical specialty

in the 19th century, pediatricians more than most physicians have been leaders in community-based medical practice. Indeed, the rising prominence of community pediatrics in the last 3 decades can be viewed as a reemergence of pediatrics' roots as a medical specialty focused on the health and well-being of the community.

For centuries, children were considered a mere economic asset of their fathers. Many young children started working in factories or as street vendors at age 8, and all children contributed substantially to household and farm work from the time they were able to walk. By the early 20th century, a new consensus emerged in which children were valued principally for their emotional value. By 1900, most Western nations had instituted laws providing compulsory education to children, protecting them against physical abuse from their parents, and outlawing excessive or dangerous labor before a certain age.

As has been described earlier in this volume, many early 20th-century pediatricians shared these broader concerns for the welfare of children. Indeed, the impetus to found the AAP originated in part out of the recognition that the scope of pediatrics extended beyond the hospital or laboratory. Nonetheless, it must be acknowledged that enthusiasm for community pediatrics waned as the 20th-century miracles of immunization and antibiotics brought new prestige to the medical profession. Infant mortality dropped from approximately 300 deaths per 1,000 live births to less than 10 deaths per 1,000 live births—a change that had more to do with improved nutrition and sanitation than to specific medical interventions.

In the last 3 decades of the 20th century, many pediatricians have rediscovered their roots in the community. This is partly due to changing disease patterns—psychosocial conditions have replaced infectious diseases as the major causes of morbidity for US children. Recently, the AAP Committee on Community Health Services defined community pediatrics as

> *"a perspective that enlarges the focus from one child to all children in the community; a recognition that family, educational, social, cultural, spiritual, economic, environmental, and political forces act favorably or unfavorably, but always significantly, on the health of children; a synthesis of clinical practice and public*

health principles directed toward providing health care to a given child, and promoting the health of all children within the context of the family, school, and community; a commitment to using community resources to achieve optimal accessibility, appropriateness, and quality of services for all children, and to advocate especially for those who lack access to care; and an integral part of the professional role and duty of the pediatrician."

Acting on this during the 1990s and continuing into the new century, the AAP Department of Community Pediatrics has supported pediatricians by providing public awareness, policies, technical assistance, programs, and leadership to help advance the field of community pediatrics.

An example of the AAP community pediatrics efforts is the Community Access to Child Health (CATCH) Program, which, in 2003, celebrated 10 years of providing funds to innovative pediatricians to develop child health initiatives in their local communities. Pediatricians have the capacity to be effective and credible leaders in their

communities. They are in a position to identify the gaps in children's services, and they have the skills and training to develop programs to meet those needs. But pediatricians, who usually do this work on a volunteer basis, typically do not have the time or staff to do the necessary research and planning to initiate a complex community-based health care program.

The CATCH Program was founded to improve children's access to health care. Its mission is to support pediatricians who work with communities to ensure that all children have medical homes and access to any other needed health care services. To achieve this goal, the CATCH Program provides pediatricians with training, technical

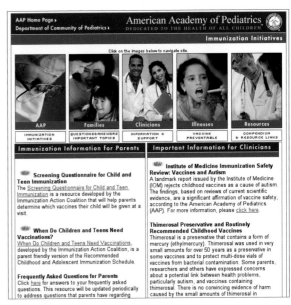

Childhood Immunization Support Program (CISP) Web site (www.cispimmunize.org).

Community Access to Child Health (CATCH) at Work: Reducing Youth Gun Violence in Miami, FL

The firearm epidemic was at its height during my residency in California, and the homicide rate in the adjacent town was among the highest in the nation. Shortly after I moved to Miami, FL, I learned that firearms were the leading cause of youth death in my community and topped the list for trauma visits as well. It was hard to imagine a more useless and preventable cause of death than youth gun violence. The public health literature recommended a multidisciplinary collaboration to address the issue. I felt that the entire community ought to be working together so that "not one more child shall die by gun violence!"

A CATCH grant and the support of the county mayor provided the impetus to form NOT ONE MORE, a coalition of leaders in law enforcement, health, education, elected office, business, community-based groups, clergy, and media all with the goal of building a plan to reduce youth gun violence. Among NOT ONE MORE's accomplishments are an incident-based violent injury statistics system, a resource center for youth violence prevention, greater cooperation among municipal law enforcement agencies, school-

based initiatives, and safer gun storage awareness campaigns. More recent activities include "Summer-Jamz," a combined violence and HIV prevention educational event attended by nearly 700 teenagers, and an art/youth development program that brings together middle school youth from historically isolated ethnic groups in the city. Now 4 years since its founding, the coalition has grown to 80 members and expanded its scope to all forms of youth violence. The initial $7,500 American Academy of Pediatrics investment has since translated into $1.5 million in new funding in violence prevention.

Gun violence has fallen nationwide. However, the systems in place have helped us identify early a recent increase in our youth homicide rate. The coalition provides a forum to share such information and to plan a collaborative response. Regardless of whether trends in violence are up or down, the coalition remains committed to continue its work until not one more child dies by violence.

— Judy Schaechter, MD

assistance, peer support, networking opportunities, and funding opportunities for project development. The CATCH Program has trained more than 1,000 pediatricians, which has led to the development of more than 500 community health projects.

— *Jeffrey P. Brosco, MD, and Thomas F. Tonniges, MD*

THE AMERICAN ACADEMY OF PEDIATRICS TODAY: AN OVERVIEW OF SELECTED ACTIVITIES

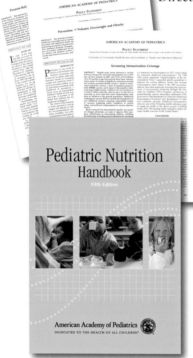

Top, policy statements; *bottom, Pediatric Nutrition Handbook,* 5th Edition, published in 2003.

While the basic purpose of the AAP has not changed in more than 70 years, the environment in which the AAP serves children and members has changed with the times. A Board of Directors, consisting of district chairs elected by AAP members in 10 geographic districts, oversees the governance of the AAP. The AAP chapters are organized groups of pediatricians and other health care professionals working to achieve AAP goals in their states and communities. Chapters are separate from the AAP national organization, with their own bylaws and methods of governance. There are 59 chapters in the United States and 7 chapters in Canada. AAP committees are made up of experts nominated by chapters and selected by advisory committees and the Board of Directors. Committees have historically been responsible for most AAP policy statements. The AAP has not only welcomed pediatric and

non-pediatric subspecialists to join the AAP, but established sections in its constitution as a mechanism for groups of members with specific interests to establish a home within the organizational structure. Sections often play an important role in developing education opportunities, and they have executive committees that are elected by the membership. The AAP staff, approximately 350 dedicated individuals, works on behalf of children's health at offices in Elk Grove Village, IL, and Washington, DC, and the organization's membership grew to 60,000 members during the 2003–2004 fiscal year. Just a few of the many activities of the AAP membership and staff are outlined below.

Policy Statements, Guidelines, and Programs

The AAP committees and sections analyze research before developing policy statements to guide pediatricians in their practices. These statements usually are a response to practical practice issues and cover a wide range of topics including obesity, breastfeeding, immunization, and injury prevention. In addition to writing AAP policies, some committees publish manuals on topics such as infectious diseases, nutrition, environmental health, and school health.

Clinical practice guidelines are evidence-based, decision-making tools for managing common medical conditions. The guidelines are developed by carefully defining the condition and identifying interventions and health outcomes that help maintain and improve the quality of care. The recommendations in the guidelines are based on

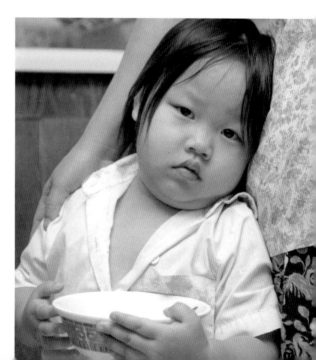

What Is a FAAP?

A FAAP is a Fellow of the American Academy of Pediatrics (AAP) who is certified in pediatrics by the American Board of Pediatrics, the American Osteopathic Board of Pediatrics, the Royal College of Physicians and Surgeons of Canada, La Corporation Professionelle des Medicins du Quebec, or a specialty board approved by the Accreditation Council for Graduate Medical Education with a minimum 50% of his or her practice devoted to the care of infants, children, adolescents, or young adults. FAAPs are the only members who are granted full privileges and benefits of AAP membership.

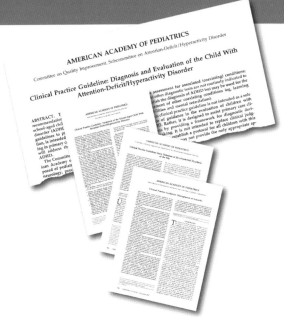

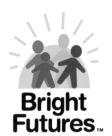

learning programs (via *Pedia*Link), and CD-ROMs, to journals and periodicals. The Neonatal Resuscitation Program (NRP) is one of the most successful AAP educational programs, and has had an enormous impact nationally and internationally (for more about NRP, see Chapter 6).

Pediatrics Review and Education Program (PREP) The Curriculum helps members keep pace with new developments and prepare for the American Board of Pediatrics recertification. More than 50,000 pediatricians worldwide make use of PREP The Curriculum, which includes PREP Self-Assessment and *Pediatrics in Review.*

The AAP National Conference & Exhibition (formerly the Annual Meeting) provides an opportunity for general and subspecialty pediatricians to explore the latest trends in pediatric medicine, improve their technical skills, interact with peers, and see the latest pediatric products. More than 10,000 attendees, including professionals, exhibitors, reporters, family members, and staff, make this annual meeting one of the highlights of the year.

extensive literature review and data analysis, and the guidelines as a whole go through a thorough peer-review process before they reach practicing pediatricians. Past topics covered by AAP clinical practice guidelines include diagnosis and treatment of attention-deficit/hyperactivity disorder (ADHD), detection of developmental dysplasia of the hip, and management of sinusitis.

The AAP spearheads or plays a key role in numerous advocacy campaigns, partnerships, and community-based programs, such as Bright Futures, Healthy Child Care America, and Buckle Up America. These campaigns, partnerships, and programs are important AAP activities. The AAP also provides pediatricians with proactive tools and information resources to cope with the ever-changing aspects of practice management, including quality improvement, insurance and reimbursement, liability, and information technology issues.

Continuing Medical Education and Conferences
The AAP is the premier source of continuing medical education (CME) for pediatricians. The AAP educational programs are diverse—from live courses held around the country, Internet-based

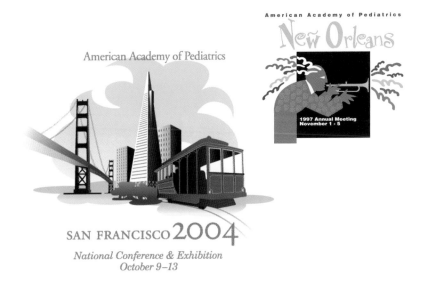

American Academy of Pediatrics

SAN FRANCISCO 2004
National Conference & Exhibition
October 9–13

American Academy of Pediatrics
New Orleans
1997 Annual Meeting
November 1 - 5

"I must point out another incredibly important part of the American Academy of Pediatrics—the staff. This organization has the most dedicated, loyal, professional, and knowledgeable staff of any organization I have ever been associated with."

KATHRYN PIZIALI NICHOL, MD

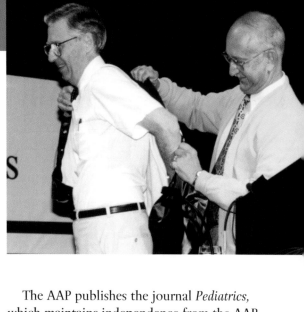

Right, Fred Rogers ("Mr Rogers") with then–American Academy of Pediatrics President George D. Comerci, MD, at the 1995 Annual Meeting.

Among the memorable speakers at the AAP annual meetings have been comedian Bill Cosby in 1980, First Lady Hillary Clinton in 1993, Fred Rogers ("Mr Rogers") in 1995, President Bill Clinton in 1999, and First Lady Laura Bush in 2002.

Publications and Periodicals

The AAP is the largest pediatric and the third-largest medical society publisher, and produces more than 480 publications and electronic products. The AAP publishes a broad range of professional references and textbooks, practice management publications, patient education materials, parenting books, and professional journals.

Red Book®: Report of the Committee on Infectious Diseases is the best-selling AAP professional clinical reference book and is used by health professionals worldwide. It has also become an essential resource for schools, public health departments, community centers, and more. The 2003 *Red Book* was published in 5 different formats: softcover, hardcover, CD-ROM, personal digital assistant, and Internet. It features several international editions (for more about the *Red Book,* see Chapter 6).

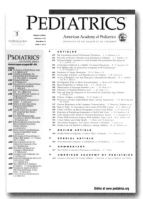

Pediatrics, March 2004, Volume 113, Number 3, Part 1 of 2 .

The AAP publishes the journal *Pediatrics,* which maintains independence from the AAP with an editorial office in Vermont. It has the largest circulation of any peer-reviewed pediatric journal, reaching more than 62,000 subscribers worldwide. *Pediatrics* publishes studies on issues covering every aspect of child health, editorials on pediatric subjects, and new policy statements from the AAP and its committees. Other AAP journals and periodicals include *Pediatrics in Review, AAP News,* and *NeoReviews.*

Millions of AAP patient education brochures reach families and caregivers each year. More than 150 brochures aimed at families are available in English and Spanish on topics ranging from breastfeeding, toilet training, and immunizations to adolescent health, substance abuse prevention, and childhood nutrition.

The AAP has also published more than 15 books for parents, including *Caring for Your Baby and Young Child: Birth to Age 5* (more than 4 million copies sold), *Your Baby's First Year* (more than 2 million copies sold), and the recently published *ADHD: A Complete and Authoritative Guide.*

Surveys and Research

The AAP conducts 4 statistically significant, random sample surveys of its membership each year to track attitudes and practices, to plan and evaluate AAP programs, and to provide information for the development of policy statements. Recent survey topics include screening for perinatal HIV transmission, direct-to-consumer advertising for prescription drugs, identification and referral of children with special needs to early intervention programs, violence prevention counseling, and use of health supervision guidelines.

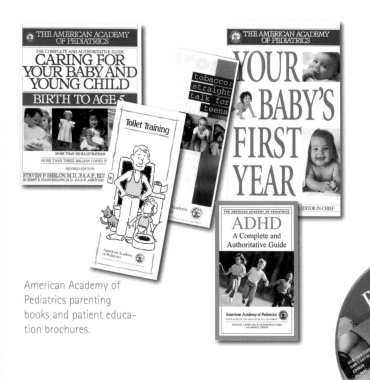

American Academy of Pediatrics parenting books and patient education brochures.

Visual Red Book on CD-ROM, 2nd Edition, published in 2003.

Pediatric Research in Office Settings (PROS) is a nationwide network of more than 1,800 AAP Fellows working in office-based practices. The PROS network conducts research on child health conditions seen in practice to determine how these conditions are treated and the effectiveness of such treatments. Issues explored in recent PROS studies include preschool vision screening, onset of secondary sexual characteristics in young girls, the treatment of pediatric patients with psychosocial conditions, febrile infants, and asthma management. PROS has proven to be an effective, grassroots, quality improvement tool. The AAP also sponsors the Center for Child Health Research based at the University of Rochester, NY, to help shape public policies and improve medical practices.

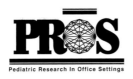

The Pediatric History Center, located in the AAP Bakwin Library, collects materials related to the history of pediatrics in the United States and Canada and the history of the AAP itself. Through its oral history program, the center conducts interviews with selected pediatricians and other leaders in the advancement of children's health care, preserving the recordings and transcripts.

Public Outreach

The AAP conducts national public information campaigns to inform the public about child health issues such as SIDS, the dangers of air bags to small children, and the back seat being the safest place for children of any age to ride. To provide support on legislative issues that affect children and physicians, the AAP Federal Advocacy Action Network (FAAN) helps to unite the voice of thousands of pediatricians in the fight for better public policies. As part of the FAAN effort, AAP members receive special alerts via e-mail on federal legislation and regulations along with sample key messages to send to Congress or other federal officials when immediate action is needed. In 2003, for example, members of FAAN helped to secure legislative successes that included passing of the Pediatric Rule, funding for SCHIP, and improving a Head Start bill in the House of Representatives.

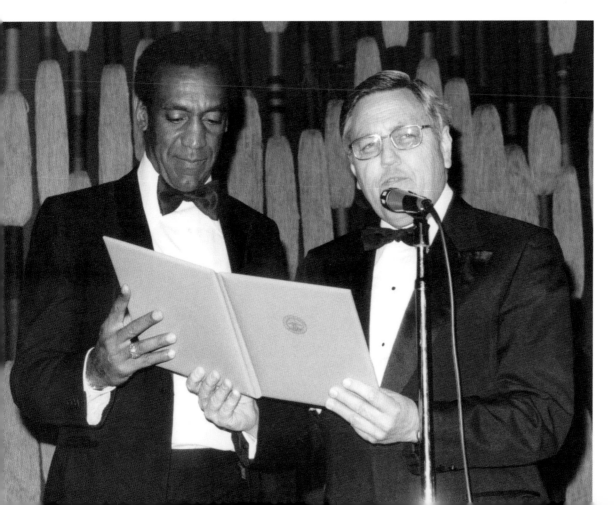

Comedian Bill Cosby with then–American Academy of Pediatrics President Bruce D. Graham, MD, at the 1980 Annual Meeting.

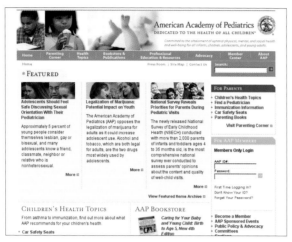

American Academy of Pediatrics Web site (www.aap.org), redesigned in June 2004.

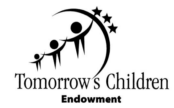

Tomorrow's Children
Endowment

The AAP Web site (www.aap.org) features breaking news and recommendations from the AAP, information and resources for parents, background on AAP programs and advocacy efforts, an online bookstore, a member center, and more. The site receives more than 500,000 visits per month, and 2 million pages are viewed each month. The AAP Web site is an excellent resource for parents, pediatricians, news makers, policy makers, and the general public to learn more about all of the numerous and ongoing activities of the AAP.

Individual and corporate contributions to the AAP annual campaign, called the Friends of Children Fund, support high-priority projects including access to child health programs, quality improvement initiatives, and public information campaigns on issues such as immunization, obesity, and tobacco use and prevention. The Tomorrow's Children Endowment was created to enhance the ability of the AAP to carry out research, education, advocacy, and community service programs and initiatives that advance pediatrics. The endowment will provide resources above and beyond operating revenues that give flexibility to address emerging issues.

American Academy of Pediatrics Friends of Children Fund

Since its establishment in 1989, the American Academy of Pediatrics Friends of Children Fund has provided nearly $3 million in grants to support AAP programs and activities nationwide, including

- Breastfeeding promotion
- Cardiology research
- Child health research
- Community Access to Child Health
- Critical care research
- Disaster relief efforts
- Future of Pediatrics Education
- Immunization awareness
- Medical student outreach
- Neonatal Resuscitation Program
- Pediatric History Center
- Resident scholarship program
- Resident international travel grants
- Resident research grants
- State Children's Health Insurance Program
- Substance abuse prevention
- Violence prevention programs

Friends *of* Children *fund*®

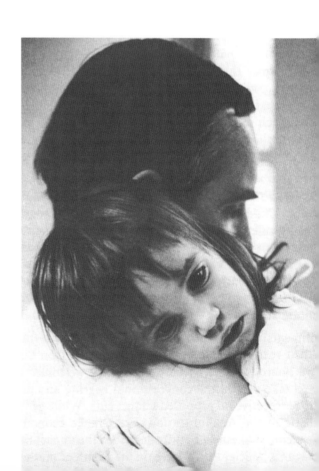

International Activities

Among the goals of the AAP international activities are to foster relationship-building with a worldwide community of health professionals, researchers, and societies; to improve the lives of children no matter where they live; and to obtain information and perspectives that will enable pediatricians to better serve the changing needs of their patients in the United States.

The AAP has programs that serve and educate more than 1,000 international members in more than 60 countries, and the AAP has held CME meetings in countries such as Italy, India, and Mexico. More than 12,000 AAP publications are shipped annually to more than 140 countries and, in a recent initiative, free electronic access to *Pediatrics, Pediatrics in Review, NeoReviews, AAP Grand Rounds, AAP News,* and *Red Book Online* has been given to child health care professionals who live in more than 60 low-income countries. Several state chapters have developed relationships and special projects with countries such as Brazil, Nicaragua, Vietnam, and Guatemala. The AAP also provides travel grants to pediatric residents who wish to complete a clinical pediatric elective in the developing world. International activities continue to be a growing aspect of AAP efforts.

NARRATIVES ON SELECTED INITIATIVES, 1980 TO 2005

The following narratives provide a glimpse (and by no means an exhaustive summary) of the many efforts of the AAP and its member pediatricians on behalf of children and adolescents over the past 25 years.

Emergency Medical Services for Children: The Formative Years

In the mid-1970s, pediatricians and pediatric surgeons began to raise concerns that emergency care for children wasn't what it should be. The problem was that the emergency medical services (EMS) system was organized around cardiac and trauma care for adults. The unique aspects of pediatric care were not incorporated into EMS and children were suffering unnecessarily as a result.

In January 1981, the AAP established the Section on Pediatric Emergency Medicine (which continues today as the Section on Emergency Medicine), and in 1988, the Committee on

Pediatric Emergency Medicine was established. Working with others, AAP pediatricians and pediatric surgeons tackled the challenge of change. Their job was to bring the principles of pediatric emergency care to numerous and varied EMS systems across the country. The movement to integrate the specialized knowledge, attitudes, skills, and equipment critical to pediatric emergency care became known as emergency medical services for children (EMSC). Advocates for EMSC started with the basics and created the first pediatric life support courses (resulting in the current Pediatric Advanced Life Support [PALS] and Advanced Pediatric Life Support [APLS] courses).

In 1984, a major boost for EMSC came from federal legislation. Senator Daniel Inouye (D-HI) and Hawaii Pediatric Society President Calvin C. J. Sia, MD, focused congressional attention on the gaps in EMSC. This resulted in the funding of the EMSC program under the Health Resources and Services Administration. Emergency medical services for children have come a long way since the 1970s, at a cost of a great deal of dedication and sweat equity of many pediatric advocates. But the results, measured in the lives of children saved, are priceless.

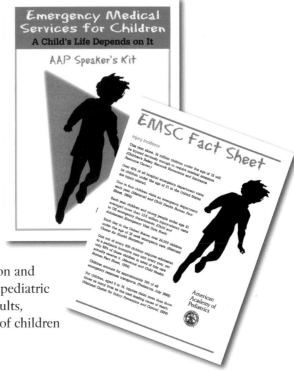

— *Jane F. Knapp, MD*

TIPP®—The Injury Prevention Program: A Brief History

In 1983, noting that "accidents cause 4 out of 10 deaths of preschool children," US Surgeon General C. Everett Koop, MD (a Fellow of the AAP), praised the AAP for launching a nationwide program to reduce childhood injuries and poisonings to assist pediatricians in their counseling of parents on the major causes of accidents. TIPP was the first initiative by a national medical organization to address accident prevention, and

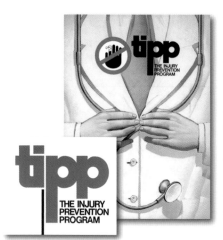

TIPP program folder and logo from the 1980s.

had its origins in 3 federally funded state projects in California, Massachusetts, and Virginia. At the completion of these projects, their directors, on the basis of their experiences, advised the AAP on the development of what became TIPP.

The guiding principle of TIPP was to focus on epidemiologically important injuries for which proven effective preventive strategies were readily available. TIPP, which emerged from this meeting, made pediatric counseling to prevent injuries a standard of care and established a schedule for childhood safety counseling. A packet of materials, including safety information sheets, was developed. The original program, focused on children from birth to age 4, received attention on national TV. In 1988, the program was expanded to include children ages 5 through 12, and a bicycle helmet component was added.

TIPP has had several updates, including 2 entirely new designs since that time. In 1993, a critical review of the literature demonstrated that primary care–based injury prevention counseling was an effective strategy, and a benefit-cost analysis in 1995 indicated that $3.4 billion in annual US injury costs could be saved if all children younger than 4 had access to TIPP. Since the program's inception, more than 40 million TIPP materials have been distributed through the AAP, making the program one of the organization's most extensive and successful efforts.

Much has changed since the first version of TIPP was released in 1983, most notably the shift from the concept of "accident"—a seemingly chance event caused by random forces, to "injury"—a scientifically understandable and avoidable occurrence. Also, as was to be expected, the hazards confronting children in 2005 and the knowledge we have about prevention have changed since 1983. TIPP has endured because flexibility to adapt to new developments was planned from the outset. It is well poised to continue to serve our young patients in the years to come.

— *Joel L. Bass, MD*

The Quiet Successes of a Primary Care Pediatrician

Primary care pediatricians like me don't often encounter the so-called "great cases" of a subspecialist researching the latest diagnostic algorithm, exploring a cutting-edge therapy, or managing the subtleties of a complicated disease. An example of one of my "great cases" this year involved a well-child visit for a 12-year-old boy. As part of this routine visit, I learned that he enjoyed biking and that he had recently been to an urgent care center after falling off his bike after sliding on gravel. He wasn't wearing a bicycle helmet at the time, and fortunately only had a leg abrasion. In this visit, he needed clearance to play football. We both agreed that he wouldn't dare play football without a helmet. Given how dangerous his biking can be, I asked him, "Why not wear a helmet while biking as well?" He agreed that he should.

I didn't see him again for a year for his routine physical examination. He told me that he'd been to the emergency department after he fell of his bike again, ultimately landing on his head on a manhole cover. This time he was wearing a helmet. He was taken to the ER and diagnosed with a concussion. He says he still wears his bicycle helmet and credits it with preventing a larger injury.

Even though there was no big emergency department workup, hospitalization, or intervention by a subspecialist or surgeon, as a primary care pediatrician, this routine well visit was a highlight of my year.

— *Michael D. Cabana, MD*

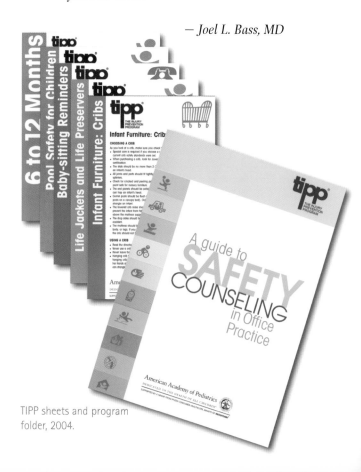

TIPP sheets and program folder, 2004.

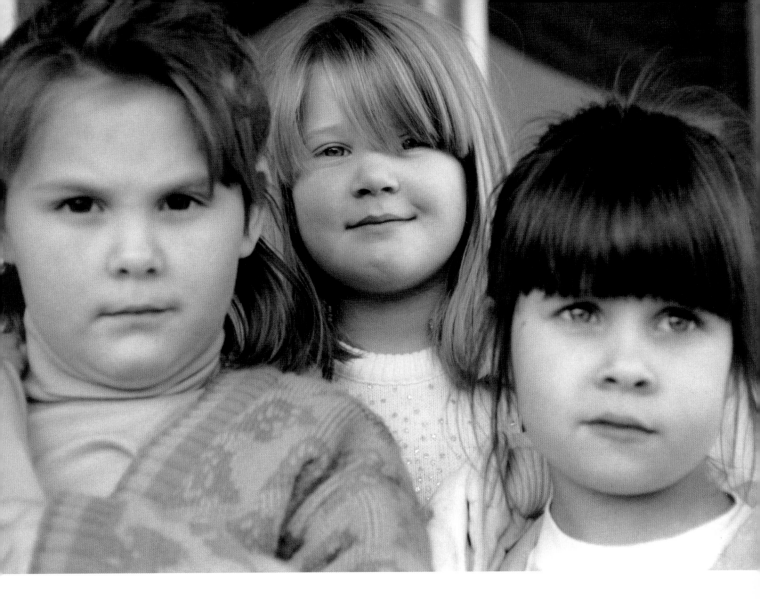

Child Passenger Safety—You Can Change the World

A child dies, a family grieves, and life for them is changed forever. The death of any child is tragic, but a death that is avoidable and occurs because the child is not protected by a car safety seat causes a special pain for the parents and the physician responsible for his care. Robert Sanders, MD, a soft-spoken pediatrician and director of the County Health Department in Murfreesboro, TN, decided that a child passenger protection law would help save lives.

Dr Sanders educated his patients, spoke to the media, organized coalitions, influenced his friends, wrote letters to the editor, made countless phone calls, and contacted legislators again and again. He became a familiar figure in the halls of the Tennessee state capital. After an unsuccessful first attempt, the law was ultimately enacted in Tennessee, and one legislator commented that Dr Sanders deserved credit for the law's passage because of "his personal attendance, vigor of persuasion, and knowledge of the facts."

By 1985, persuaded by the successes in Tennessee, all 50 states had passed laws to protect children as passengers in motor vehicles. Dr Sanders, though he has been described as "the last person you would think of as a rabble rouser for controversial causes," is an excellent example of how one person can make a difference and even change the world.

— *Marilyn J. Bull, MD*

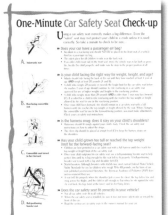

One-Minute Car Safety Seat Check-up fact sheet, first published in 1996.

Every Child Deserves a Medical Home

The phrase, "Every Child Deserves a Medical Home," originated as part of Hawaii's Child Health Plan in 1979. This concept lay on the drawing board until 1986, when a Maternal and Child Health Bureau grant enabled physician leadership to spearhead the implementation of the first medical home training in Hawaii. The success of the Hawaii project led to the development of similar projects in many other states.

The medical home concept recognizes the important role of primary care pediatricians in facilitating quality health care for all children, especially those with special health care needs. Pediatricians become partners in sharing responsibility with families and coordinating medical care with all related support services. The medical home provides primary health care that is accessible, family-centered, community-based, coordinated, continuous, culturally effective, compassionate, and comprehensive in addressing the needs of the whole child.

Based on the AAP commitment to attain optimal physical, mental, and social health for all infants, children, adolescents, and young adults, the medical home has a priority within AAP strategic plans. The AAP officially adopted the medical home concept in a 1992 policy statement, and reaffirmed this in a more definitive statement in 2002. "Every Child Deserves a Medical Home" is official AAP policy.

— *Calvin C. J. Sia, MD*

A Tribute to Calvin C. J. Sia, MD, and the Medical Home

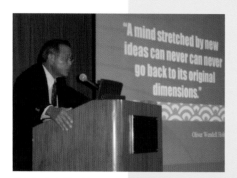

Calvin C. J. Sia, MD, lecturing.

Dear Dr Sia,

On June 7, 1990, our son John graduated from high school...we'd like to take this moment to thank you for all of your assistance and support that made this occasion possible...We came to you as anxious parents when he was born prematurely in the hospital and you cared for him during his acute breathing difficulties and feeding problems...You watched him grow and develop in his early years and were concerned about his hyperactivity and inattentiveness...Without your assistance in getting proper testing and your influence to enroll him in early therapy and special education, he would not be the person he is today. We will never forget your concern and help with all his many "not-so-normal" behavior problems...that seemed to go on and on...Well, he outgrew his funny habits, his peers grew up to accept the way he was and, attending high school, things started to look better and better...He will attend Community College in the fall and try to transfer to the University later. That's pretty good for a kid who was labeled "severely learning disabled," don't you think? We wanted to share this news with you, since you had such a BIG part in this sweet success story! We thank you so much and will never forget what you've done for us!

Sincerely,
John's parents

— *Letter to Calvin C. J. Sia, MD, shared by Kenn Saruwatari, MD, and Sharon Taba, MEd*

Health and Safety in Child Care Centers

House calls had always been a familiar function for me. As a teenager in the mid-1940s, I frequently drove my doctor-father to his "visits" to have the opportunity to drive. I would hear some of the details of the visit as we drove off. When I went on to medical school and spent a month making calls in East Boston, MA, under the guidance of a preceptor, I had an opportunity to observe an environment and learn the importance of follow-up.

One evening, after I became a private practitioner, a young working mother and her child with a very high fever confronted me. "And where has she been all day?" I asked. "In a day care center," was the answer. This was in 1965 and I really didn't know about day care centers—what were they? Remembering my house call experiences, I visited my patient at the day care center the following day. What an education! Cribs all over. Many children in the basement. Only *one* overworked person caring for all the children. When I left and called the health department, I learned that the only thing that licensing inspectors were concerned with was the temperature in the refrigerator!

The following year, I went back to school to get a masters in public health degree, and for my thesis I wrote about child care facilities in Manchester, NH—the staffing, the fees, and the characteristics of the families whose children were registered. I began to share my concerns with members of the New Hampshire Pediatric Society and was appointed to a national committee. That committee made public its concerns about health and safety in child care centers. The committee edited the 1980s edition of *Health in Day Care* and then, working with the American Public Health Association and the National Resource Center for Health and Safety in Child Care, developed standards for *Caring for Our Children* (now in its second edition).

The AAP has had a profound influence on health care issues in this increasingly important out-of-home site for children. Home visits got me started, but the AAP kept me at it!

— *Selma R. Deitch, MD*

(Editors' note: Dr Deitch passed away in February 2004 before her account for this history was published. We are pleased to present you with what was surely one of her final reminiscences on this topic.)

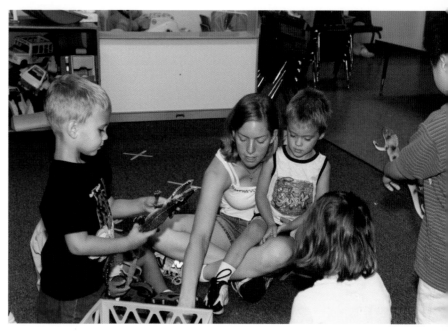

Child care facility, 2002.

Dramatic Advances in the Care of Children With Spina Bifida

When I was a child in the 1960s, I rarely saw children who were not able-bodied. Many children with spina bifida didn't survive infancy, and those who did were raised in isolation and educated in special schools. As a medical student in the era of "selective treatment," I waited helplessly with parents and nurses as a baby boy with spina bifida was left to die.

Today, there is a boy with spina bifida in my own child's classroom. Education laws have established the rights of children with disabilities to attend school alongside their able-bodied peers, and to receive the services necessary to enable them to do so. Not only are disabled children gaining access to educational opportunities, but there is increasing access to social and recreational opportunities. Summer camps, adaptive skiing, and wheelchair basketball are testaments to the profound changes that have occurred in the past 2 decades.

The care of children with spina bifida has seen dramatic advances in clinical management, in scientific research, and in policy. The ventriculo-peritoneal shunt, developed by engineer John Holter in a courageous effort to save his son Casey, has saved the lives of countless children. The advent of clean intermittent catheterization

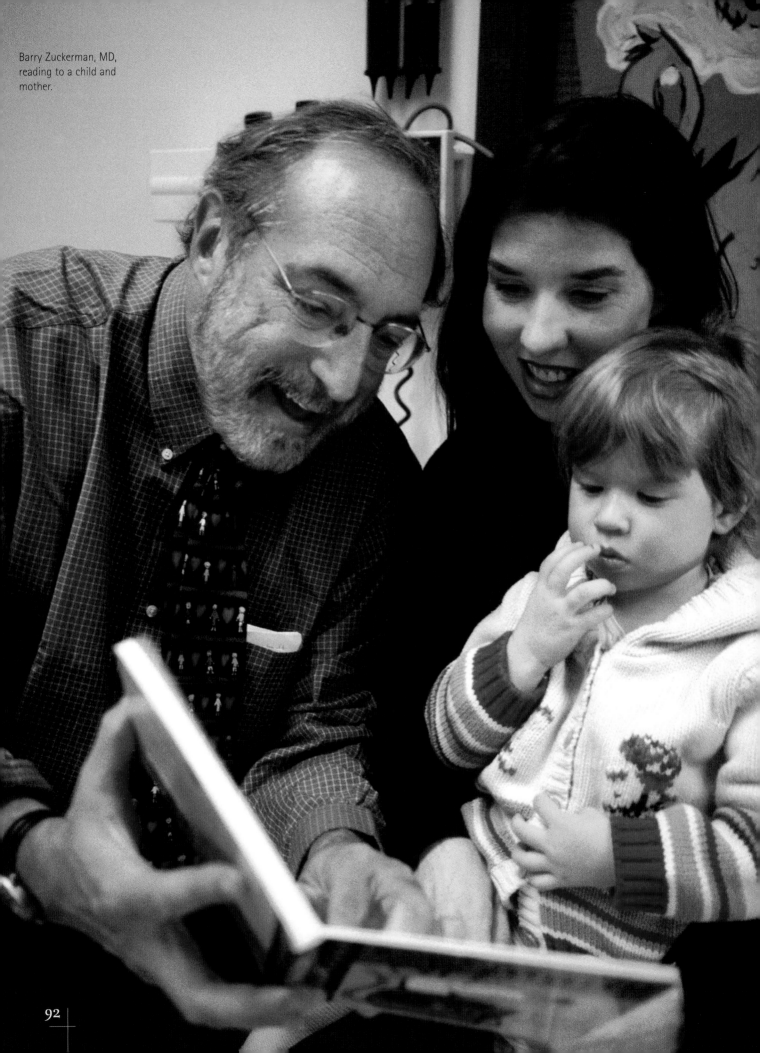

Barry Zuckerman, MD, reading to a child and mother.

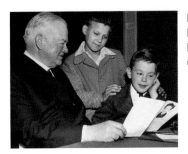
Historical photo of President Herbert Hoover reading to children.

has protected survivors from renal failure. Folic acid supplementation has been very effective in preventing neural tube defects. Pediatricians have been instrumental in all of these advances, preventing disability and promoting the health of individuals with spina bifida.

— *Adrian Sandler, MD*

Promoting Literacy in Primary Care (Reach Out and Read)

The past 2 decades have seen an increasing national focus on brain development, as educators have emphasized the crucial role that school readiness plays in ultimate school success. In addition, there has been a growing understanding of the economic burden of 23 million illiterate adults in the United States. Pediatricians, whose own professional imperatives have drawn them steadily toward the fostering of healthy child development, have found a role in literacy promotion that builds on the brain research, improves school readiness, and may, by helping children acquire literacy skills on schedule, help break family cycles of illiteracy, poverty, and dependency. Reach Out and Read was a program developed to meet this challenge.

Most pediatricians read aloud to their children—and many would probably name this as a favorite family activity. Until the late 1980s, however, few brought this emphasis across the line from personal life to professional practice. Reach Out and Read, which celebrated its 15th anniversary in 2004, has been instrumental in bringing an awareness of the importance of books and reading aloud in the lives of young children into standard pediatric practice.

Reach Out and Read begins in the pediatrician's waiting room with volunteers reading aloud to children and modeling book-sharing strategies for parents. The model continues in the examination room, where the pediatrician provides age-appropriate anticipatory guidance

about books, book sharing, and literacy. The child is then given a developmentally and culturally appropriate book to take home at every visit from ages 6 months to 5 years. Research supports clinicians' impressions of the value of this effort for low-income children; parents participating in the program are more likely to read to their children, and children's language development is significantly enhanced—in one study, an average developmental gain of 6 months for a 2-year-old child. By the end of 2003, Reach Out and Read had grown from the single founding site in 1989 to more than 1,900 pediatric sites in all 50 states. Pediatricians gave more than 3 million books annually to approximately 1.8 million children, with appropriate guidance and modeling for parents.

Books do more than promote literacy. They provide a framework for positive interactions with young children and thereby promote social and emotional development, in addition to language, cognitive development, and memory. Pediatricians have found that observing the child's behavior with a book can provide important information about attention span, fine motor abilities, and language. Literacy promotion and books at the health supervision visit, following the Reach Out and Read model, should become as routine as giving immunizations; both are important for the healthy growth and development of young children.

— *Barry Zuckerman, MD; Perri Klass, MD; and Robert Needlman, MD*

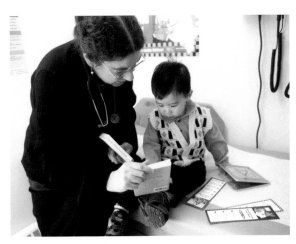
Perri Klass, MD, reading to a young boy.

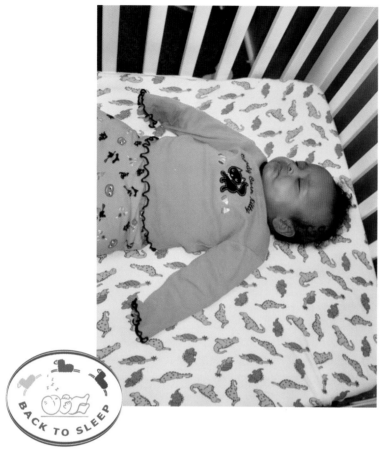

Sometimes Things Turn Out Right: Sudden Infant Death Syndrome and the Back to Sleep Campaign

In 1991, several AAP members from the Seattle, WA, area contacted the AAP, saying that a number of articles had appeared in the Seattle newspapers citing reports from Australia and New Zealand that suggested that the incidence of SIDS was reduced when babies slept supine rather than prone. This was a rather distressing possibility since, at the time, stomach sleeping was the predominant position used for infants in the United States and most other Western societies. The Seattle pediatricians asked what the AAP position was on this matter. Obviously there was none! The usual AAP approach would have been to refer this to one of the AAP committees. However, the usual time for a committee to write and issue a position paper was 2 to 3 years, and the Seattle pediatricians wanted a prompt answer.

In November 1991, AAP Executive Director Dr James E. Strain suggested an alternative approach. Rather than referring this issue to one of the AAP committees, Dr Strain facilitated the appointment of a task force consisting of John

Brooks, MD; David Myerburg, MD; and me (John Kattwinkel, MD). We were asked to examine the evidence, and given a 3-month deadline to accomplish this. Dr Brooks led our task force through a careful examination of the literature and we concluded that the evidence showing a reduction of SIDS by prone sleeping was indeed compelling. In April 1992, at the AAP Spring Meeting in New York, NY, as part of a previously scheduled roundtable on SIDS, we presented our report that recommended that infants should be placed down for sleep on their backs, rather than their stomachs.

The recommendation caused quite a stir! The national television networks reported the story widely on the evening news, the prime-time news shows debated the controversy, and editorials were written. Some pediatricians, being questioned by their hospital nursery nurses, complained that the AAP had "blindsided" them and that they should have been given advance warning. Grandmothers said that babies would aspirate their vomitus; gastroenterologists warned that gastroesophageal reflux would become rampant; pulmonologists felt that oxygenation would become a problem; developmentalists expressed concern about delaying motor milestones; and primary care practitioners predicted that there would be a dramatic increase in problem sleepers.

A majority of experts at a meeting held by the National Institutes of Health (NIH) at about the same time endorsed our conclusions, although this was far from unanimous. However, the participants warned that such a radical change required careful monitoring. The NIH wisely responded by instituting an annual national survey of sleep practices. Both the NIH and our task force monitored the appropriate morbidity and mortality statistics from the National Center for Health Statistics on a monthly basis. As the SIDS rate began to fall coincident with a measured decrease in prone sleeping, the NIH and the AAP recruited other public and private national organizations in 1994 to join cosponsorship of the aggressive national Back to Sleep campaign to educate the public.

While, previously, more than 70% of mothers in the United States placed their babies down to sleep prone, now fewer than 14% do so. Over the past decade, the SIDS rate has been cut in half and nearly 3,000 fewer babies are dying each year from this horrendous tragedy. At the same time, there have been no measurable adverse consequences. We still don't know the mechanism(s) responsible, but this is an example of careful observations made by alert clinicians and epidemiologists leading to an effective societal change, which has resulted in an important improvement in health over a relatively brief period of time. It also is a terrific example of private and public organizations working together effectively to develop and implement recommendations that are based on scientific evidence.

— *John Kattwinkel, MD*

Advocacy Efforts in Nutrition: Folic Acid, Breastfeeding, Obesity, and Beyond

The AAP has consistently promoted efforts to improve the nutritional issues of children and adolescents. One example is the supplementation of flours with folic acid. Back when I was a house officer, many children with osteomyelitis had spinal defects. We have since learned that supplementing the diet of women before pregnancy with folic acid can dramatically reduce the incidence of spinal defects. The Centers for Disease Control and Prevention issued recommendations for folic acid intake during pregnancy in 1992 in response to landmark studies conducted during the previous 2 decades. Flour is now supplemented with folic acid in many developing nations and, since 1998, all enriched-grain products manufactured in the United States must be fortified with 140 micrograms of folic acid per 100 grams of grain.

One of the most gratifying changes over the past quarter century is the resurgence of breastfeeding in the United States and worldwide. Although rates of breastfeeding at birth and during the first year of life declined during the mid-20th century, there has been a very significant resurgence in breastfeeding over the past 15 years.

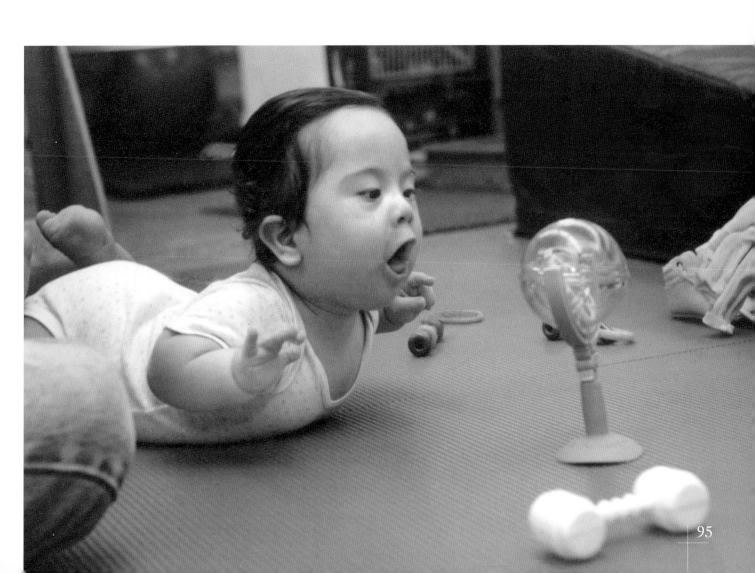

This reflects, to no small degree, the sustained and consistent campaigns and efforts by the AAP Committee on Nutrition and Section on Breastfeeding to highlight the benefits of breastfeeding. These efforts are further supported by extensive research during the past 25 years that extend our understanding of the benefits of breast milk, both for immediate and long-term health. In the United States, infant formulas are also better and safer now, thanks to the Infant Formula Acts of the 1980s that mandated quality controls and specified the content of many nutrients added to the formulas.

It has taken us 25 years to recognize the public and individual implications of obesity during childhood, and to finally react to the steadily rising and now alarming prevalence of a health issue that characterizes 30% to 40% of children today. Perhaps most gratifying is the evolution of our understanding of the molecular biology of control of appetite and energy expenditure. This has grown exponentially at the same time that efforts to change behaviors at the population level have reached new and impressive levels. The AAP has played a substantial role in supporting research at the practice level and promoting a healthier lifestyle for children to reduce the risk of overweight during childhood.

— *Ronald E. Kleinman, MD*

Consumer Product Safety for Children

The AAP has long recognized injury as a leading public health problem for children. Since its creation in 1950, the Committee on Injury, Violence, and Poison Prevention has been a leader in national initiatives to prevent childhood injuries, including those associated with consumer

Breastfeeding and the American Academy of Pediatrics

From its inception, the American Academy of Pediatrics (AAP) has been a staunch advocate of breastfeeding as the optimal form of nutrition for infants. Although advocacy for breastfeeding was included in some AAP publications and policy statements, creation of the Work Group on Breastfeeding in 1993 marked the beginning of a formal effort by the AAP to promote breastfeeding and to develop comprehensive policies and educational programs in support of breastfeeding. In 1997, the Work Group on Breastfeeding developed a policy statement, "Breastfeeding and the Use of Human Milk," which has been widely recognized as a major declaration regarding the importance of breastfeeding and set forth a series of recommendations to pediatricians and other health care professionals about how to succeed with breastfeeding. By 2000, the Work Group had evolved to become the current AAP Section on Breastfeeding.

Since 2000, the Section on Breastfeeding has produced a policy statement on vitamin D and a breastfeeding book for mothers entitled *New Mother's Guide to Breastfeeding* (published by Bantam Books in 2002).

The section presents about 6 sessions on breastfeeding at each of the annual National Conferences & Exhibitions and conducts an annual section research and education program. In a period of 10 years, the AAP has demonstrated its commitment to breastfeeding and has made a major impact on this field for pediatricians,

other health care professionals, and the world's children and their mothers. The AAP can take credit for being one of the major contributors to the dramatic increase in breastfeeding initiation and duration that has occurred during the past 10 years.

— *Lawrence M. Gartner, MD*

products. Advocacy efforts by the AAP and other groups, federal legislation, advances in product design, and changes in injury prevention paradigms have contributed to a 40% decline in the unintentional injury death rate for children aged 0 to 4 years old during the past 2 decades. However, many children, particularly children younger than 5 years old, are still injured or die each year in their own homes due to consumer product–related drownings, fires, burns, gunshots, falls, and poisonings.

One of the most defining governmental actions to protect the public from consumer product–related hazards was the Consumer Product Safety Act (CPSA) of 1972. This act created the US Consumer Product Safety Commission (CPSC), a federal regulatory agency committed to protecting consumers and families from injuries associated with the more than 15,000 types of products under its jurisdiction. Although the CPSC does not have the authority to test products before they are marketed to consumers, it plays an important role in recognizing hazardous consumer products and developing standards to reduce or eliminate risks. The CPSC also has authority to pursue recalls for products that present a substantial hazard and to inform the public and retailers about the recalls.

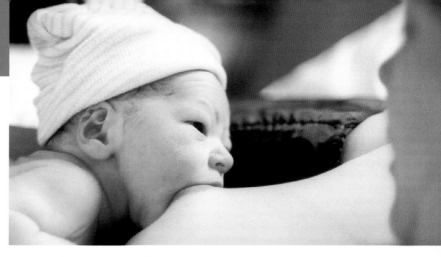
Baby breastfeeding moments after birth.

Predating the CPSA, another legislative milestone in consumer product safety occurred in 1960 with the passage of the Federal Hazardous Substances Act (FHSA). The FHSA requires hazardous household products to be labeled and gives the CPSC authority to ban substances if that labeling will not sufficiently protect the public. The FHSA was amended in 1994 by the Child Safety Protection Act, which requires choking-hazard warning labels on packaging for small balls, balloons, marbles, and toys containing small parts, when these items are intended for use by children aged 3 to 6 years old.

One of the most notable consumer product safety success stories relates to the baby walker. The AAP first issued a policy statement

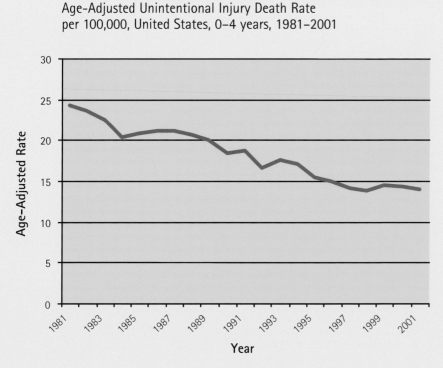

Age-Adjusted Unintentional Injury Death Rate per 100,000, United States, 0–4 years, 1981–2001

Source: Web-based Injury Statistics Query and Reporting System (WISQARS), Centers for Disease Control and Prevention.

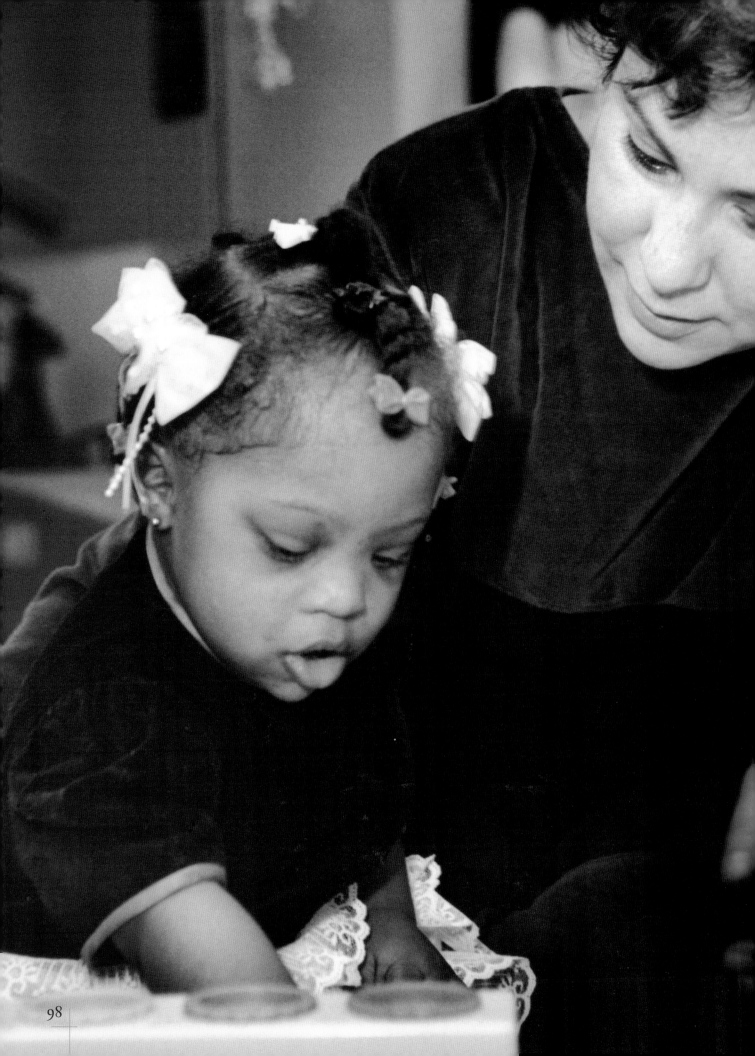

Does your baby Smoke?

recommending against the use of baby walkers in 1995 and has continued to be a catalyst in the creation of public policy that has lead to a significant decrease in injuries related to this product. Overall, there was a 76% decrease in the number of injuries during the period from 1990 to 2001.

Another example of success is the AAP-supported safety standard for cigarette lighters that became effective in 1994, requiring that disposable cigarette lighters be resistant to operation by children younger than 5 years old. According to a recent study, an estimated 3,300 fires, 100 deaths, 660 injuries, and $52.5 million in property loss were prevented by the standard in just 1 year.

Consumer product safety has made great advances during the past 50 years, but challenges remain. Many recalled and/or banned products remain in homes and continue to pose a threat to safety. Efforts to remove these products from environments where children live and play must persist. The AAP continues to provide leadership nationally to protect children from the important public health problem of consumer product–related injury.

— *Gary A. Smith, MD, and B. Christine Beeghly, MPH*

Advances in Environmental Medicine

The Committee on Environmental Health (COEH) had its beginnings during the Cold War, at a time when nuclear weapons testing was at its peak. In 1954, weapons testing in the South Pacific produced radiation injury to a cohort of children living near Bikini Island. This led the AAP, in 1957, to establish the committee now known as the COEH.

Since its creation, the COEH has played a role in identifying the most important environmental threats to children, with the goals of assisting pediatricians through education and policy recommendations, assisting parents by providing pediatricians with information needed for anticipatory guidance, and assisting government in creating legislation that limits the exposure of children to a broad array of environmental threats.

A look back over the past 25 years highlights many of the committee's most important activities. The prevalence of childhood lead poisoning has fallen by more than 80%, in part because of the unending AAP advocacy. Other environmental toxicants, including environmental tobacco smoke, ambient air pollution, mercury, ultraviolet radiation, and arsenic have become focal points of the AAP advocacy efforts. Recognizing that acts of terrorism using chemical/biological/nuclear weapons are environmental disasters, the COEH has closely examined the effect of terrorism and other disasters on children. Finally, in 1999, the COEH published the first edition of the *Handbook on Pediatric Environmental Health* as a resource for pediatricians, educators, and policy makers. Containing 33 chapters that largely define the current scope of children's environmental health, the handbook had its second edition released in November 2003.

— *Michael W. Shannon, MD*

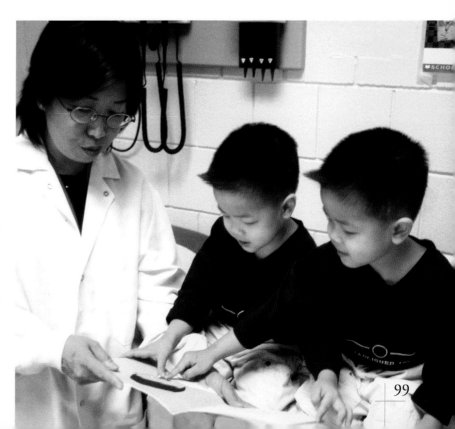

Dr Schreiber giving a typhoid
inoculation at a rural school
in San Augustine County, TX,
in April 1943.

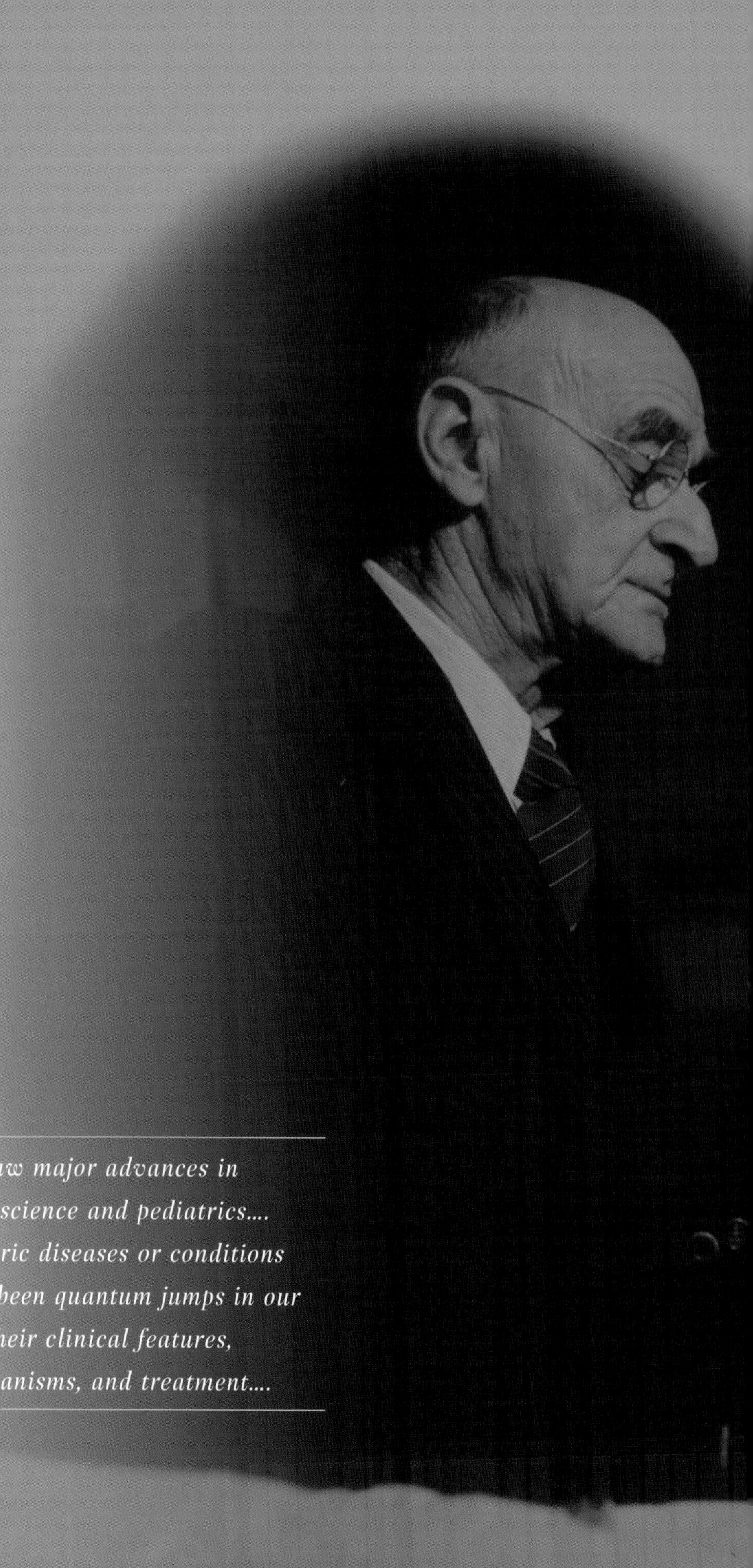

*The 20th century saw major advances in
all aspects of medical science and pediatrics....
It is hard to find pediatric diseases or conditions
in which there have not been quantum jumps in our
understanding of their clinical features,
pathophysiologic mechanisms, and treatment....*

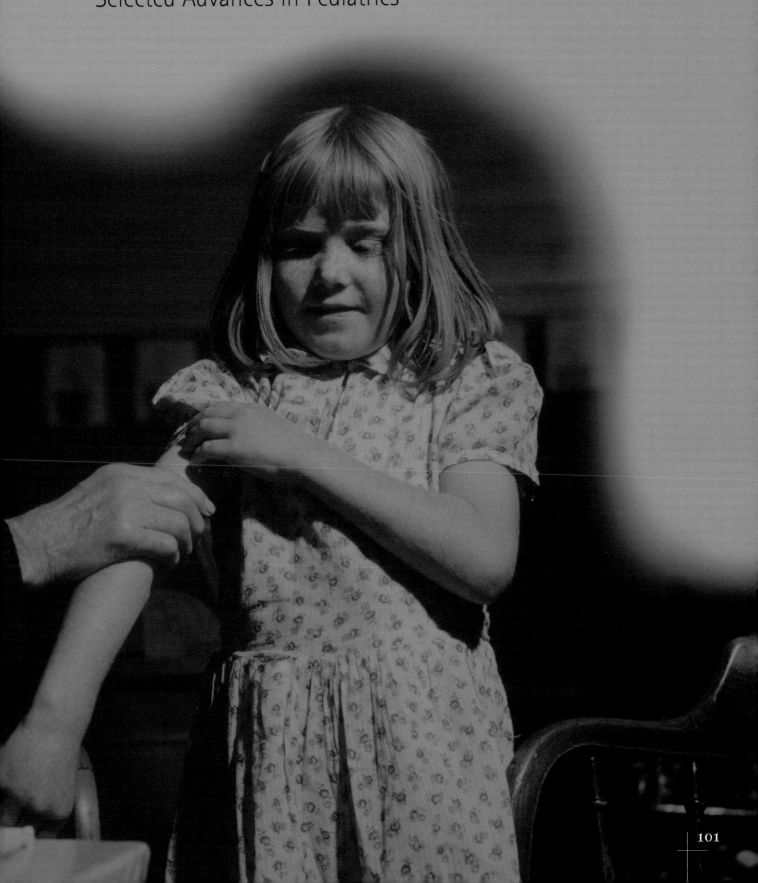

Chapter 6
Selected Advances in Pediatrics

SEVENTY-FIVE YEARS OF MAJOR ADVANCES

The 20th century saw major advances in all aspects of medical science and pediatrics. New information became available at an exponential and sometimes overwhelming rate. It is hard to find pediatric diseases or conditions in which there have not been quantum jumps in our understanding of their clinical features, pathophysiologic mechanisms, and treatment. Some diseases have disappeared and, sadly, new diseases have emerged. Any list of major pediatric advances during the 75 years of the American Academy of Pediatrics (AAP) would certainly include the following:

- Infectious diseases—the eradication of some of the great infectious scourges of childhood such as smallpox and polio by immunizations, and the control of many childhood diseases by an increasing number of effective antibiotics.

- Erythroblastosis fetalis—the definition, treatment, and prevention of a disease that was an important cause of death and mental retardation.
- Leukemia and cancer—the control and cure of leukemia and other malignancies that were once nearly inevitably fatal.
- Pediatric surgery—the emergence of safe and effective treatment for many acute and chronic diseases as well as the correction of severe and complex congenital anomalies, including cardiac defects.
- Newborn screening for genetic diseases—the neonatal diagnosis of an increasing number of metabolic and genetic diseases has enabled early institution of lifesaving interventions.
- Care of newborn and premature infants—the rise of newborn intensive care and the ever-changing frontier of viability have resulted in a dramatic decrease in neonatal morbidity and mortality.

These advances illustrate the ideal progression from recognition, to diagnosis, to treatment, and, in some instances, to prevention. There have been many other significant advances, but to include all of them would have required a virtual encyclopedia! The editors accept responsibility for their rather arbitrary selection of these advances, apologize for omissions, and gratefully acknowledge the pediatricians who submitted their experiences and comments.

IMMUNIZATIONS AND THE BATTLE AGAINST INFECTIOUS DISEASES

Overview

By the time of the founding of the AAP in 1930, great strides had already been made in the arena of childhood infectious diseases. Improved living conditions, cleaner water, and pasteurized milk eliminated the great epidemics of summer diarrhea that once stalked American cities. Tuberculosis rates were declining during the most ambitious health education campaign thus far in US history. Immunization against diphtheria was introduced on a large scale in New York, NY, during the 1920s, and was fast becoming the first childhood vaccination to be used routinely other than smallpox.

Yet in the 1930s, infectious diseases remained a great danger and consumed much of the day-to-day

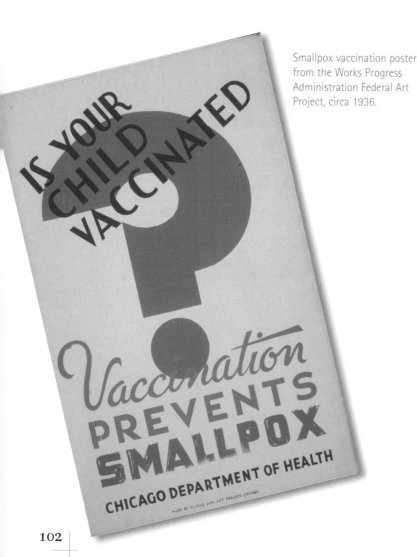

Smallpox vaccination poster from the Works Progress Administration Federal Art Project, circa 1936.

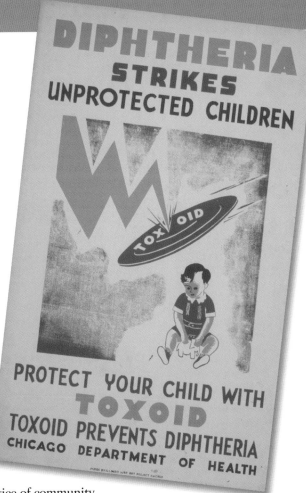

Diphtheria poster from the Works Progress Administration (WPA) Federal Art Project, circa 1936.

practice of community and hospital pediatricians. Recurrent tonsillitis presented frequently prior to antibiotics, making tonsillectomy a routine part of growing up for many children. Rheumatic fever remained common, leaving many children with permanent heart disease. Whooping cough and measles caused significant morbidity and mortality. There was little to offer children with most infectious diseases beyond supportive care and, in some cases, bacterial antiserums.

The introduction of antimicrobials marked the beginning of a new era of bacterial therapy. Sulfa drugs, introduced in 1935, were modified from the brilliant red dye Prontosil after it was shown that the compound inhibited the growth of bacteria. Penicillin, discovered somewhat serendipitously by the Scottish bacteriologist Alexander Fleming in 1928, was forgotten until a team of investigators, led by Howard Florey, appreciated its potential during World War II. Initially restricted largely to the military, penicillin entered civilian life (and pediatrics) after the war and soon became the archetype of the postwar "miracle drug." In short order, other antibiotic families were discovered as well—a fortunate development since bacterial penicillin resistance soon became widespread.

Remembering Pertussis

In 1946, I was a resident at the Charles V. Chapin Hospital for Contagious Disease in Providence, RI, arguably the oldest such institution in America. Pertussis patients were housed in a separate building containing 30 rooms, each with 2 bassinets. Many babies had serious complications ranging from hemorrhages of the brain to pneumonia that caused most of the deaths in these infants. Rarely we saw rectal prolapse, umbilical herniation, or toxic encephalitis. If the front lower incisor teeth had erupted, lacerations of the frenulum occurred. And babies died.

It was a horrendous disease that was called a 6-week disease: 2 weeks coming, 2 weeks staying, and 2 weeks going. To watch these infants whooping in spasms and screaming in between was frightening, frustrating, and unforgettable. We held our breath with them, waiting for the next inhalation. Pertussis vaccine reduced the incidence of pertussis dramatically but there are still several thousand cases in the United States each year, usually occurring in babies who were not vaccinated either because of lack of access to medical care—or because of parental fears about possible side effects.

— David Annunziato, MD

Remembering Smallpox

In February 1947, a 47-year-old American business-man who had lived in Mexico returned to New York and checked into a midtown hotel. In spite of some malaise, he was able to conduct his business, but, after 5 days, he went to the emergency room of a municipal hospital complaining of fever, headache, and a pustular rash. He was admitted to the Willard Parker Hospital for Communicable Disease where he died a few days later. He died of smallpox, but this diagnosis was only made retrospectively when 11 other individuals who had contact with him also developed smallpox. Once the diagnosis was made, health officials launched an extensive public information campaign, and mass vaccination was begun in April. Hospitals, health centers and clinics, schools, and police stations were used almost nonstop.

I was an intern at St John's Hospital and worked three or four 24-hour shifts providing vaccinations. When you're a young house officer, nothing bores you. We processed 40 to 50 people an hour. They rolled up their sleeves, had their arms prepped with acetone by the nurses who then handed me a vial of vaccine and a needle, and then they were gone. It was an assembly line. In less than a month, more than 6 million of the city's 7 million residents were vaccinated. Without this mass effort, 4,000 people would probably have been infected and nearly a thousand would have died. Instead there were only 2 deaths from smallpox, plus 6 deaths linked to the vaccine.

— *David Annunziato, MD (with additional background from Robert Grayson, MD)*

By this point, a revolution in vaccine development was also underway. The components of the diphtheria-tetanus-pertussis (DTP) vaccine had evolved before the Second World War. The development of tissue culture techniques by the team led by John F. Enders in the late 1940s set the stage for a succession of new discoveries. The introduction of the inactivated Salk vaccine against polio in 1955 was arguably the single most anticipated American medical breakthrough of the 20th century. Live attenuated vaccines against polio, as well as measles, mumps, rubella, and varicella, were subsequently developed. The AAP began making recommendations on immunizations in 1938 and, over time, its Committee on Infectious Diseases (the "*Red Book* Committee") has played a central role in setting standards for immunization as well as the treatment of many infectious diseases.

By the 1970s, most life-threatening infectious diseases were increasingly regarded as things of the past, but the human immunodeficiency virus (HIV) epidemic in the 1980s brought a halt to

New Yorkers line up in front of Morrisania Hospital, Bronx, NY, April 14, 1947, waiting for inoculation against smallpox. City residents were being vaccinated at an estimated rate of 8 per minute!

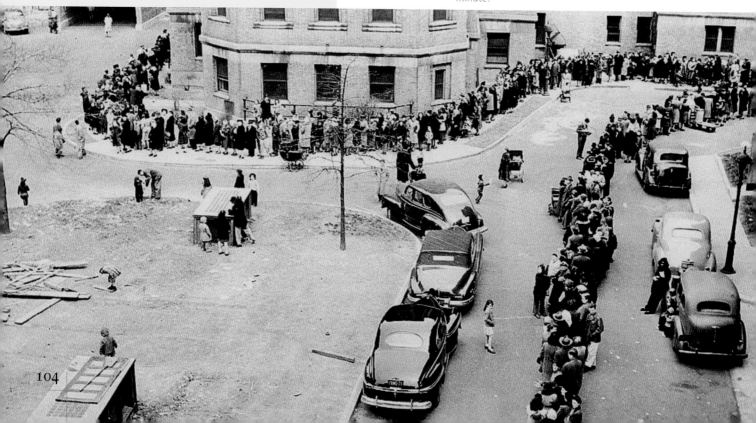

such optimism. Pediatric investigators played critical roles in elucidating antiviral agents to treat children with HIV and, most importantly, prevent transmission from mother to child. Other pediatricians became engaged in efforts to maintain the successes of past immunization, as public anti-vaccine sentiment and litigation reemerged in the 1980s. The first conjugated vaccine against *Haemophilus influenzae* type b (Hib) was introduced in 1990, followed by a precipitous decline in the incidence of Hib meningitis and epiglottitis.

It is surely too simplistic to tell the story of the decline of infectious diseases solely in terms of antibiotics and vaccines. Over the course of the entire century, improved living conditions played a major role in the decline of mortality from childhood infection independently of effective treatment. War, poverty, immigration, and global communication continue to raise new challenges. Still, as the accounts that follow illustrate, pediatricians may, with much justification, be proud of the fact that they have contributed to not only the treatment but also the prevention of a score of childhood infectious diseases.

Poliomyelitis: Terror in America in the 20th Century
The Polio Era
Poliomyelitis (infantile paralysis) made its first significant appearance in the United States as an epidemic in New York in the summer of 1916 that ultimately paralyzed 27,000 people and killed nearly 6,000 patients nationwide, mostly children. Thereafter, until 1954, it occurred as annual summer epidemics with peak incidences in July and August. Investigation in many laboratories around the world showed that poliomyelitis was caused by a "filterable agent," a virus with 3 different strains, and was spread by fecal/oral transmission through the food and water supply or by direct physical contact. It is hard to appreciate today, the panic and fear of American parents about polio in the 1930s and 1940s. Some parents kept their children isolated at home during the entire summer. Many movie houses and swimming pools were closed and other activities that involved large groups of children were curtailed. Any febrile illness in the summer caused great anxiety.

During the summer, the isolation wards in city hospitals were filled with children with acute poliomyelitis. There were few effective interventions. Orthopedic surgeons applied plaster casts

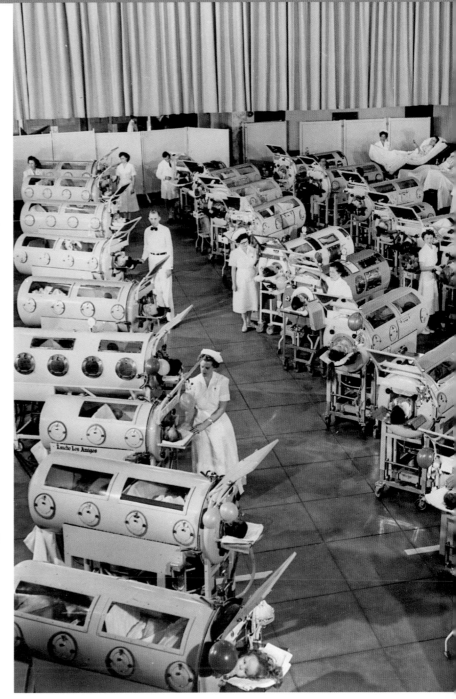

Bulbar polio patients at Rancho Los Amigos in Honda, CA, 1952.

to immobilize the extremities in a vain attempt to control spasms and prevent deformity, but many children were permanently paralyzed. Some children developed bulbar polio with respiratory insufficiency from respiratory muscle paralysis. They were placed in a tank respirator, the "iron lung," with only their heads protruding. A system of bellows intermittently reduced air pressure within the tank to facilitate inspiration.

In 1940, Sister Elizabeth Kenny, an Australian nurse, revolutionized the treatment of acute polio. Working independently, she had designed a treatment system involving hot packs and massage as early as possible to reduce pain and spasm. The polio wards of the 1940s could be recognized by the odor of Kenny packs made from heated moist wool blankets applied neck to toe for 20 minutes, 4 times daily.

The acute phase of polio accompanied by fever lasted 7 to 10 days. When the fever abated, the children were thought to be noninfectious and their paralysis no longer progressed. At that point, they were usually transferred to rehabilitation units for intensive physical therapy. Braces and splints were made to facilitate ambulation. Children in respirators were cared for in rehabilitation centers where attempts were made to wean them from respiratory support. Many children gradually regained the ability to breathe but most of those who could not, died.

The months of hospitalization were a tremendous financial burden for families. The National Foundation for Infantile Paralysis, and its fundraising arm, the March of Dimes, which were organized in response to the efforts of President Franklin D. Roosevelt, assisted in covering the hospital costs of many stricken children. The National Foundation also became a major sponsor of the research that finally resulted in the discovery of the polio vaccine.

In 1948, John F. Enders; Frederick C. Robbins, MD; and Thomas H. Weller, MD, discovered that polioviruses could be successfully grown in monkey kidney cell cultures. Soon thereafter, Jonas Salk, MD, prepared an inactivated polio vaccine (IPV), which performed favorably in pilot trials. In 1954, the National Foundation launched the largest field trials of the Salk vaccine conducted on more than 1.8 million children. The results, dramatically announced in a press conference by director Thomas Francis, Jr, MD, led to the rapid licensure and release of the vaccine. Yet a major setback soon followed when contaminated lots of IPV manufactured by Cutter Laboratories led to the paralysis of 260 individuals. Standards for vaccine production were tightened, and enthusiasm for IPV was quickly restored, leading to its

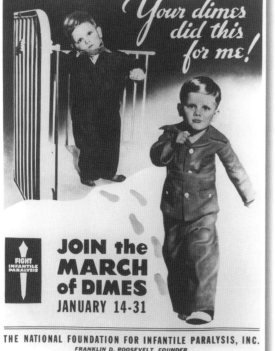

Your dimes did this for me!

JOIN the MARCH of DIMES
JANUARY 14-31

THE NATIONAL FOUNDATION FOR INFANTILE PARALYSIS, INC.
FRANKLIN D. ROOSEVELT, FOUNDER

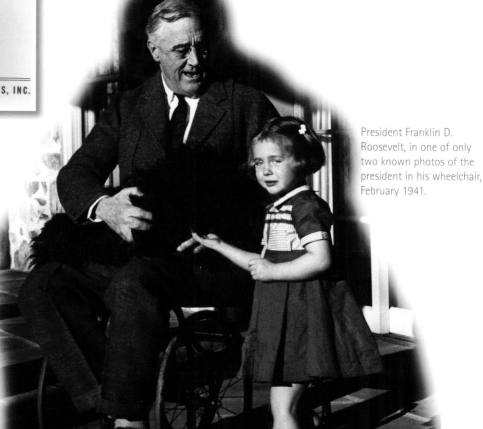

President Franklin D. Roosevelt, in one of only two known photos of the president in his wheelchair, February 1941.

Polio Pioneers

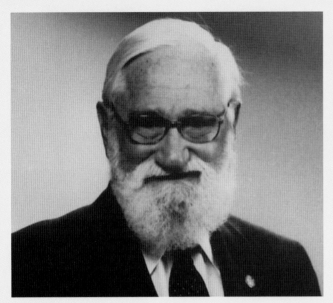

Albert B. Sabin, MD.

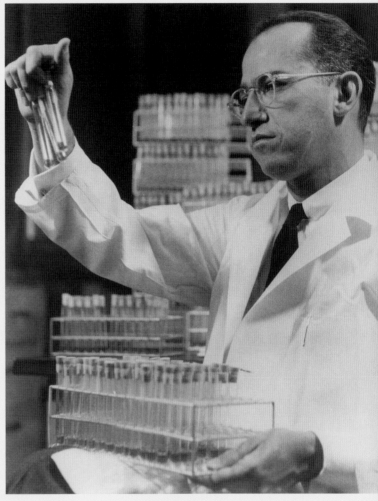

Jonas Salk, MD.

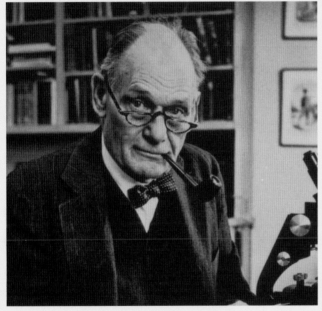

John F. Enders.

The Impact of Polio

As an intern in Rochester, NY, in 1950, I was sent to Utica to assist local doctors with an epidemic of polio. When I arrived I found more than 100 children hospitalized in a small children's hospital meant for 25. A month of around-the-clock caring for these children, many requiring tank respirators, made me an "expert" in a disease I was beginning to hate. Later, as chief resident at Children's Hospital Boston in 1955, we saw more than 3,000 patients with possible polio and had to convert the 350-bed hospital to one almost entirely devoted to this disease. The personal toll was great. I was able to get home only 3 nights in 2 months—once to give my wife, who was pregnant with our third child, a dose of gamma globulin in an effort to protect her from the disease.

— *Robert J. Haggerty, MD*

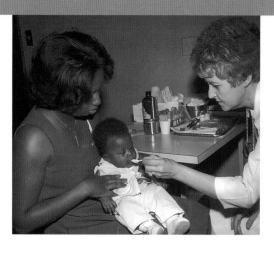

Above left, consent form for the national March of Dimes polio vaccine trials, 1954; *above right*, polio immunization at the Well-Baby Clinic in Dekalb County, GA, 1977.

widespread utilization and the decline of poliomyelitis in the United States and Europe.

Working separately from Dr Salk, Albert B. Sabin, MD, developed an attenuated live oral polio vaccine (OPV) that, after successful trials of millions of children in the Soviet Union, was recommended in the United States in 1961. "Sugar Cube Polio Sundays" were conducted throughout the country and millions were immunized at schools, churches, and public health facilities. The last case of polio caused by wild strains of the virus in the United States was reported in 1979, and, in 1994, the World Health Organization reported the elimination of poliomyelitis from the Western Hemisphere. The Sabin vaccine

continued to be used throughout the United States until 2000 when the Advisory Committee on Immunization Practices and the AAP recommended a return to IPV because, by this point, the only remaining cases of polio were the 6 to 8 immunosuppressed children who annually contracted the disease following OPV.

The conquest of polio was accomplished in less than 50 years. It is gratifying to know that today's families never have to experience the fear, bordering on panic, of polio that was so prevalent in the first half of the 20th century.

— *James E. Strain, MD*

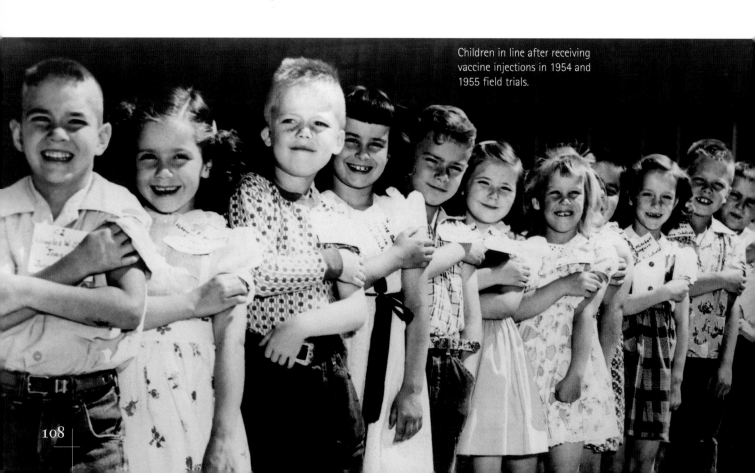

Children in line after receiving vaccine injections in 1954 and 1955 field trials.

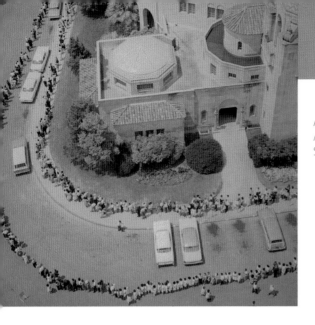

An aerial view of a crowd of children and families in San Antonio, TX, lining up for polio immunization with the live Sabin vaccine in 1962.

The Kenny Treatment

The standard treatment of polio in the United States prior to 1940 was complete bed rest, and patients were often placed in splints or casts and were given medicine for muscle pain. Sister Elizabeth Kenny changed both the treatment and prognosis of polio patients through her unorthodox approach. I first met and got to know her during her visit to the University of Minnesota when I was a medical student. Sister Kenny was a very impressive and caring person, and when she entered a patient's room, the patient felt better. She had served as a nurse in the Australian bush country and, in that capacity, had treated many patients with polio during Australia's recurrent epidemics. She believed that the most significant problem during the acute phase of polio was muscle "spasm" and, for this, she advocated hot, moist compresses and passive movement of the limbs to prevent distortion of the joints. Her strong ideas were a turnoff for most physicians and if she was asked a simple question to explain what she meant, it started off a tirade of invectives. I learned to say nothing and just observed it all.

— *Forrest H. Adams, MD*

Polio Outbreak in New York

I was a resident at the Babies Hospital of Columbia University in the summer of 1944 when an outbreak of polio occurred in New York. It quickly became the largest epidemic in the city's history, and an entire floor of the hospital was set aside for polio patients. In a back ward we had 4 cumbersome Drinker respirators (the so-called iron lung machines) and they were fully occupied for almost 6 weeks.

The weather that summer was brutally hot and humid. In those days, hospitals were not air-

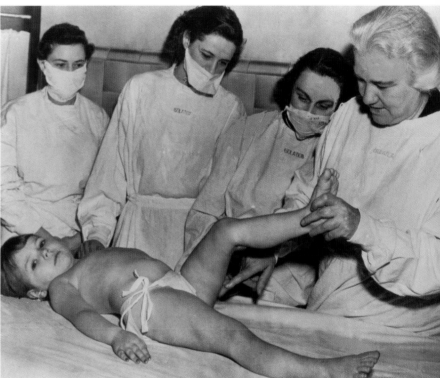

Sister Elizabeth Kenny (far right) at Minneapolis General Hospital, circa 1942.

conditioned and ambient conditions on the polio wards were made even more uncomfortable by huge copper vats of water, boiling day and night to keep the Kenny packs steaming hot. At night during that harrowing summer, I remember the ward nurses wearing masks and floor length isolation gowns. They seemed to be suspended a few inches above the floor in the darkened ward as they glided silently in a continuous shuttle between the steaming cauldrons and the naked patients lying in the ward beds.

— *William A. Silverman, MD*
(Excerpt from Silverman WA. *Where's the Evidence?* Oxford, England: Oxford University Press; 1998, by permission of Oxford University Press.)

Polio on the Loose in a Rural Practice

It was a warm, lazy Sunday morning in late August 1943. A worried-looking couple carrying a small boy came to my door. The mother related that the child had had slight diarrhea and a runny nose, but wasn't really sick until the day before when he complained of a headache and didn't want supper. The next morning when he tried to get out of bed, his legs gave out and he fell. I was not surprised when he resisted my bending his head forward, had no knee jerk reaction, and couldn't move his feet. I had the parents put the child in the back seat of their car and I followed to the local community hospital. I performed a spinal tap, noting that the fluid was turbid. I made arrangements to have the child transported by ambulance to the special polio unit in New Haven, CT.

Two weeks later, I got a phone call from the mother who wanted to talk to me. No, this was not about the child. He was doing all right. His legs were getting stronger, he was learning to walk with braces, and it was hoped that he would be coming home soon. Something else was bothering her. When I saw the parents a half hour later, it all spilled out—their world was falling apart. The mother had been told that she was not needed for a while as a volunteer at the Red Cross blood bank. The father's shared ride to work was canceled and he was told to take time off from his job at the post office to protect his coworkers. Their 2 older sons had been ostracized from the town ball field and were moping around the house. Sunday at church, the family was left alone in the pew. I listened and commiserated over the foolish and exaggerated behavior of "friends" whose unfounded fears seemed even more contagious than the disease itself. I assured them that time and patience would eventually cool the unreasonable hysteria.

— *Elinor Fosdick Downs, MD*

Polio Strikes a Pediatric Resident

I finished my internship in 1954, and I was classified as I–A by my Draft Board, which meant that I could be taken by the services whenever they elected, with only 10 days' notice. I started my second year of residency at the Children's Hospital Boston, MA, but, in August, I developed weakness and difficulty swallowing and was found to have polio. I was seen by a world-famous neurologist who attempted to do a lumbar puncture. After several misses, he called in a resident who was successful. (Moral: Never let an attending attempt a resident's job!)

Initially, I was unable to swallow and had severe weakness of both arms and my right leg. I managed to keep my respiration just above the iron lung requirement. I was initially fed fluids by

Polio affected parents as well as children. Shown here, a mother with polio and her 3 children, Goldwater Memorial Hospital, Roosevelt Island, NY.

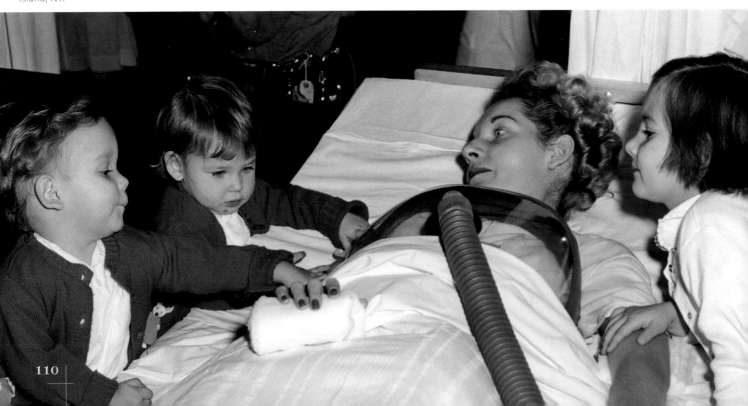

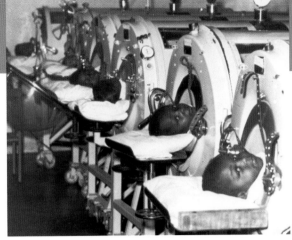
Children in iron lungs, Lutheran Hospital, Vicksburg, MS.

nasogastric tube but, after 2 to 3 weeks, I had progressed enough that I could swallow baby food and liquids. Being in the hospital was boring—no television, and I was so weak that I couldn't hold a book. After 2 months, I improved to the point that I could walk with a brace, but I still could only swallow liquids and baby food. I started back to work, but only from 9:00 to 5:00, 5 days a week. For this "half-time" job, my pay was reduced from $88 to $44 a month. I lost more than 70 pounds during the next year. While I was in the hospital, my call from the armed services finally came through, but I was reclassified as 4-F until the end of my residency. Then I entered the Public Health Service, still wearing a brace, but able to eat soft, mushy food.

— *Thomas F. Dolan, MD*

The Antibiotic Revolution
An Early Prontosil Trial
In the fall of 1936, during my fourth year of medical school at Johns Hopkins, I had a sub-internship at Sydenham Hospital, a 100-bed infectious disease hospital affiliated with Hopkins. I was unprepared for the variety and severity of the diseases I saw—scarlet fever, measles, mumps, diphtheria, whooping cough, and even meningitis. Many children had

complications such as pneumonia or septicemia. Some would get well, but many died or were left with permanent damage. There was no effective therapy for most of these diseases.

One morning, during my second week at Sydenham, Perrin Long, MD, a professor at Johns Hopkins, joined us for rounds. He had just returned from visits to hospitals and pharmaceutical firms in Europe where he learned of a new medication called Prontosil, which could reduce the mortality of streptococcal infections of women after childbirth. Dr Long was anxious to promote its use but, first, he wanted to find out whether it was effective against other streptococcal infections such as scarlet fever. From a small paper bag, Dr Long took a tightly closed glass bottle containing an innocuous-looking white powder—Prontosil. It looked harmless, but could it really help our patients or might they get sicker? Was there a risk?

The hospital's medical director, Horace Hodes, MD, quickly silenced these kinds of questions by consenting to an immediate test trial of the new drug—no fuss, no request for permission from the parents of 5 of our sickest patients with scarlet fever selected for treatment. One-gram doses of the powder were weighed out on the laboratory scales and wrapped in packets of wax paper. One packet of the powder, mixed in orange juice, was given to each child, 4 times a day for 5 days. We all watched and waited, nervously at first and then incredulously. Within a few hours of the first dose, the infants stopped fussing, their temperatures began to drop, and the raw, scarlet coloring of their skins began to fade. We noticed that their urine turned orange because of the drug. When the Prontosil was stopped on the fifth day (because there was none left), the children were smiling. Although their skin was peeling, they were well enough to be discharged home. Amazing! As

"On September 8, 1982, the polio era poignantly came to a symbolic end for me when the Children's Hospital maintenance forces deposited the last 'iron lung' in the trash heap. This diabolical, if lifesaving, machine should have been bronzed like baby shoes, or planted with geraniums, or put in the hospital lobby for dollar donations through its ports."

SEYMOUR E. WHEELOCK, MD

reports of success in Europe mounted, American pharmaceutical firms began producing and improving Prontosil, changing its name to sulfanilamide—the first of the sulfa drugs. Eventually large-scale studies confirmed its effectiveness against many infectious diseases, saving countless lives; and I was there at the very beginning!

— *Elinor Fosdick Downs, MD*

The First Use of Penicillin in New Hampshire: "An Undeniable Air of Drama"

One dark winter night in 1944 during my rotating internship at the Mary Hitchcock Memorial Hospital in Hanover, NH, I got a call from chief of medicine Sven Gundersen, MD, asking me to pick up THE PENICILLIN that had been sent in response to a formal grant request to the central agency in Washington, DC, several months before. The penicillin had just arrived at White River Junction on the night train to Montreal. I went to White River, passed the requested $50 cashier's check, and received a small package containing the maximum amount available—50,000 units!

The next morning, the hospital operator announced over the public address system, "Dr Gundersen will be mixing the penicillin at 7:30 am. Anyone interested is invited to watch him." Twenty-five people were on hand as Dr Gundersen, with an undeniable air of drama, drew up saline and injected it into the small bottle from Washington. The resulting solution was a deep yellow in color with dark particulate matter floating about. It was administered as a continuous infusion from a syringe actuated by the mechanism of a discarded Big Ben alarm clock into the vein of the first patient ever to receive penicillin in the state of New Hampshire (a 30-year-old farmer). He received 5,000 units a day until the precious material was gone.

— *Seymour E. Wheelock, MD*

Early Use of Penicillin: "A Miracle Drug"

When World War II ended in 1945, penicillin became more available to the general public. To access supplies of the drug, a senior attending physician had to request permission from a central bureau in Boston. It was released only for serious illnesses such as meningitis and pneumonia. We gave what were considered to be "massive" doses of aqueous penicillin, 5,000 units

every 3 hours. To expand the limited supply, we collected the urine of the patients being given penicillin and sent this to the laboratory where the penicillin was harvested for reuse—that's how precious it was. As an intern, I was assigned to make "penicillin rounds." I made rounds with 2 nurses throughout the hospital. The nurses checked the patient's identification, calculated the dose of penicillin, and filled a syringe that was given to me for injection. It usually took about 3 hours to complete penicillin rounds. We would then start all over again because penicillin had to be given every 3 hours. We rotated injection sites—deltoids, buttocks, triceps, and thighs—in a specific sequence. Sometimes we even had time for a cup of coffee between rounds! Penicillin rounds were rewarding because we knew that many patients who would have died could be made well. It was truly a miracle drug!

— *David Annunziato, MD*

Penicillin and Congenital Syphilis

In 1945, 8 small, very sick newborn infants with florid congenital syphilis were assembled in the Babies Hospital in New York for the first experimental use of penicillin in this form of the infection. The new agent was given to all of these babies and the results were apparent almost immediately: spirochetes from skin and mucous membranes disappeared within hours and, in a day or 2, all of the infants were miraculously improved. The results were strikingly different from anything ever seen. The unstated yes/no form of the question of efficacy in our minds at the onset of the experiment was answered with complete certainty: Penicillin "works" in the treatment of congenital lues, despite the fact that there were no parallel observations in a comparable control group of conventionally treated infants with syphilis. We had complete confidence of its benefit based on our experience with only 8 babies.

— *William A. Silverman, MD*
(Adapted from Silverman WA. Foreword. In: Sinclair JC, Bracken MD. *The Effective Care of the Newborn Infant.* Oxford, England: Oxford University Press; 1992, by permission of Oxford University Press.)

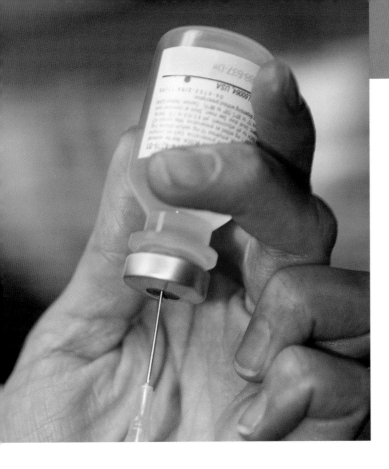

Fighting the Staphylococcal Pandemic

During the 1950s, multidrug-resistant staphylo-coccal disease was a palpable threat to the children and newborns on the pediatric wards. Even the students and house officers were not exempt from the disease. At a grand rounds during my pediatric clerkship, a resident presented his personal experience with staphylococcal pneumonia showing his own chest x-ray with multiple abscesses. I had recurrent staphylococcal abscesses during my third-year clerkship and the day before my wedding in June 1956 I needed drainage of an abscess on the middle finger of my right hand. Disaster was near when I took the ring from my best man and it got caught in the threads of the bandage! Thankfully, my luck held and somehow I was able to release the ring and get it onto Linda's finger.

The pandemic continued unabated as I began my infectious diseases fellowship in 1961 with Maxwell Finland, MD, at the Boston City Hospital. Because of Dr Finland's reputation, drug companies sought his help in assessing promising new drugs. New penicillin compounds were being created by attaching various side chains to the penicillin nucleus, and penicillinase-resistant drugs soon became available. I was assigned to do the in vitro studies that determined the minimum concentrations of drugs needed to inhibit or kill the bugs. Setting up hundreds of tubes for multiple assays of many strains was tedious but it was

a revelation when, after overnight incubation, the clear tubes indicated effective concentrations of the drug. My second role was to recruit patients in clinical trials. There were no institutional review boards. I'm not sure that we obtained consent and the trials were not randomized. However, we showed that the new penicillins were effective for treating a variety of staphylococcal infections.

The epidemic of staphylococcal disease diminished in the mid-1960s for reasons that remain uncertain. Perhaps it was the efficacy of the penicillinase-resistant penicillins or a change in virulence of the organism or some other mystery of the microbial world. Since we don't know why the staphylococcal pandemic began or ended, we don't know if and when it may return.

— *Jerome O. Klein, MD*

Great Milestones in the Prevention of Measles
Overview

Until the mid-1960s, measles was a nearly inevitable infection of childhood with severe morbidity and some mortality in the US population. Between 500,000 and 800,000 cases were reported annually but, since there was no requirement for reporting, this was a gross underestimate and the true incidence was probably in the 3 to 4 million range. By the time US children reached the 2nd grade, nearly all had experienced measles, unless they grew up in an isolated environment.

Measles virus is one of the most highly communicable of infectious agents. The reliable sequence of fever, cough, coryza, and conjunctivitis, followed by a specific maculopapular rash, was well-known to parents and was unlikely to require a physician's visit. However, an astute clinician dealing with a febrile, toxic youngster before the onset of the rash could often diagnose measles by noting Koplik spots on the inner cheek, which appeared 1 or 2 days before the rash. Serious respiratory or gastrointestinal complications occurred in 5% to 15% of patients in the United States. Encephalitis (inflammation of the brain), the most dreaded effect, was limited to about 0.1% of cases.

With the licensure of live-attenuated measles virus vaccine in early 1963, and its incorporation into the routine childhood immunization schedule, measles cases rapidly declined and, even with the enhanced reporting, there were fewer than 100,000 cases per year in the United States in 1970 and a continuing decline thereafter. In 1989 and 1990, there was a resurgence of cases that emphasized the need for immunization of infants in the second year of life. A "routine" 2-dose schedule was implemented and, as a result, there are now fewer than 100 cases of measles annually in the United States. Many of these cases have proven to be imported, principally from Japan, which still has several hundred thousand cases of measles annually.

In the United States today, few physicians and even fewer parents have ever seen measles. Measles has become a "rare" disease, although the virus persists globally and is only a jet-plane ride away from any locale. Recent examples have been outbreaks in Hawaii and in the Marshall Islands, both results of importations by Japanese travelers. In some other nations, misinformation about the measles virus vaccine's responsibility for infantile autism led to markedly decreased immunization, and serious outbreaks have occurred. In Dublin, Ireland, alone, there were more than 350 cases in 2000 to 2001.

In contrast to the experience in the United States, measles still exacts a heavy toll in nations with poor resources, with mortality rates ranging from 5% to 10%. Prior to the availability of the measles vaccine, there were 8 million annual measles deaths among children, most common in sub-Saharan Africa and the Asian subcontinent. Because of active immunization programs, the number of cases declined and efforts are underway to decrease this even further. The World and Pan-American Health organizations and the International Red Cross have embarked on programs to reduce measles throughout the world. Success will depend on continuing efforts to attain a 2-dose immunization rate of more than 90%. This will be a major challenge in many countries in the face of war, civil strife, migrations, poverty, and other inhibitory factors.

— *Samuel L. Katz, MD*

Tissue Culture and the First Isolation of the Measles Virus

I became a research fellow in the laboratory of John F. Enders in July 1953. I learned basic laboratory virology and the tissue culture techniques and Enders assigned me to work on measles. In late January 1954, a mini-epidemic of measles began in the Fay School in Southborough, MA, and I traveled frequently to the school to collect specimens for inoculation in tissue culture. On February 10, I collected specimens from a 10-year-old boy with full-blown measles and transferred his blood to roller tubes within 24 hours of the onset of rash, indicating that the virus was on the move throughout his body. I watched the array of kidney cell culture tubes periodically but saw nothing promising at first.

Five days later, however, I began to observe strange happenings! Here and there, in the sheets of normal-appearing kidney cells, areas that looked like patches of lace or foam were visible, and there were many giant cells within these areas. Enders thought that this phenomenon was

The varicella vaccine (licensed in 1995) has virtually eliminated chickenpox in the United States.

probably an artifact; however, when I transferred culture liquid from the original tube to a new human kidney cell roller tube, I noticed the same effects, while none appeared in the uninoculated control tubes. It now started to become clear that this was a change induced by the virus. It was a very exhilarating time—I would close my eyes at night and see giant cells in my dreams!

We infected monkeys with the virus and recovered the virus from them, and witnessed a rise in antibodies as the disease subsided. These observations were crucial in the subsequent development of the measles vaccine.

— *Thomas C. Peebles, MD*

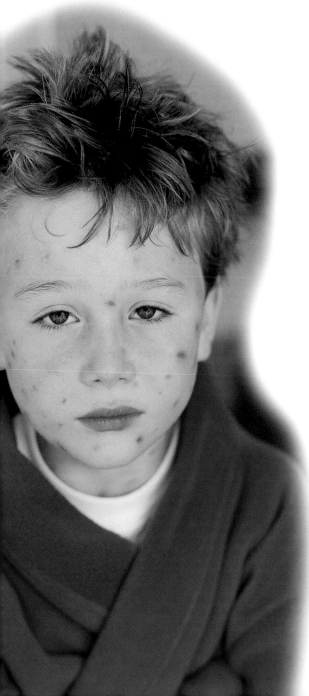

Conquering *Haemophilus influenzae* Type B

Until the early 1970s, invasive, systemic infections with Hib were major, serious diseases of children. Hib meningitis occurred in approximately 1 of 250 children younger than 5 years, resulting in about 12,000 cases annually in the United States. Although antibiotic therapy reduced the mortality of about 95% to 5%, central nervous system sequelae occurred in approximately 30% of "cured" cases, making Hib meningitis a leading cause of acquired mental retardation and deafness.

The identification by Margaret Pittman of Hib as a polysaccharide capsulated bacterium, and the descriptions by Leroy Fothergill and Joyce Wright of an inverse relation between the incidence of Hib meningitis and the presence of serum antibodies to this pathogen, provided the rationale for vaccine development. Newborns and infants up to the age of 3 months were effectively protected against meningitis by placentally acquired antibodies. As these maternally acquired antibodies waned, the incidence of Hib meningitis gradually increased to a peak at 9 to 15 months. Thereafter, antibodies began to reappear in the childhood population and the incidence of Hib meningitis decreased to low levels by 6 years and thereafter.

These observations were the impetus for vaccine development in the 1960s in the laboratories of Albert Einstein College of Medicine and then the National Institutes of Health (NIH) by John B. Robbins, MD, and Rachel Schneerson, MD; and at Harvard University and then the University of Rochester by David H. Smith, MD, and Porter Warren Anderson, Jr, MD. Both groups developed a polysaccharide vaccine that was safe, but didn't provide the desired immunity in children younger than 18 months. The original polysaccharide vaccine was introduced in 1985 and recommended for children at 2 years of age, even though this was an age by which most Hib infections had already occurred. Both groups then developed methods to chemically bind the Hib polysaccharide to proteins, forming conjugates. Notably, protein conjugate Hib vaccines elicited protective levels of antibodies at 2 months of age. The Hib conjugate vaccines were introduced in 1990 and included in the routine vaccination schedule. The impact of Hib conjugate vaccines has been dramatic. The incidence of meningitis and other invasive systemic infections caused by Hib decreased by more than 98%. Today's pediatric house officers may never see a case of Hib meningitis or epiglottitis.

The conjugate polysaccharide-protein technology has also been adapted to other pathogens. Conjugate vaccines of pneumococcal, meningococcal, typhoid Vi, and group B streptococcal polysaccharides are effective and are becoming a part of routine immunization throughout the world. The development of conjugate technology for Hib began a modern triumph in the never-ending war on infectious diseases.

— *John B. Robbins, MD*

The Emergence of HIV/AIDS and the Pediatric Response

Overview

HIV infection was first recognized in the population of men having sex with men. That fact dramatically influenced the public health policies and the management of the disease. Medical providers were frightened and discrimination against infected persons was rampant. The communicable nature of the illness, including the risk of blood and blood products, heterosexual transmission, and mother–to–child transmission, was understood only after several years of study. Antiretroviral medications were developed and tested in adults but, early on, our hope was, "If they work in adults, they should do something for children." The first effective antiretroviral, zidovudine, was approved for use in children only 3 years after its approval for adults.

It was our privilege to be the first group to administer zidovudine to children. We will always remember the incredible clinical differences that we observed during these first studies. Although HIV could be a rapidly fatal disease, more often it took months or a few years of debilitating illness before it killed. With the advent of zidovudine, instead of a small baby with failure to thrive, developmental delay, frequent infections, and death in the first years of life, we observed treated children with better growth and cognitive development, fewer opportunistic infections, and longer survival. It was a miracle for affected families and also for us.

In 1994, we learned to substantially decrease transmission of the virus from mother to child by administering zidovudine perinatally. Combination antiretroviral treatment has further reduced transmission rates to 1% to 2%. Healthy babies, and now healthier mothers and fathers, receiving effective antiretroviral therapy have transformed the disease to a chronic illness in the United States. The number of newly infected babies has decreased by an estimated 90% and our clinics have students in elementary school through college age.

However, HIV continues to be an overwhelming problem in the developing world where an estimated 1,800 to 2,000 infants infected with HIV are born daily. Programs implementing prevention of mother-to-child transmission have only begun there. Every trip to Africa takes me back to 1983. We have the knowledge to decrease the disparity between our country and the Third World. Let us hope the future will bring these advances to the parts of the world that have 90% of the HIV infections in children.

— *Catherine M. Wilfert, MD*

No Greater Gift Than Hope

1987 was a sad and tragic time for HIV-infected children and their families. Effective therapy was a distant dream and society imposed its own special punishment—segregation in portable classrooms, teachers in space suits, banishment from swimming pools, and even torched homes. By 1995, antiretroviral therapy was helping some children but benefits were modest at best. No matter how much we denied it, HIV/acquired immunodeficiency syndrome (AIDS) remained a death sentence. Only a year later, new medications, the protease inhibitors, were revolutionizing the therapy of adults infected with HIV; but what about children? The protease inhibitors had not been given to children. No one knew the right dose or the potential risks. In August 1996, 12 children infected with HIV were the first to receive protease inhibitor therapy at the Texas Children's Hospital. Ten of the 12 are still alive, including one girl, 6 years old at the time we

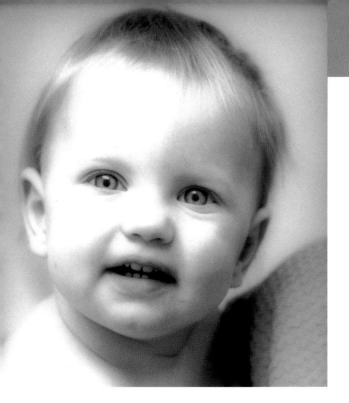

The first *Red Book* in 1938, officially titled *Report of the Committee on Immunization Procedures of the American Academy of Pediatrics*, was 8 pages long and considered the following 18 diseases:

- Common cold
- Diphtheria
- Epidemic encephalitis
- Erysipelas
- Epidemic meningitis
- Epidemic parotitis
- Pertussis
- Pneumonia
- Poliomyelitis
- Rabies
- Measles
- Scarlet fever
- Staphylococcus infections
- Tetanus
- Tuberculosis
- Typhoid fever
- Varicella
- Variola

began treatment, who was literally on her deathbed in home hospice care. Today she is a beautiful, thriving 13-year-old, far more interested in clothes and boys than HIV and AIDS.

— *Mark W. Kline, MD*

Red Book®: Report of the Committee on Infectious Diseases

The AAP established a Committee on Immunization Procedures in 1936 to make recommendations concerning management and prevention of pediatric infectious diseases. This committee was the antecedent of today's Committee on Infectious Diseases. The committee issued a yearly report to the Executive Board of the AAP that would ultimately be edited and published as a separate document to be distributed to all members. From its first publication in 1938, the report was sent out under a red cover and quickly became known as the "Red Book," a name that was officially adopted as the title in 1994. The *Red Book* became an authoritative source of information on the current management and prevention of infectious diseases.

Left, AIDS ribbon; *right*, first *Red Book*, published in 1938.

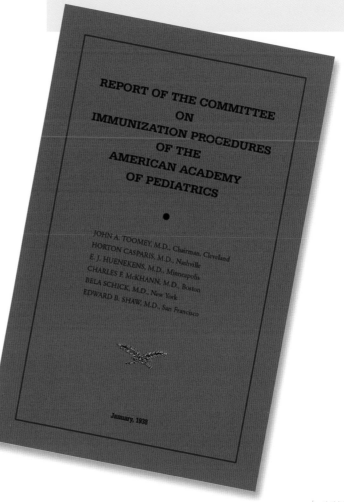

REPORT OF THE COMMITTEE
ON
IMMUNIZATION PROCEDURES
OF THE
AMERICAN ACADEMY
OF PEDIATRICS

•

JOHN A. TOOMEY, M.D., Chairman, Cleveland
HORTON CASPARIS, M.D., Nashville
E. J. HUENEKENS, M.D., Minneapolis
CHARLES F. McKHANN, M.D., Boston
BELA SCHICK, M.D., New York
EDWARD B. SHAW, M.D., San Francisco

January, 1938

The publication provided a clinical guide for the practicing pediatrician and shared new information from academic laboratories and clinical studies with them. The second edition in 1939 included a discussion of the use of sulfonamides, the first antibiotics for clinical use. In 1945, when penicillin came into general use, the *Red Book* made recommendations for its use. After 1945, an explosion of newly discovered antimicrobial agents and newly developed (and increasingly effective) vaccines made the *Red Book* even more relevant. In 1961, an index was added, making new topics such as hospital-acquired staphylococcal infections, appropriate dosages of gamma globulin, and recommendations for use of rabies and typhoid vaccines more accessible.

The *Red Book* continued to evolve as new advances came about through the years—the development of the measles, mumps, and rubella (MMR) vaccines in the 1960s; the rise of antibiotic drug resistance in the 1970s; and the onset of the newly identified HIV virus in the 1980s. At the turn of the century, the *Red Book* included chapters on "new" infectious diseases such as hantavirus pulmonary syndrome and mad cow disease.

A CD-ROM containing hundreds of images and the establishment of the *Red Book Online* Web site (www.aapredbook.org) have enhanced the content and availability of the *Red Book's* trusted information as we move into the 21st century.

— *Larry K. Pickering, MD*

The National Childhood Vaccine Injury Act: Averting a Crisis

There have been many phenomenal advances of pediatrics in the 20th century, yet in terms of lives saved and morbidity prevented, nothing has equaled the record of the national immunization programs against infectious diseases of childhood. Before the 1970s and 1980s, there were no serious concerns about supply or cost of childhood vaccines. There were 7 producers of DTP, 3 producers of OPV, and 6 manufacturers of MMR vaccine.

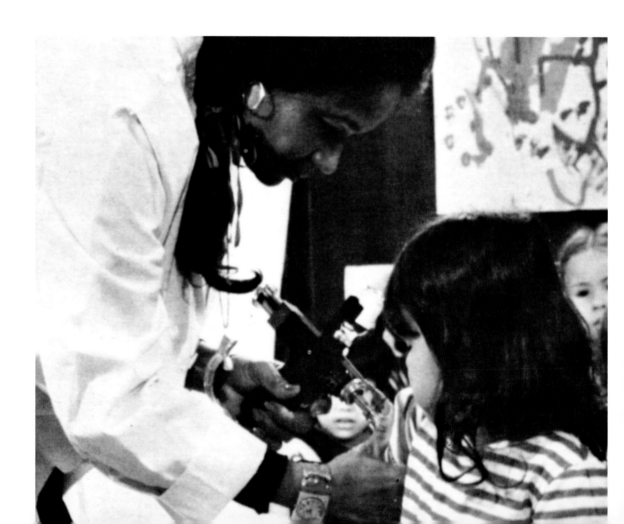

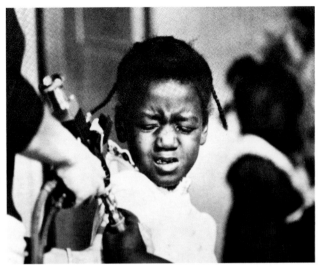

By the 1980s, vaccines were in danger of becoming victims of their own success, as fewer parents could remember the infectious diseases they prevented.

The cost of these vaccines was relatively low for pediatricians, and still lower in bulk purchases by public health departments. Liability for vaccine-related injury was not a significant issue.

In 1974, a child in Texas who had developed polio shortly after receiving polio vaccine in a public health clinic was awarded a judgment against the manufacturer of the vaccine *(Reyes v Wyeth Laboratories)*. Despite the fact that wild-type, rather than vaccine, virus was the cause, the court held that when a vaccine was given in a public program without the presence of a physician, the manufacturer had a duty to inform patients about possible adverse reactions. This judgment cast doubt on whether there could be any mass immunization programs in the future, and de facto implicated manufacturers in vaccine-associated injuries. It was about this time that discussions concerning the creation of a vaccine compensation system began.

Following a sensationalized television report in 1982, *DPT: Vaccine Roulette*, a group of parents of children thought to have vaccine-associated injuries united to form a lobbying organization, Dissatisfied Parents Together. The possible dangers of vaccination soon became the focus of a major national controversy, first in the press and later in Congress. This publicity was associated with a great increase in the number of lawsuits filed against manufacturers, escalating the cost of the vaccine and persuading some manufacturers to discontinue production. Shortages of DTP occurred in a number of areas around the country, resulting in a need to delay booster doses to conserve the dwindling supply.

By the summer of 1984, only 2 companies (Lederle Laboratories and Connaught Laboratories) were still producing DTP and, within a year, Lederle announced that it was discontinuing production. This would leave only one remaining firm as the sole producer of DTP, and that firm did not have the production capacity to meet national requirements. This could be a potential national disaster, comparable to the experience in England and Japan, where epidemics of pertussis, with 30 to 40 deaths each year, occurred in those countries shortly after they discontinued mandated DTP immunization. Fortunately, the Lederle decision was not implemented, but the price of a vial of DTP increased from $60 to $170.

In the early 1980s, vaccine injury legislation, crafted by the AAP and its legal counsel, began to be created. The proposed legislation recognized that the usual tort process was a difficult and prolonged way to settle alleged vaccine injury compensation cases, but it also recognized that any legislation had to provide justice for a child truly harmed by a vaccine. The AAP proposed a no-fault system that would move these cases to the US Court of Claims where they would be judged by an experienced judge, rather than by a jury. The formal National Childhood Vaccine Injury Act was introduced in the House of Representatives by Congressman Henry Waxman and in the Senate by Senators Paula Hawkins and Orrin Hatch, and was passed as the last act of Congress before it adjourned in October 1986.

Now all the effort had to shift to the White House to prevent a veto of the bill by the president. We knew that President Ronald Reagan

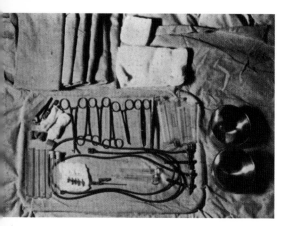

Materials included in sterile pack for exchange transfusion.

wanted to veto the legislation because he had promised in his election that there would be "no new taxes." Because the program would be funded by a levy on each dose of vaccine to create a trust fund, out of which awards could be paid, he considered it to be a new tax. In contrast, the AAP held that this was a "user's fee" because it only applied to users of the vaccine.

By coincidence, the AAP Annual Meeting took place in Washington at just the same time we were trying to ensure the president's signature. Several times during that meeting, the phone number at the White House was flashed on the screen with the message asking members to call the White House and ask the president to sign the law. Members did call, and in such large numbers that additional phone lines had to be installed at the White House!

Shrewd political maneuvering contributed as well. In the final passage of the bill, Congressman Waxman created what he called a "medical package," containing all pending bills having a medical implication. Ironically, the package also contained a bill funding research into Alzheimer's disease; though the president probably had no strong feelings on that bill at that point in time! He was strongly in favor of another bill, the Drug Exports Bill, that would allow the export of drugs not approved by the FDA to other countries. He could not veto the vaccine legislation without vetoing all of the bills in the package. He finally signed the package with the expectation that the next congress would not fund it. Nonetheless, Congress did fund the bill when it reconvened, and the act became law in 1987.

This legislation, the culmination of a decade of intense and effective AAP activity, ensured that national immunization programs that had been close to collapse only a few years before were safe and could continue, ensured of an adequate supply of vaccines and the prospect of controlling their cost.

How has the system worked in its 15 years of operation? Claims are now adjudicated quickly, usually within 1 year, instead of the 6 to 8 years under the tort process. Settlements are fair. The number of vaccine manufacturers is increasing, new vaccines are being developed, and these vaccines are reducing disease and saving lives. It is a tribute to the AAP and its members, the Washington office, and the worthiness of the cause, that we prevailed and a national crisis was averted.

— *Martin H. Smith, MD*

ERYTHROBLASTOSIS FETALIS AND EXCHANGE TRANSFUSION

Overview

In 1932, Louis K. Diamond, MD; Kenneth D. Blackfan, MD; and James M. Baty, MD, proposed that anemia of the newborn, icterus gravis familiaris, and hydrops fetalis were all manifestations of a disease process they designated erythroblastosis fetalis. In 1938, pathologist Ruth Darrow, MD, postulated, "The mother is actively immunized against fetal red blood cells, or some component of them....The antibodies formed in the maternal organism may then pass through the placenta and cause destruction of the fetal red blood cells." Several of Dr Darrow's own children had died of severe erythroblastosis.

In 1939, Philip Levine, MD, and Rufus E. Stetson, MD, reported that the serum of a woman who had recently given birth to a hydropic infant contained a "new" antibody, which agglutinated her husband's red blood cells. In 1940, Karl Landsteiner, MD, and Alexander Wiener, MD, produced an antibody that they called anti-rhesus (Rh), which agglutinated the red blood cells of about 85% of white individuals. Dr Levine showed that the serum of the mother of the hydropic baby contained Rh antibody, establishing the etiology of erythroblastosis fetalis. It became standard practice to transfuse affected infants with Rh-negative red blood cells, but mortality rates did not change.

It was not until 1946 that exchange transfusion was introduced as a treatment for erythroblastosis. In New York, Harry Wallerstein, MD, used the sagittal sinus for removing blood while infusing Rh-negative blood through a peripheral vein. Dr Wiener and Irving B. Wexler, MD, used cannulation of the radial artery for removal of blood and simultaneous infusion of blood through the saphenous vein. These invasive procedures were replaced by a method introduced by Dr Diamond in 1946 that used cannulation of the umbilical vein with polyethylene catheters to alternatively remove the infant's blood and then replace it with Rh-negative donor blood. Exchange transfusion was also an effective treatment of the hyperbilirubinemia that caused kernicterus. The risk of neurological damage was quite low if the level of serum bilirubin did not exceed 20 mg/dL. By the early 1950s, pediatricians were doing exchange transfusions in their own hospitals and the mortality of erythroblastosis in the United States decreased from 70 per 100,000 to 60 per 100,000 live births.

Most infants with hydrops fetalis were stillborn or died shortly after birth. In 1963, Sir Albert William Liley, MD, of New Zealand, using spectrophotometric analysis of amniotic fluid,

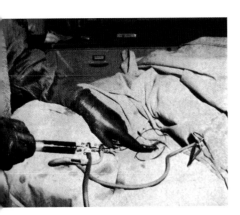

Exchange transfusion through the umbilical vein.

showed a correlation between the amniotic fluid optical density at the peak spectral absorption of bilirubin and the severity of erythroblastosis in fetuses. Amniotic fluid spectroscopy became standard for antenatal assessment and the indication for early induction of labor. Also in 1963, Dr Liley described intrauterine, intraperitoneal transfusions to mid-trimester fetuses to prolong their intrauterine life. Between 1963 and 1968, deaths from erythroblastosis in the United States decreased from about 60 per 100,000 to 45 per 100,000 live births.

In the 1980s, percutaneous umbilical blood sampling made it possible to insert a needle through the uterus into the umbilical vein under ultrasound guidance to obtain a fetal blood sample as early as 22 to 24 weeks, allowing direct assessment of severity. If indicated, a transfusion and, later, exchange transfusions, of Rh-negative red blood cells could be given through the same needle. Large series of intrauterine exchange transfusions have been reported with a 60% to 90% survival in fetuses with hydrops.

In London, England, in 1958, Richard J. Cremer, MD, reported that exposure of large areas of the skin of jaundiced infants to blue fluorescent light reduced serum bilirubin. Phototherapy became an accepted treatment of neonatal hyperbilirubinemia.

The optimal way to prevent Rh erythroblastosis fetalis would be prevention of primary sensitization of Rh-negative mothers. In 1963 and 1964, teams in Liverpool, England, and New York showed that primary Rh sensitization could be prevented by giving anti-Rh immunoglobulin to non-immunized Rh-negative pregnant women within 72 hours after delivery. After Rh immunoglobulin was approved for general use in 1968, mortality from erythroblastosis fetalis in the United States decreased from 45 per 100,000 live

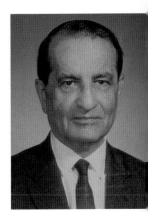

Louis K. Diamond, MD.

"Rarely has it been our good fortune to have a disease recognized, its cause clearly determined, its treatment successfully developed to an extent, and its prevention found, all in one generation."

LOUIS K. DIAMOND, MD, ON ERYTHROBLASTOSIS FETALIS IN 1968

births in 1965 to 10 per 100,000 in 1975, and Rh immunization in pregnant women was reduced by 90%.

Exchange Transfusion: The Race Was On

The year was 1947 and babies were still dying of erythroblastosis fetalis. After discovery of the Rh factor, the usual treatment of this problem had been multiple transfusions with Rh-negative blood. But the mortality remained about 30% and many survivors developed kernicterus. In 1946, Dr Harry Wallerstein described the first exchange transfusion by simultaneously withdrawing blood from a baby's sagittal sinus while administering Rh-negative blood through a cannulated, peripheral vein. The race was on to see who would be the first to do this in Brooklyn, NY. Our first case was a 4-lb premature boy, born to a 30-year-old mother with sickle-cell disease who was Rh negative and had received many transfusions over the years.

Bill Doyle, MD, the chief resident, and I, an intern at the time, did an exchange transfusion in the treatment room of the neonatal unit. Following Dr Wallerstein's technique, I extracted 20 cc of blood from the baby's superior sagittal vein while Dr Doyle injected 20 cc of Rh-negative blood via a cutdown in the saphenous vein at the ankle. We did this 20 times, achieving what we had calculated to be an 80% exchange. The baby did well. The next day a picture of the baby, a nurse holding him, and an unidentified intern (me) appeared on the front page of the now-defunct *Brooklyn Eagle* newspaper.

— *David Annunziato, MD*

Unexpected Erythroblastosis Fetalis

In 1949, a female radiology resident in her first pregnancy was found to be Rh negative and had high Rh antibody titers. Her father was the chief of medicine at our hospital. After the baby was born, I exchange transfused him and he did very well. Of course, all of us were trying to figure out how the baby's mother had been sensitized. She had never had a transfusion or previous pregnancies. About a week later, her father called me and said he knew how she had been sensitized. While at dinner, he and his wife discussed the dilemma of sensitization of their daughter. The mother immediately said, "Don't you recall that you gave her some blood intramuscularly when she had the

measles when she was about 2?" We learned that it had been common medical practice in the 1920s to treat measles with intramuscular blood. The pediatricians of that day believed that this resulted in a milder disease the same way that gamma globulin did in later years. Of course, they were unaware of the Rh factor.

— *David Annunziato, MD*

In Utero Treatment of Erythroblastosis

As a senior resident while in the Army Medical Corps, I was chosen to be the leader of a group that was doing intrauterine transfusions (IUTs) on severely affected Rh babies. Any military physician who had an Rh-sensitized mother would fly the mother to us. If the baby had signs of congestive heart failure, such as scalp edema, we would do an IUT immediately. Since we didn't have ultrasound, we had to determine scalp edema by injecting opaque material into the amniotic fluid so we could see the thickness of the fetal scalp. Under fluoroscopy, we inserted a needle through the mother's abdominal wall, into her uterus through the amniotic sac and hopefully, from there, into the baby's peritoneal cavity. We put the red blood cells directly into the baby's peritoneal cavity, from which they were absorbed by the lymphatics and then into the circulation. Sometimes a fetus would actively move out of the way, and it was necessary to manually secure the head and put pressure on the legs before injecting the blood into the peritoneal cavity. It was dramatic! We were saving babies that previously would have been lost.

We did as many as 3 IUTs to get a baby old enough to survive after delivery. After delivery, we often would have to do multiple exchange transfusions. The most I ever did on one baby was 3 IUTs and 6 exchange transfusions after birth. I tell the house staff now that, in 1 month, I did 39 exchange transfusions. Now if we do an exchange transfusion, we call all the residents that we can find to come to watch.

— *William L. Gill, MD*
(Adapted from Waring WW, Washington L. *Pro Parvulis: On Behalf of the Little Ones. A History of the Department of Pediatrics, Tulane Medical School, 1834–2003.* New Orleans, LA: Tulane Medical School; 2003.)

Overview

The 20th century has seen tremendous advances in the surgical treatment of children with acute surgical conditions, congenital anomalies, cardiovascular defects, malignancies, and trauma-related injuries. American surgeons have played a preeminent role in these quantum advances.

At first, surgeons were mostly involved in the treatment of traumatic injuries and the drainage of abscesses but, with the discovery of anesthesia in the mid-19th century and later the introduction of antiseptic surgery, attention could be given to other pediatric surgical conditions—sometimes with disastrous results. By the beginning of the 20th century, European surgeons had attempted to correct a number of surgical conditions, but with high mortality from blood loss, anesthesia-related complications, and infections. A majority of hernias were managed nonsurgically with large, uncomfortable trusses. If hernia surgery was performed, the typical operation would start with an incision 3 to 4 inches long. After the hernia sac was ligated, the skin would be closed with heavy sutures. The child was then placed in a muslin girdle, confined to a hospital bed for 1 to 2 weeks, and, after discharge, was kept on restricted activity for 6 or more weeks. As William E. Ladd, MD, commented:

> *"At the turn of the century, little distinction was made between the treatment of surgical diseases of the child and those occurring in the adult. It was soon discovered, however, that the mortality rates in the younger groups were extraordinarily high and that if improved results were to be expected, the infant or small child could not be treated as though he were a diminutive man or woman."*

In the United States, the development of pediatric surgery undoubtedly can be ascribed to Dr Ladd, who joined the surgical staff at Children's Hospital Boston in 1910 and in 1927 became chief of surgery. At that time, general pediatric surgery was largely restricted to hernia repairs, appendectomies, drainage of abscesses, and the treatment of injuries. In most instances, surgeons were part-time consultants. At this time, there were only 2 other full-time pediatric surgeons in the entire country: Herbert E. Coe, MD, of Seattle, WA, and Oswald Wyatt, MD, of Minneapolis, MN.

Dr Ladd remained chief of surgery until his retirement in 1945 when he was succeeded by his brilliant student Robert E. Gross, MD. Dr Ladd's enormous contribution to pediatric surgery in the United States is perhaps illustrated by the recognition in 1997 of a "direct line of descent" from Drs Ladd and Gross to 75% of pediatric surgeons with official training and 73% of pediatric surgery training directors. Many young surgeons came to Boston to work with and learn from Drs Ladd and Gross, and then returned to their home

William E. Ladd, MD.

"[I]f improved results were to be expected, the infant or small child could not be treated as though he were a diminutive man or woman."

WILLIAM E. LADD, MD

Robert E. Gross, MD.

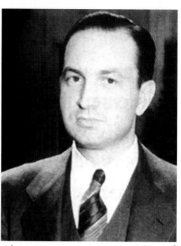

hospitals bringing their surgical skills to children around the country. These new leaders of pediatric surgery soon began to train another generation of pediatric surgeons.

The special skills of trained pediatric surgeons were recognized by pediatricians who increasingly referred their patients to established pediatric surgery services, often in children's hospitals. In these services, there were major advances in the management of children. Surgical instruments that were appropriate for small patients were designed. Anesthesia became much safer as pediatric anesthesiologists concentrated their practice on infants and children. Open drop ether was supplanted by cyclopropane and other improved anesthetic agents usually administered through endotracheal tubes. The special features of metabolic, pharmacological, and fluid and electrolyte problems of infants and children were studied, better understood, and addressed. Blood transfusion became safer. An increasing number of effective antibiotics became available. All of these advances resulted in very low rates of surgical complications and deaths and permitted the addressing of an increasing number of conditions that could be improved or corrected by surgical interventions that were increasingly more complicated.

In addition to the safe surgical correction of imperforate anus, esophageal atresia and tracheoesophageal fistula, intestinal obstruction, pyloric stenosis, Hirschprung disease, and many others, pediatric surgeons began to address congenital heart disease. In 1938, Dr Gross ligated a patent ductus arteriosus for the first time. In 1944, Alfred Blalock, MD, at the suggestion of Helen B. Taussig, MD, performed a palliative procedure for "blue babies," cyanotic children with tetralogy of Fallot (a complex congenital heart abnormality), which involved an anastomosis between the subclavian and pulmonary arteries. With the invention of cardiopulmonary bypass equipment, it became possible to correct a wide variety of congenital cardiac lesions that were previously inoperable.

In the 1960s, more advances emerged that led to better outcomes for children. The recognition of necrotizing enterocolitis, a lethal intestinal condition of the preterm infant, led to successful surgical treatment. Modern intensive care, including appropriate ventilatory management of patients and intravenous nutrition to provide long-term support during the recovery period, led to an increasingly improved survival. During this time, the number of children requiring open surgery for injuries of the spleen and liver dropped as pediatric surgeons recognized that nonoperative management was possible. Kidney, liver, and heart transplantation was being increasingly used. In 1969, the first multi-institutional, randomized control trial for the treatment of Wilms tumor (of the kidney) provided the prototype for similar studies on other childhood tumors and have led to increased survival rates.

The forefront of pediatric surgery today includes the expanding indications for minimally invasive treatment procedures such as laparoscopy and thoracoscopy. The objectives of minimally invasive surgery are to reduce cost, pain, and length of hospitalization, while still providing good, long-term results. Randomized control trials are underway to study new alternative treatments of a variety of surgical conditions as evidence-based medicine becomes the standard of care.

Despite an increasing number of surgeons trained in, and exclusively practicing, pediatric surgery, and despite tremendous improvement in their results, pediatric surgery was at first only grudgingly accepted by the American College of Surgeons and the American Board of Surgery as a distinct discipline. Many general surgeons believed that there had already been too much fragmentation of the specialty—ophthalmology, urology, orthopedics, neurosurgery, colon/rectal, and plastic surgery had been granted special recognition—and there was great reluctance to add pediatric surgery to that list. With their paths blocked to recognition by the surgical establishment, pediatric surgeons, led by Dr Coe, petitioned the AAP to set up a Section of Pediatric Surgery within the AAP, which was accomplished in 1948. The section continues to meet in conjunction with the annual meetings of the AAP and owes a debt of gratitude to the AAP that gave pediatric surgeons their "first home."

— *Robert J. Touloukian, MD*

The First Blalock–Taussig Operations

In 1944, when I was a first-year student at Johns Hopkins Medical School, some of my classmates tipped me off to an important presentation scheduled in the hospital auditorium. Dr Alfred Blalock, chairman of the Department of Surgery, presented his first 3 patients on whom he had created subclavian-pulmonary artery anastomoses for tetralogy of Fallot. All 3 were brought into the room; all were acceptably pink. After presentations of the 3 patients, Arnold Rich, MD, chairman of the Department of Pathology, was asked

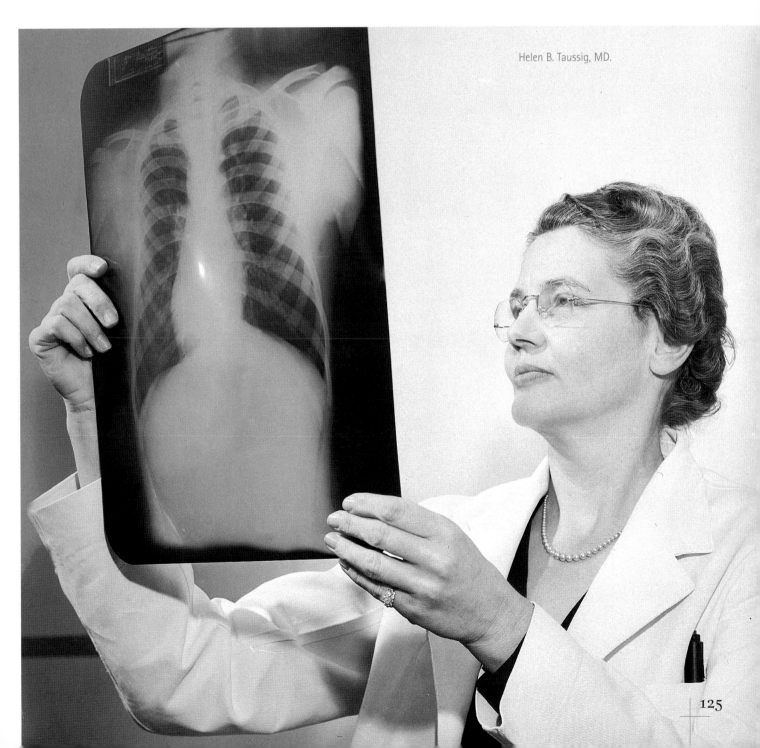

Helen B. Taussig, MD.

to describe his research in dogs, studying the effects of connecting a systemic artery to the pulmonary artery.

Dr Helen Taussig had learned about Dr Rich's work and recognized that this might be a way to increase pulmonary blood flow and palliate "blue babies" with tetralogy. Some cardiology historians say that Dr Taussig first went to Boston and asked Dr Robert Gross to perform the procedure. Dr Gross's response was that he *closed* ductus rather than *creating* them. Dr Taussig then returned to Baltimore and convinced Dr Blalock, and the first Blalock-Taussig operation was performed soon thereafter. In any event, it was appropriate for Dr Rich to be asked to make the first comments, and he said, "I feel like Adam being asked to comment on the Creation." Such praise, following such an epochal presentation, fixed that occasion in my memory permanently.

— *Avrum L. Katcher, MD*

Pediatric Liver Transplantation

In May 1981, a 2-year-old boy with biliary atresia was brought to Children's Hospital of Pittsburgh, PA, in the hope that transplant pioneer Thomas E. Starzl, MD, with the use of the new immune-suppressing medication cyclosporine A, might give him a new liver and a new life. "The bile is flowing!" was alleged to have been said by a member of the team during that first pediatric liver transplant surgery in Pittsburgh. This successful transplant opened an era of hope for children with end-stage liver disease, and a period of tremendous energy and enormous growth ensued.

The liver transplant program at Children's Hospital grew exponentially, accepting children from all over the United States and many countries around the world. The program's success, however, taxed the support systems of both the hospital and the city. There were many long-term admissions of patients being evaluated for transplantation, waiting for surgery, and recovering postoperatively. Laboratories were inundated

with the huge volume of tests necessary to monitor these patients. The large volumes of blood required during the 18-hour surgeries stressed the city and regional blood banks. Operating room staff and anesthesiologists often had to delay elective procedures.

Dr Starzl advanced knowledge of transplantation in every domain. Cyclosporine A increased the hope that children would not reject their new livers and we learned critical information on dosage, complications, and monitoring. Pediatric surgeons from around the world came to learn and carried this knowledge back to their home institutions around the nation and world.

Research continues in all phases of liver transplantation. Insights into immune system function have permitted some transplant patients to be taken off immunosuppressive drugs, and induction of immune tolerance to transplanted organs may someday make immunosuppressants unnecessary. A great deal has been learned and accomplished since Dr Starzl's first liver transplant in Pittsburgh more than 20 years ago. Our first patient is now a handsome, healthy young man.

— *Basil J. Zitelli, MD*

LEUKEMIA AND CANCER

Overview

In 1940, Harold W. Dargeon, MD, stated that the average survival of a child after diagnosis of acute lymphoblastic leukemia (ALL) was less than 3 months. Long-term survivals were sometimes attributed to "miracles." The modern era of chemotherapy, which changed the grim prognosis for childhood malignancies, began when Sidney Farber, MD, at Children's Hospital Boston, observed what he believed was accelerated growth of pediatric tumors, including ALL, induced by folic acid. Based on this observation (which was probably incorrect!), Dr Farber hypothesized that folic acid antagonists might inhibit tumor growth. He obtained aminopterin,

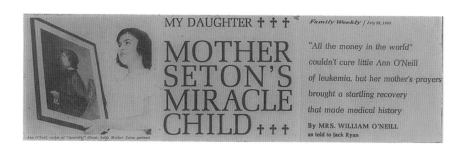

MY DAUGHTER † † †

MOTHER SETON'S MIRACLE CHILD † † †

Family Weekly / July 28, 1963

"All the money in the world" couldn't cure little Ann O'Neill of leukemia, but her mother's prayers brought a startling recovery that made medical history

By MRS. WILLIAM O'NEILL as told to Jack Ryan

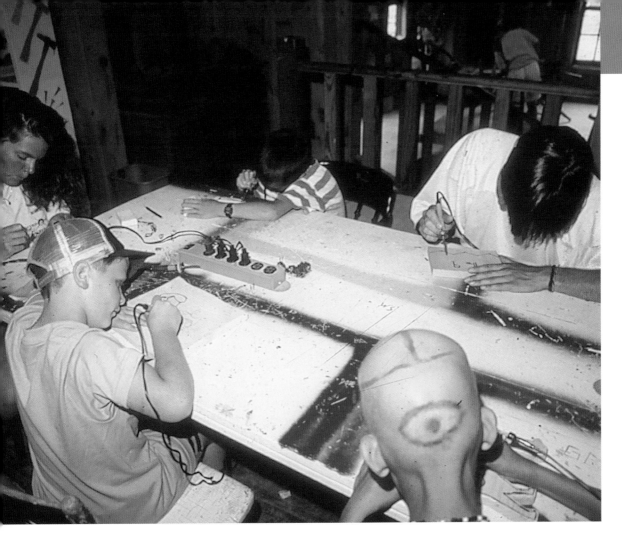

a folate antagonist, and in 1948 he reported inducing temporary remissions in 10 of 16 children with ALL with aminopterin. Following Dr Farber's report, numerous new antileukemic drugs were introduced and used in sequence.

Combination drug chemotherapeutic regimens were devised for ALL that resulted in better survival when compared to sequential treatment with the individual drugs. A major advance in the treatment of ALL was made by Rhomes J. A. Aur, MD; Joseph V. Simone, MD; Donald Pinkel, MD; and associates at St Jude Children's Research Hospital in Memphis, TN, who hypothesized that relapses in ALL occurred because of persistent leukemic cells that were protected in "sanctuaries" in the central nervous system. Methods were developed to eliminate these cells, and modern therapeutic protocols have increased the cure rate of ALL to more than 90%.

Notable successes have occurred in the management of other pediatric malignancies using multimodal protocols that include surgery and radiation to control local disease when possible, integrated with combination chemotherapy given in maximal tolerable doses. Many of the advances in the therapy of childhood malignancies have

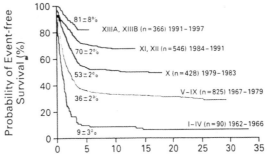

Improving survival of acute lymphoblastic leukemia, 1982–1997, St Jude Children's Research Hospital, Memphis, TN.

been made possible because of the establishment of large, national, multi-institutional cooperative therapy groups. These groups developed common therapeutic protocols and, because of the relatively large numbers of enrolled patients, were able to rapidly assess effectiveness of therapy and treatment toxicities, even in low frequency malignancies. The National Wilms Tumor Study was organized in 1969 and, within a decade, demonstrated that local radiation was not necessary for totally removable tumors and that surgery combined with multiagent chemotherapy resulted in a more than 90% survival rate with a low incidence of treatment-related morbidity.

In the 1960s, the long-term survival and cure of all children's malignancies was about 20%; in the 1990s, survival and cures had increased to 70%. Acute lymphoblastic leukemia cures increased from 5% to about 90%; Wilms tumor cures increased from 30% to 90%; and malignant bone tumor cures increased from 10% to 60%. Cures can be attained even in some children with metastatic disease, which was previously associated with nearly inevitable death.

First Light on the Horizon: The Dawn of Chemotherapy

Before 1947, the management of children with leukemia was that of supportive care. Neither radiation therapy nor surgery was applicable to leukemia, and there was no chemotherapy. The mortality of childhood leukemia was essentially 100% and death almost inevitably occurred within weeks or a few months after diagnosis. I was a pediatric hematology fellow at Children's Hospital Boston when Dr Farber initiated his epochal clinical trials for the treatment of leukemia. Dr Farber observed what he believed was acceleration of the leukemic process in children who received folic acid, and hypothesized that a folic acid antagonist might be effective as therapy. He enlisted the help of a biochemist at the Lederle Laboratories, Yellapragada SubbaRow, to synthesize several folic acid conjugates with antimetabolite activity, and one of them, aminopterin, was used in the pioneer study.

I was one of 3 Fellows involved in the investigations. Between December 1947 and April 1948, we treated 16 children with acute lymphoblastic leukemia with intramuscular aminopterin. All of them were seriously ill at the start of treatment. Ten children showed significant clinical and hematological improvement lasting several months. You can imagine our elation as we observed this improvement and then the sadness we felt when the relapses and deaths occurred. Because of the reluctance of referring physicians to refer leukemia patients for therapy because they believed there was no hope for these children, recruitment was difficult; it became more difficult as severe toxic effects of aminopterin became apparent. The investigation also met strong resistance from some of the house staff who believed that it was cruel to do repeated blood tests and bone marrow examinations in children whom they believed were dying. Despite

an early undercurrent of disapproval, as some children went into remission, the obvious benefits overruled these objections and we gained enthusiastic support.

The first report of these studies appeared in the *New England Journal of Medicine* in June 1948, giving detailed data of temporary remissions in 5 children. This publication roused widespread interest throughout the world. Early in 1948, another folic acid antagonist, later called methotrexate, which was less toxic and more effective than aminopterin, became available. On reflection, the passage of 50 years has not diminished the heady excitement that accompanied these groundbreaking investigations. For me, there were many satisfactions, especially the realization that even back then, we very likely had started down a path that would benefit future generations of children.

— James A. Wolff, MD
(Adapted from Wolff JA. Chronicle: first light on the horizon: the dawn of chemotherapy. *Med Pediatr Oncol.* 1999;33:405–407. Used with permission.)

Those Were Exciting Times! (Early Use of Actinomycin D)

I still have vivid memories of the mid-1950s as a Fellow at the "Jimmy Fund" in Boston, headed by Dr Farber. Although cure of childhood cancer was a rarity in those days, there was much we could do and we were a young and enthusiastic group. Two of my best memories are associated with the early use of actinomycin D (AMD). Shortly before Christmas, a patient came from Maine with a large Wilms tumor with spread of the tumor to the lungs. We persuaded a reluctant surgical service to remove the kidney tumor and gave a 1-week course of AMD before sending him home for Christmas, presumably to die. Some weeks later, he returned in good health and with a clear chest x-ray film. This was probably the first "cure" of metastatic cancer with a single course of AMD. About 2 years later, another child came with a history of a previously removed Wilms tumor and a snowstorm of secondary tumors in the lungs. He, too, was cured by several courses of AMD. These were exciting times!

— Audrey E. Evans, MD

NEWBORN SCREENING FOR GENETIC DISEASES

Overview

In the mid-1950s, several reports described clinical improvement of children affected by phenylketonuria (PKU) when the amino acid phenylalanine was restricted in their diet. It became obvious that a simple screening test in the newborn period might make it possible to prevent the inevitable cognitive impairment of this disease. Because of the infrequency of PKU (estimated at 1 per 10,000 births) it would be necessary to perform universal neonatal screening to identify all affected infants so that early dietetic intervention could be instituted.

In 1963, Robert Guthrie, MD, introduced his "microbial inhibition assay" for rapid, accurate, and inexpensive detection of elevated levels of phenylalanine in capillary blood specimens taken from newborns. This method permitted large-scale newborn screening for PKU, which was rapidly accepted and instituted throughout the country.

Other genetic diseases could be detected in the newborn period and guidelines for screening were formulated for those that cause disease or disability when early diagnosis would permit institution of effective therapy. An important characteristic of such tests was applicability to large numbers of samples that could be easily obtained, inexpensively analyzed, and quickly processed. The tested needed to have no false-negative results and few false-positive results. Fortunately, it was possible to use capillary blood collected on filter paper for most of the tests. The list of candidate diseases grew and by the end of the 20th century, universal newborn screening was possible for a number of genetic conditions, including PKU, galactosemia, cystic fibrosis, and sickle cell anemia. In addition, although it is not usually a genetic disease, screening for congenital hypothyroidism became possible. Although there is some interstate variability in the diseases that are screened, all 50 states have active programs.

The latest major breakthrough in newborn screening has been the introduction of tandem mass spectrometry (MS/MS), a method that permits simultaneous measurement of many analytes that signal 20 or more biochemical genetic disorders. The spectrum of disorders includes most of the amino acid disorders currently screened, along with disorders of fatty acid and organic acid metabolism. Twenty-five states are now using MS/MS in their newborn screening programs.

The outcome of patients with diseases identified by newborn screening and entered into appropriate management has been strikingly successful. The IQs of children with PKU are within a few points of their unaffected siblings, if they are treated with the special diet in the first few weeks of life. In children with sickle-cell anemia diagnosed at birth and treated with prophylactic penicillin, mortality from overwhelming pneumococcal sepsis in the first few years of life has fallen to less than 1% from a historical 10% to 20%. Early diagnosis and treatment of children with congenital hypothyroidism regularly prevent the severe mental retardation and other complications. Newborn screening is one of the great success stories in pediatrics in the last half of the 20th century—one that has prevented significant morbidity and mortality of a large number of children in the nation and world.

— *Margretta Reed Seashore, MD*

The Second Case of Galactosemia

Of all my patients during my training at the Harriet Lane Home in the mid-1940s, one stands out in my memory. His name was Mac, a 3-week-old baby, who was referred to us by his family doctor across the bay because of vomiting, diarrhea, and failure to thrive. My resident took him into the treatment room while I explained to the mother that we would begin to treat him right away because he was all dried out. In the treatment room, his severe dehydration was obvious. His anterior fontanel was sunken and when his tummy was pinched, the skin stayed humped up. After receiving intravenous fluids, the baby perked up and wet his diaper for the first time in 24 hours.

The parents very reluctantly had to go home and to their work as fishermen. We cultured every orifice and body fluid but found no infection. We drew many, many blood tests, but could find no clues to his diagnosis. One morning, our chief resident came to rounds in an ecstatic mood because he had just read a case report in the latest *Journal of Pediatrics* describing the case of a patient, very similar to Mac, who was found to be unable to metabolize galactose. We tested for this and showed that, indeed, Mac was the second case of galactosemia. It was then the job of the lowly intern, me, to see that he took the unusual formula that the dietitians came up with. Many a night I was on the floor at the time of his 2:00 am feeding, so Mac often had his nighttime cuddling while I fed him. These were days when doctors were not supposed to be friendly or playful with their patients. We were to be scientific, true *Medical Deities*!

Mac stayed with us for 4 months. His liver decreased in size, he was much less whiney, and he gained weight. Every Friday, Mac's mother would ride the bus from across the bay to see him and to give me a quart of fine, freshly shucked oysters. This was great pay for our work, for our only pay from the hospital was 3 meals a day, a bed to sleep in, and the chance to work and learn there. After he went home, I received a letter from his mother saying that he was doing well. She also told me that while she knew our scientists were the best, it was the concern and care of the nurses and the lowly intern that convinced her to leave her baby there. It sometimes doesn't matter how much you know, it's how much you show that you care that counts.

— *Sylvia Morris, MD*

CARE OF NEWBORN AND PREMATURE INFANTS

Overview

Though intensive care nurseries did not emerge until the 1960s, physicians' efforts to reduce the mortality from premature birth began in the late 1800s. At that point, French obstetricians, using simple incubators, were able to reduce the mortality rate of premature infants weighing between 1,200 and 2,000 grams by nearly half. Great excitement followed this announcement, and incubators became one of the first 20th-century

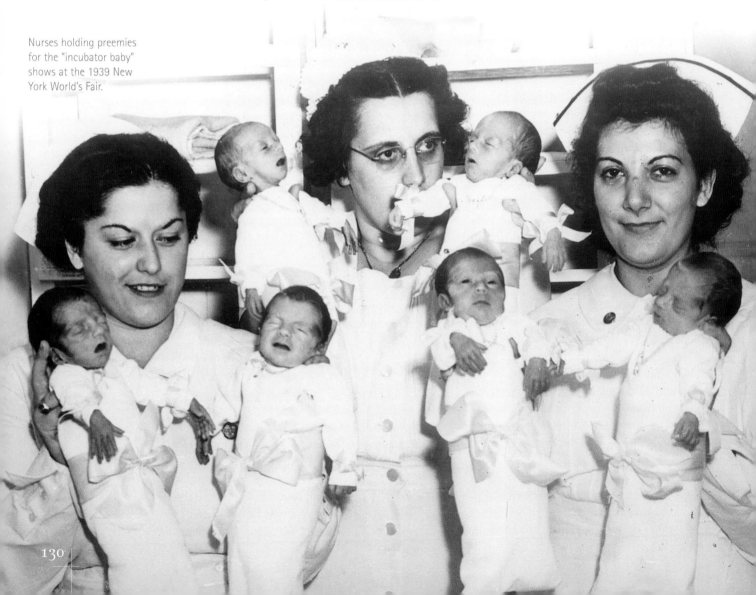

Nurses holding preemies for the "incubator baby" shows at the 1939 New York World's Fair.

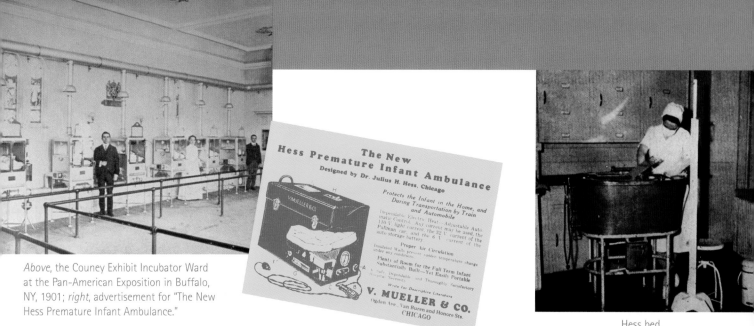

Above, the Couney Exhibit Incubator Ward at the Pan-American Exposition in Buffalo, NY, 1901; *right*, advertisement for "The New Hess Premature Infant Ambulance."

Hess bed.

medical technologies to become a popular sensation. "Incubator baby" shows, featuring live infants on display in the midway, attracted huge crowds at world fairs and expositions as late as the 1939 New York World's Fair. Pediatric leaders such as L. Emmett Holt, Sr, MD, and Thomas Morgan Rotch, MD, took great interest in the devices, and in 1900, obstetrician Joseph B. DeLee, MD, opened the first US hospital-based "incubator station" in Chicago, IL, featuring elaborate ventilated incubators, trained nurses, and a transport service. It barely lasted 8 years before succumbing to financial losses.

By the time of the First World War, however, this early enthusiasm had waned. At the turn of the century, most babies were born at home; mothers tended to be fearful of entrusting their newborns to a hospital except as a last resort. Even as childbirth shifted to the hospital as the century progressed, premature babies became lost in a kind of no-man's-land between obstetrics and pediatrics. Although obstetricians had pioneered the use of incubators, they found less and less time available to care for the babies. It was not uncommon for premature infant deaths to be recorded as "stillbirths," even when occurring several days after birth. Pediatricians had great trouble gaining access to newborns and, as a result, often failed to appreciate that rearing premature babies involved more than good nutrition. Many openly disdained the thought of placing premature babies in incubators, which struck them as little more than warm boxes. Finally, even those individuals who did try to promote good premature infant care found it expensive and unappealing

to hospital boards at a time when society in general remained ambivalent about the long-term outcome of "weakly" newborns.

Despite these obstacles, Chicago pediatrician Julius H. Hess, MD, opened the nation's first permanent incubator station at Sarah Morris Hospital in 1922. He developed a metal water-jacketed heated bed to warm the infants, the "Hess bed," which worked efficiently but rendered close observation of the infant all but impossible. This was, in part, by design, because Dr Hess promoted a hands-off philosophy of neonatal care that assumed premature infants should be handled as little as possible so as not to be depleted of their minimal energy reserves. Nurses, not doctors, ruled the nursery and were responsible for almost all of their day-to-day care. Of course, this emphasis on minimal handling of the infant had the effect of selecting for the relatively "fit" babies at a time when eugenic concerns obsessed many Americans. Dr Hess conducted extensive research during the 1930s showing the IQs of children born prematurely to be comparable to that of other children, dispelling the common notion that premature birth was nature's way of expelling a defective fetus.

In the late 1930s, Ethel Collins Dunham, MD, the first woman accepted by the American Pediatric Society, led a sustained drive by the Children's Bureau to improve premature infant care around the country. Thanks both to her efforts and the nation's rising prosperity, premature nurseries became increasingly common in hospitals around the country during the following decade. Their centerpiece was no longer the

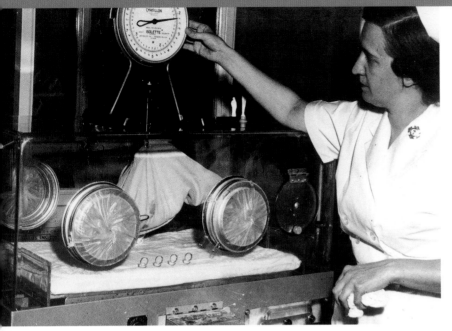

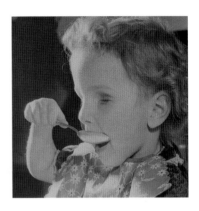

Left, weighing a newborn in an Isolette; *below*, a young girl at the Lighthouse, an institution for the blind in New York, NY, 1944.

clumsy Hess bed, but the Chapple incubator or Isolette. Charles C. Chapple, MD, had designed the Isolette to reduce the risk of airborne infections by having an air intake from outside of the nursery. Featuring clear side panels with portals giving nurses access to the baby, the new incubator allowed physicians to actually see the premature infant—and to recognize phenomena such as periodic breathing and labored retractions. Pediatricians found that oxygen often ameliorated these symptoms, and modified the Isolette to accommodate oxygen concentrations approaching 100%. As will be discussed, this was the main reason for the epidemic of retrolental fibroplasia (RLF) that followed. Though the hands-off philosophy remained in other ways intact, and nurses continued to play a dominant role in the premature nursery, a revolution in neonatal care was quietly gaining force.

The postwar baby boom brought new changes to neonatal care. By that point, childbirth routinely took place not only in the hospital, but also with the aid of anesthesia. Newborns often were born with depressed respirations and, in turn, attracted the attention of anesthesiologists in the delivery room. In 1952, Virginia Apgar, MD, developed her scoring system to rate newborn asphyxia. Neonatal resuscitation became more aggressive. The rise of antibiotics brought great benefits for mother and child. Breastfeeding, on the other hand, reached its nadir in the postwar hospital, segregating nursery infants from their mothers. Experiments such as Yale's

mother-baby "rooming in" unit remained the exception.

The most promising therapy for the premature infant of the time, oxygen, came to epitomize both the potential benefits and dangers of the new technology. By 1942, a number of reports had convincingly demonstrated that clinical cyanosis as well as periodic breathing and apnea could often be corrected by oxygen administration. Oxygen, which previously had been administered for the symptomatic relief of apnea and cyanosis, now was given continuously. Modifications in the Isolette allowed its provision at concentrations approaching 100%, far higher than had been possible with the Hess bed. By the late 1940s, such therapy had become routine for premature infants.

There followed perhaps the most tragic setback in the history of neonatology. In 1942 a Boston ophthalmologist, Theodore L. Terry, MD, described the first case of a premature infant blinded by a condition that he called retrolental fibroplasia (today re-designated as retinopathy of prematurity, or ROP), which quickly became the most common reason for blindness in children. It was a postnatal disorder, seen only in premature infants, especially those of lowest birth weight. Its incidence varied from 0% to 20% in different institutions around the United States and seemed to be more prevalent in infants cared for in large nurseries with the most modern facilities. Most disturbingly, the cause of the epidemic was unclear. Numerous theories of etiology were advanced, but none were proven to be causative. It was only through a major collaborative randomized trial in 1953 and 1954 that oxygen was implicated. The study was highly controversial, as oxygen was widely regarded as an extremely beneficial therapy.

The RLF story thus marks a milestone in the history of what has become known as "evidence-based medicine." Randomized controlled trials were just beginning to penetrate medicine at the time, and played a role in unmasking other previously unsuspected toxicities or mistaken therapies in the premature nursery. Sulfa antibiotics were linked to kernicterus, chloramphenicol to gray baby syndrome, and the common tendency to keep premature infants' temperatures on the low side was shown to contribute to mortality.

Limiting oxygen to 40% did reduce the incidence of RLF, but with an unacceptable trade-off in the form of a rise in cerebral palsy. To contemporaries, the only way to scientifically employ oxygen treatment was to develop a way to *monitor* oxygen concentrations in the blood and control its levels precisely. Measuring concentrations of blood gases and chemistries using tiny volumes of blood was a major technical feat in itself in the late 1950s, and perhaps did more to inaugurate neonatal intensive care than did the more visible technological companions. Although mechanical resuscitation devices by this time had been introduced in delivery rooms, prolonged use of a

Ethel Collins Dunham, MD: A Prime Mover in Setting the Stage for the Neonatal Revolution

Ethel Collins Dunham, MD, was a member of a small, informal band of American pediatricians in the second quarter of the 20th century who had a particularly keen interest in the problems of prematurely born infants. (This was many years before the term *neonatology* was coined by Alexander J. Schaffer, MD, of Baltimore, MD, in the 1950s.) At Dr Dunham's request in the early 1930s, the Children's Bureau surveyed 105 hospitals to determine the methods used in the management of premature neonates and the mortality rates in these hospitals. There was marked variation in the quality of treatment, convincing Dr Dunham that there was an urgent need for establishing premature infant stations throughout the country, and a need to train a large number of nurses and physicians to provide specialized care in these units.

When Dr Dunham became director of research at the Children's Bureau in 1935, she saw the issue of premature birth as a national problem. She lectured throughout the United States, calling attention to conditions in pregnancy such as infections, toxemia, heart disease, and overwork that needed remedial attention to reduce the risk of premature delivery. She stressed the need for special facilities to care for the fragile neonates and, in 1943, wrote a manual, *Standards and Recommendations for Hospital Care of Newborn Infants, Full-term and Premature,* that quickly became a standard book on the subject and was reprinted 7 times through 1977 (the AAP became the publisher in 1949). Dr Dunham died on December 14, 1969, just as the revolution she sparked was beginning to accelerate beyond anything she could have imagined.

— William A. Silverman, MD

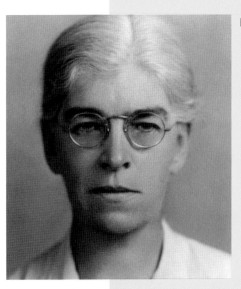

Ethel Collins Dunham, MD.

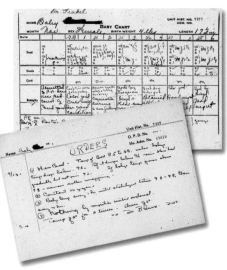

Handwritten orders and charts from the first recorded case of retrolental fibroplasia at the Boston Lying-in Hospital, 1942.

133

Because premature infants were thought to be very susceptible to staphylococcal airborne infections, units for premature infants at the time consisted of isolated individual cubicles. These impeded access to the babies and hampered their care. My research had shown that these infections were primarily the result of poor hand washing rather than being airborne. In 1960 I opened a neonatal intensive care unit (NICU) that was a wide-open area with oxygen and electrical outlets that dropped from the ceiling. This design violated an array of state rules and regulations. When I presented my design to an official of the Connecticut State Board of Health for approval, he responded, "You academic people have to do your research. Go ahead and open your unit, but if anything goes wrong, I never met you."

— *Louis Gluck, MD*
(Adapted from Pearson HA. History of the Department of Pediatrics Yale University School of Medicine. *Yale J Biol Med.* 1997;70:201–208. Used with permission.)

The first neonatal intensive care unit, designed by Louis Gluck, MD, at the Yale-New Haven Hospital, CT, 1960.

ventilator was unthinkable to most investigators without blood gas monitoring.

During the 1960s, many of the elements of what would become known as newborn intensive care began to emerge, not always neatly or logically. They did so in a close but complex relationship with advancing basic science. The description of the pathogenesis of hyaline membrane disease as a manifestation of surfactant deficiency by Mary Ellen Avery, MD, was clearly of great importance in the long term. It later was shown by Louis Gluck, MD, that maturity of the fetal lung could be assessed by measuring phospholipids in the amniotic fluid, and that treatment of the mother with corticosteroids could enhance lung maturity.

Yet the route forward was by no means clear in the 1960s. Paul Swyer, MD, of Toronto, Ontario, Canada, developed positive-pressure ventilators, which, in their early days, often had to be secured by tracheostomy. Mildred Stahlman, MD, at Vanderbilt, treated premature babies in miniature negative pressure ventilators, similar to the iron lungs used a decade earlier for polio victims. Robert Usher, MD, championed an approach to respiratory distress syndrome relying on alkalosis and metabolic control. It was not until 1971

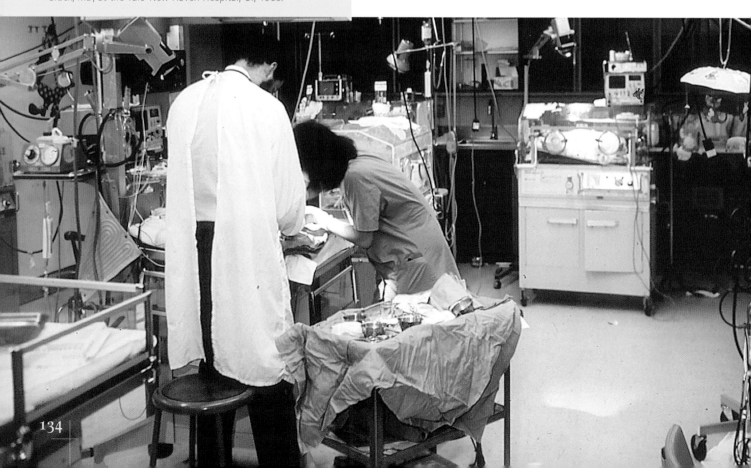

that George A. Gregory, MD, and his colleagues at the University of California, San Francisco, introduced a continuous distending pressure. Appearing at a point where many of the other elements of neonatal care (umbilical artery lines, cardiorespiratory monitors, feeding techniques, and many others) were coming into alignment, this technique (continuous positive airway pressure) struck contemporaries as a particularly notable breakthrough.

At last, in the 1970s, newborn intensive care came into its own. Dr Gluck had introduced the first neonatal intensive care unit (NICU) in 1960 and, over the course of the next 10 years, numerous premature nurseries were converted as well. The federal government provided powerful impetus by coordinating regional perinatal and neonatal care through regionalized networks served by air and ground transport systems. Neonatology became organized as a board-certified subspecialty within pediatrics. Premature infants born at 28 to 32 weeks' gestation, who once would have succumbed to respiratory distress syndrome, now survived in astonishing numbers. The threshold of viability was pushed back ever further to well under 1,000 grams.

As babies became smaller and smaller, questions about who should make ethical decisions concerning their treatment brought a great deal of attention to the NICUs in the late 1970s and early 1980s. Interestingly, public debates centered less on small premature infants than term newborns with congenital conditions such as Down syndrome and spina bifida. These came to a climax with what became known as the Baby Doe controversy. Provoked by a 1982 incident in which the parents of an infant with Down syndrome had refused to authorize operative repair of esophageal atresia, the Reagan administration developed a system to investigate and compel treatment of any newborn allegedly denied life-sustaining therapy. An 800 phone number was introduced to allow anonymous reporting. The AAP played a key role in resolving this controversy, and the ethics of newborn intensive care became less of a publicly contentious issue in the 1980s.

Compared with their stormy preceding decades, the late 1980s and 1990s were a stabilizing period for neonatology, in which previous gains were consolidated and adverse effects curtailed. The most notable single advance of the

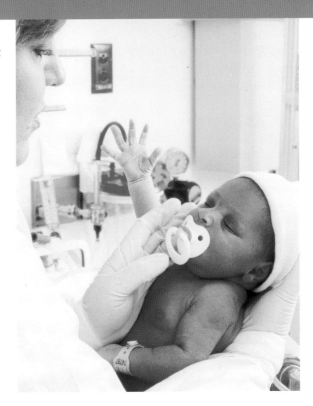

period was the synthesis of artificial surfactant, which greatly reduced the need for ventilating babies in the "classic" hyaline membrane disease range accompanying 30 to 33 weeks' gestation. Combined with other improvements in ventilatory management, surfactant therapy has contributed to a reduction in incidence of bronchopulmonary dysplasia. Intraventricular hemorrhage, in contrast, remained a significant threat, limiting efforts to save the smallest premature babies. The ethical challenges raised in the 1970s continue to be worked out daily in newborn intensive care nurseries, though in a less public manner than before. The record of accomplishment of neonatal care over the past 3 decades is, nonetheless, a little short of astonishing when judged against the background of what came before.

Neonatal Medicine in the Hands-off Days

When I was a medical student and in pediatric training, newborns were not given medical care. They were given nursing care. Newborns were handed to the nurse who washed them, wrapped them, and put them in their bassinets where they made it or not. We did not provide intravenous fluids, and we did not do chemistries or x-rays. Microchemistries were not available. X-rays were useless because the slow machines of the time could not stop the breathing at 60 to 80 breaths per minute of infants with respiratory distress. Infants weighing less than 1,000 grams were considered nonviable and no effort was made to save them.

At the University of California, San Francisco, during 1943 to 1946, students were not allowed in the nurseries because of the fear of infections, and there were no antibiotics as yet. My first night on call as a pediatric intern at UC Hospital, I had to relieve the house officer assigned to the nursery. When I told him that I had never been in the nursery, he waved at the adjoining 2 rooms and said, "That's the normal nursery and that is the premature nursery. Good luck." Then he vanished down the hall, leaving me with my heart in my mouth. As it turned out, I did not need to be so apprehensive, as the experienced night nurses knew exactly what to do with the limited options available.

For my pediatric residency from 1948 to 1950, I came home to the Los Angeles County General Hospital. The hospital had a large delivery service of about 15,000 deliveries per year. There were premature nurseries but they had no ventilators or monitoring equipment. Gordon Armstrong incubators were used for the smaller infants, but to access the infant, the lid needed to be raised, allowing the heat and oxygen to escape. Standard rectal temperatures were taken with a thermometer that registered only down to 94°F. The routine temperature notation for babies on admission was NR, which stood for not registered, and many babies were undoubtedly hypothermic. Babies were not fed immediately, and very small infants were not fed for as long as 72 hours, for fear that they would vomit and aspirate. Some very small infants actually died of starvation and dehydration. My major responsibility each morning as a resident was to sign out the stack of charts of half a dozen or so infants who had died during the night.

— *Joan E. Hodgman, MD*

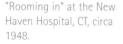

"Rooming in" at the New Haven Hospital, CT, circa 1948.

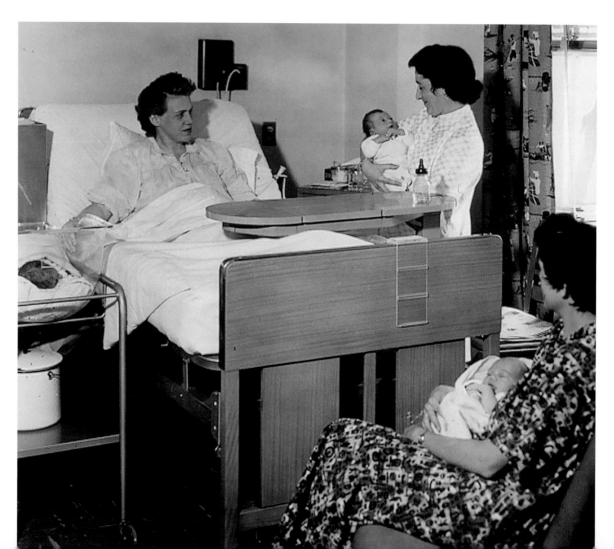

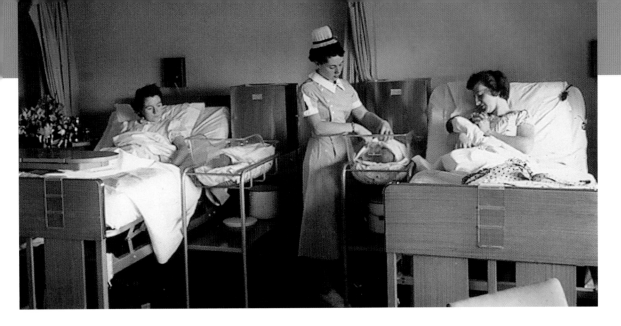

"Rooming In" at Yale in 1946

The "Rooming In Project" at Yale was initiated by Grover F. Powers, MD, in 1946 in response to the requests of mothers who wanted to participate in the direct care of their babies while they were in the hospital, including feeding them by individual demand rather than by rigid nursery schedules. At that time, the usual postpartum stay was 5 to 7 days. Ten years earlier, Dr Powers had set up a program for pediatric interns assigned to the newborn nursery in which they would continue to follow babies that they had cared for during the rotation. They would make a house call shortly after discharge and then continue to see them in the well-baby clinic during the next year. This was probably the first involvement of pediatric house staff in longitudinal care—now called the "continuity clinic." The interns reported that some of the mothers seemed to be afraid to handle their infants and many had difficulty maintaining the rigid feeding schedules that they believed had been recommended in the hospital. It became clear to Dr Powers that rooming in arrangements during the lying-in period could enhance the infant-mother relationship and reduce tensions. It would also enable pediatricians to examine the baby at the mother's bedside frequently, in the presence of the father.

Dr Powers assigned Edith Jackson, MD, to meet with representatives from obstetrics, nursing, and the hospital to discuss the design, construction, and staffing of a facility on the maternity floor for rooming in. The concept was not universally accepted at first. The head of the hospital was quoted as saying, "That's as crazy an idea as I have ever heard!" but the persuasive powers of Dr Powers prevailed. He received a grant from the Mead Johnson Company to "study the interrelations between maternal attitudes and the development of behavior patterns in children." Thus, from the start, rooming in was considered to be a research project—and was so designated. A 4-bed unit with an adjacent small nursery for the babies during rest periods was constructed in a little used solarium on the maternity floor. A charge nurse and student nurses provided 24-hour coverage. Pediatric coverage was provided by a full-time rooming in Fellow, supervised by Dr Jackson. (I was that Fellow from 1949 to 1951.)

Rooming in was almost immediately successful and soon was oversubscribed. In 1948 there was growing popular and professional pressure to expand the program. Additional funds were obtained from the Children's Bureau for a second unit. The units were in continuous operation until 1953, when the maternity service was transferred into a new hospital facility where rooming in was included as part of standard care. There is little doubt that the Rooming In Project at Yale humanized the birth experience for families and was a direct antecedent of today's birthing centers.

— *Morris A. Wessel, MD*

Virginia Apgar, MD, and Newborn Resuscitation

When I was a house officer in the 1940s, obstetricians ruled imperiously in the delivery rooms. I was told, "We don't attempt to save newborns weighing less than 1 kg because they are previable." In academic institutions on both coasts of the United States, I saw this dictum carried out in actual practice. A neonate weighing less than 1 kg was unwrapped and placed in a cold corner of the delivery room and ignored until the infant stopped breathing. The agonal gasping seemed endless, much to the discomfort of everyone in the room, but no one made a move to interfere or even question the "rule." Parental consent was not solicited, the nurse baptized the marginally viable newborn, and the outcome was recorded as "stillborn." There was much head shaking, but as the delivery room personnel conceded, "It was just as well."

This widely accepted discriminatory practice changed dramatically in the 1950s. I saw the first example of this change in 1951, when a very energetic anesthesiologist named Dr Virginia Apgar first came into the delivery rooms. She was a very effective teacher who taught activism by example—"No one ever stops breathing on me!" Dr Apgar was horrified when she encountered the practice of allowing marginally viable neonates

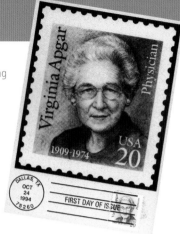

Postage stamp featuring Virginia Apgar, MD, issued in 1994.

to die with no effort made at rescue. She lost no time in launching a vigorous campaign to change the culture of the delivery room, doing away with the fiction of labeling marginally viable premature infants as "stillborn."

— *William A. Silverman, MD*
(Adapted from Silverman WA. Compassion or opportunism? *Pediatrics.* 2004;113:402–403. Used with permission.)

A National Study on Retrolental Fibroplasia

In the 1950s there was a sharp upsurge in attention to the possibility that supplemental oxygen was responsible for the alarming epidemic of blindness then spreading throughout the world. By early 1953, controversy about the causal relationship of oxygen rose to a fever pitch. Finally, the US Public Health Service convened a conference to devise a plan that might put an end to the international disaster—by this time, 10,000 infants throughout the world had been blinded. It was immediately clear that there were 2 highly vocal opposing camps. One side argued that a randomized trial of oxygen restriction must be carried out to assess 3 outcomes: blindness, brain damage, and death. The opposition maintained that there was sufficient evidence extant to prove oxygen was the cause of RLF blindness, and a controlled trial was not only unnecessary, it was immoral! A compromise was hammered out.

Eighteen hospitals participated in a randomized study for 3 months, recording week-by-week mortality among infants weighing 1.5 kg or less under 2 policies: "routine oxygen" (FiO2 over 50% for 28 days) compared with "curtailed oxygen" (supplemental O2 administered only for cyanosis or respiratory difficulty, FiO2 under 50% and discontinued as soon as possible). If there was no increase in mortality at the end of this preliminary stage of the study, the next 9 months would be used to carry out a prospective survey, solely

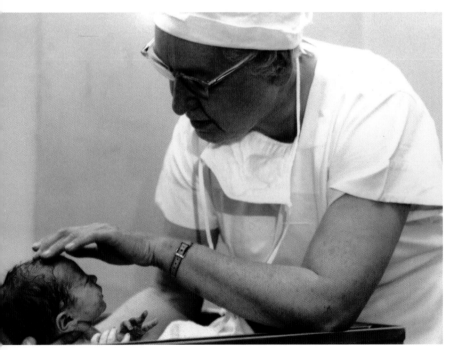

Virginia Apgar, MD.

under a policy of curtailed oxygen, to measure the size of an expected decrease in the frequency of cicatricial RLF.

On September 19, 1954, the preliminary results of this pioneering national study were presented in New York. The outcomes appeared to be clear-cut: there was no appreciable increase in mortality under oxygen curtailment and the rate of cicatricial eye disease was reduced by two thirds. After 12 years of bewilderment, the cooperative study results seemed to provide a final answer.

Following this report, there was an abrupt decrease in the use of high concentrations of oxygen in premature infants, and its use in concentrations more than 40% was restricted to severely symptomatic infants. At the same time there was a dramatic reduction of ROP. However, with the more restricted use of oxygen, there was an increase in neonatal mortality, perhaps as a consequence of hypoxia-related deaths of sick infants in the first few days of life.

ROP still occurs, even with restricted oxygen use. Its incidence is highest in very low birth weight infants who rarely survived in the past. It is possible that even normal ambient oxygen levels may be toxic for some of these infants.

— *William A. Silverman, MD*
  (Adapted from Silverman WA. A cautionary tale about supplemental oxygen: the albatross of neonatal medicine. *Pediatrics.* 2004;113:394–396. Used with permission.)

Huey Helicopters as a Transport for High-Risk Newborn Babies

In the early 1970s, rapid changes were taking place in the care of high-risk newborns. Increased knowledge and technology were improving the ability of the NICU to treat respiratory distress and to meet the infant's basic needs of temperature stability, metabolic and glucose support, and nutrition. It was recognized that the outcome for these infants was improved when they received intensive care and stabilization as soon as possible after birth.

The NICU at the University of Oregon Medical School was a referral center for all of Oregon, southern Washington, and parts of Idaho. For years, a limited neonatal transport system had existed for transports in the greater Portland area, using a nurse to warm and observe the infant in a car or taxi. In the late 1960s, a station wagon was used to carry a nurse and a physician to the referring hospital with improved, but still limited, equipment for infant stabilization. In about 1970, it became apparent that a more sophisticated system was needed to provide the care that these infants needed as early as possible, even at distances of 50 to 200 miles.

In 1971, S. Gorham Babson, MD, head of the NICU, persuaded the hospital to buy a new battery-powered transport incubator and, in the same year, a new van was donated. This van, built to NICU specifications, was equipped with the transport Isolette, oxygen, a heart rate monitor, and equipment for respiratory, fluid, and resuscitation support. The transport team, consisting of a neonatologist, nurse, and respiratory therapist, could now travel up to 100 miles to provide effective stabilization of the distressed infant at the referring hospital before transport.

But what about the more distant, smaller hospitals and their need to have the team there promptly? Dr Babson, with the support of the medical school dean and the governor, persuaded the Oregon Air National Guard to provide Huey helicopters for emergency transport, and adaptations were installed so that the helicopters could securely carry the transport incubator, oxygen tanks, equipment, and the neonatal transport team. Transports between 50 and 200 miles away were now possible. The first baby transported by

> *"This disorder [retrolental fibroplasia]
> is caused primarily by prematurity and only
> secondarily by oxygen."*

THOMAS F. CONE, JR, MD

How to Be Sure You're Right When You're Surely Wrong: An Example of a "Baby Doe" Situation

The boy was born at a community hospital weighing 5.5 lb. The pregnancy and delivery had been smooth and the 1-minute Apgar was 9. The mother and father were delighted and everything seemed rosy. However, the baby spit up his first sugar water feeding and, after tests, I determined that the baby had esophageal atresia with a tracheoesophageal fistula. I gave the parents my presumptive diagnosis and explained that the prognosis was excellent after surgical correction. I then hesitated because the baby's slanted eyes, rounded head, full nape, and transverse palmar crease had raised my suspicion that the child had Down syndrome.

After genetic confirmation of the diagnosis, I told the parents and they decided they did not want surgery on their son. I explained that although I was under legal obligation to report their "withholding of consent," I would not do so because I felt they had the right to make the decision. After a week on the ward without any intravenous hydration, the boy's weight had fallen to 3.5 lb.

At this point, someone—probably a nurse—called the district attorney and told him about the child being left to die. Almost immediately, urgent calls from the district attorney went out first to the father and then to me. The father was told that if he did not sign consent, he would be immediately imprisoned. "Please," he asked me, "operate on the child, otherwise, I'll go to jail!" The baby was transferred to a university hospital and, the next day, I operated on him. The procedure went well, and when he was ready for discharge, the parents put him up for adoption. In the end, I was not sent to jail, nor was the father. On the basis of my experience with other children with Down syndrome, he may very well be making his foster family or, even better, his adopted family happy with his sunny disposition.

— *Kenneth Kenigsberg, MD*

Huey, on June 7, 1972, was a 2-lb, 7-oz girl from John Day, OR, approximately 150 miles away. Over the next few years, the Army Hueys did approximately 1 to 3 neonatal transports per month (a total of about 126). The support by the Oregon Air National Guard was an important step in the development of a neonatal transport system, which, after 1976, began to depend more on fixed-wing transport aircraft.

— *Katharine Simpson, RN*
  (with S. Gorham Babson, MD)

The Legacy of Baby Doe: An Overview

In April 1982, Baby Doe, an infant with Down syndrome and tracheoesophageal fistula, died in Bloomington, IN. The parents had made a decision to forego lifesaving surgery and the Indiana Supreme Court upheld this decision. The Reagan administration reacted by invoking provisions of Section 504 of the Rehabilitation Act of 1973, which prohibited discrimination against the handicapped in education, transportation, employment, and medical care. The Department of Health and Human Services (HHS) issued an Interim Final Rule on March 7, 1983, that required immediate posting of large posters in a conspicuous location in all newborn nurseries and intensive care units. These posters called for anonymous reporting through an HHS toll-free hotline by anyone who believed that an infant was being deprived of food or customary care. The posters stated,

> *"Discriminatory failure to feed and care for handicapped infants in this facility is prohibited by federal law."*

The government also organized Baby Doe squads to review, on-site, allegations about the care given to disabled, hospitalized infants. In the 6 weeks that the Interim Final Rule was in effect, approximately 600 calls were received over the hotline. Twenty percent of these calls were wrong numbers or the callers hung up. Most of the rest were for information or comment only. Only 16 of the callers made a specific allegation. The HHS thought 5 of these merited investigation, after which none were found to warrant further action. One particularly disturbing incident occurred at the Vanderbilt Hospital in Nashville, TN, where an anonymous caller reported that 10 infants were being deprived of food. Within hours, an HHS investigative squad appeared at the hospital and conducted an all-night investigation, tying up medical staff and medical records. It turned out that most of these infants had not been fed because of surgery scheduled for the following day.

On April 14, 1985, the Interim Final Rule was nullified by an injunction by Judge Gerhard A. Gesell in the District Court in Washington, in a suit filed by the AAP, the Children's Hospital National Medical Center, and the National Association of Children's Hospitals and Related Institutions. A number of ethical issues were raised, including (1) the rights of the handicapped child, (2) the parent's authority to decide for the child, (3) the physician's responsibility, and (4) the role of the federal government in the protection of the rights of handicapped infants.

A compromise approach to the Baby Doe controversy was introduced in the Senate and supported by the AAP, other medical organizations, and several disability and pro-life groups. An amendment was passed to the Child Abuse Prevention and Treatment Act, which defined a new category of medical neglect and assigned oversight responsibility to the State Child Protective Services. This legislation moved the Baby Doe controversy from being a civil rights issue to one of child abuse.

The new law specified that every baby, regardless of disabilities, should receive nutrition, hydration, and medication. It did provide for selective nontreatment when, in the judgment of the responsible physicians, (1) the infant was chronically and irreversibly comatose, (2) the treatment would only prolong the act of dying or otherwise be futile, (3) the treatment would not be effective in ameliorating the infant's life-threatening conditions, and (4) the treatment was futile or inhumane.

The AAP recommended in-hospital infant care review committees, made up of interested lay individuals and medical personnel. They would educate families of infants who were disabled with life-threatening conditions about resources for treatment, counseling, and rehabilitation; make policies and guidelines concerning the care of infants who were disabled; and review cases involving disabled infants with life-threatening

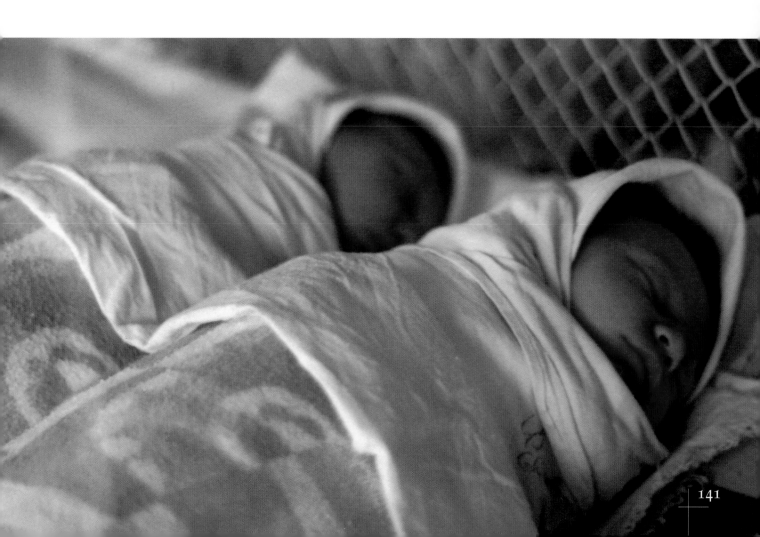

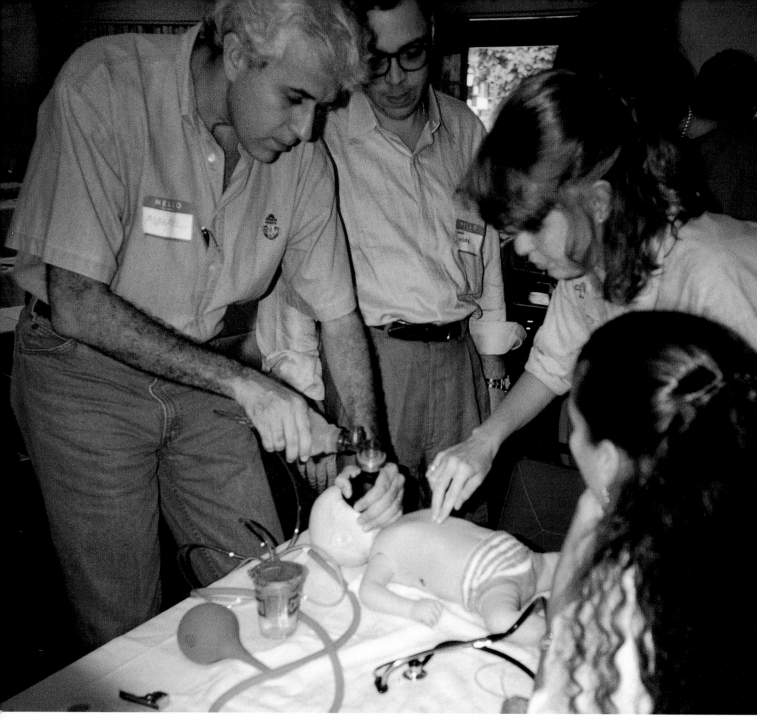

Physicians learning neonatal resuscitation at an American Academy of Pediatrics course in Rio de Janeiro, Brazil, 1994.

conditions. If there was disagreement about management, the State Child Protective Service would be asked to intercede.

Three years to the day after Baby Doe died, HHS issued final regulations that implemented the compromise amendment to the child abuse legislation. This legislation and its regulations continue in effect today.

— *James E. Strain, MD*

The Neonatal Resuscitation Program

The Neonatal Resuscitation Program (NRP) is the official educational program of the AAP and the American Heart Association (AHA) for neonatal resuscitation education and training. This train-the-trainer program was developed in the 1980s with support from the NIH and introduced nationally in 1987. National, regional, and hospital-based instructors were trained to ensure widespread dissemination. There are more than 25,000 instructors in the United States alone.

The NRP is so influential that, in only 16 years, more than 1.5 million health care professionals in the United States have received training. The NRP has become the recognized standard of care for treatment of newborns at birth in the United States and many developed countries. Essentially all professional groups responsible for perinatal care in the United States have endorsed the NRP. In addition, many pediatric societies worldwide have accepted the NRP as their official educational program for neonatal resuscitation.

The NRP aims to have a person appropriately trained in neonatal resuscitation present at every delivery. The lack of appropriate resuscitation at birth was one of the leading causes of infant mortality and long-term morbidity in the United States. In the decade following the introduction of the NRP, US deaths due to asphyxia (breathing complications) at birth decreased by 42%, although this improvement cannot be ascribed exclusively to the NRP.

The NRP course participants not only complete self-directed and self-assessment exercises, but also participate in hands-on practice scenarios with resuscitation equipment, under the guidance of a trained instructor. Other features include a self-instructional format that allows completion of the course through self-paced self-instruction or group meetings. The program is designed so that various levels of personnel working in delivery rooms and nurseries can complete only the modules consistent with their job responsibilities and needs.

The NRP is based on the "Guidelines for Cardiopulmonary Resuscitation and Emergency Cardiovascular Care" developed jointly by AAP and AHA volunteers. The educational materials that accompanied the new guidelines set a new bar of excellence for continuing medical education materials. The NRP educational materials have been translated into 22 languages and the program has been introduced in 71 countries. The NRP is one of the largest programs of the AAP. Countless lives are saved every day by pediatricians and other health care professionals trained in this lifesaving and life-giving program.

— *Waldemar A. Carlo, MD*

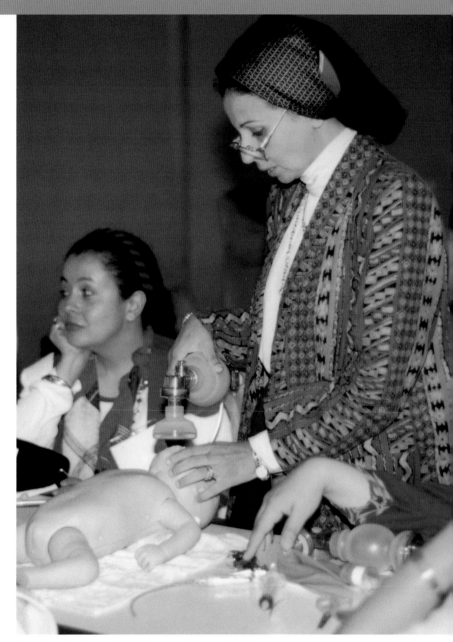

American Academy of Pediatrics neonatal resuscitation course in Cairo, Egypt, 1996.

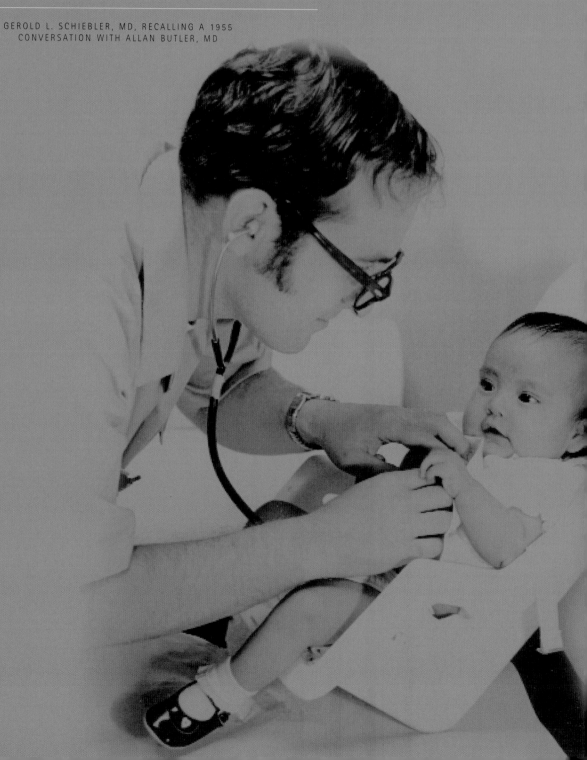

"Dr Butler said to me in the first week of my pediatric training, "Gerry, we have a new policy at the Mass General now. We're going to pay you." I said, "Oh boy, what will the pay be?" He said, "$25 a month." As I was leaving, he asked, "Gerry, are you married?" When I said, "Yes, sir," he told me that there was a different pay scale for married house officers—$28 a month!"

GEROLD L. SCHIEBLER, MD, RECALLING A 1955
CONVERSATION WITH ALLAN BUTLER, MD

Chapter 7
Snapshots in Time

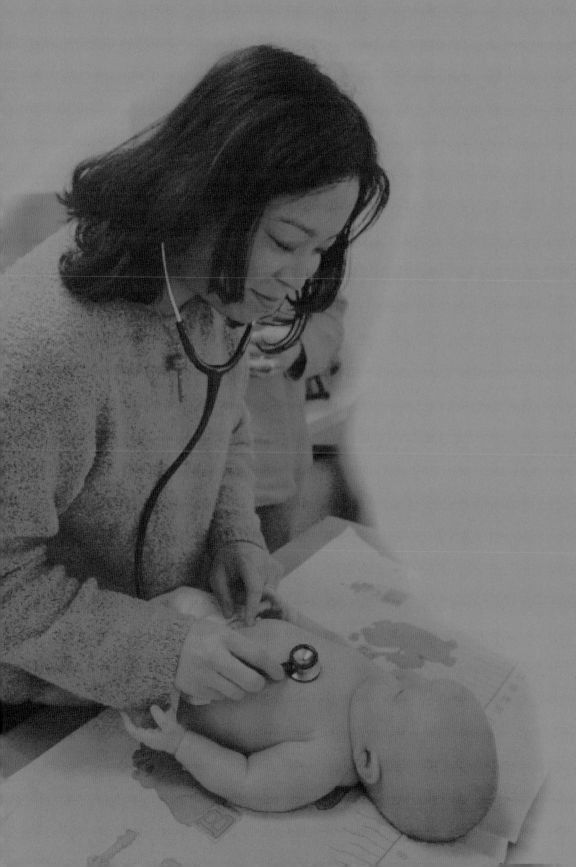

The preceding chapters have presented a chronicle of pediatrics and the American Academy of Pediatrics (AAP) over the past 75 years. This has been a time of growth, progress, and extraordinary scientific discoveries. But these great advances also required the efforts of the many thousands of pediatricians who translated these discoveries into better care for their patients. We believe that these stories are best told through pediatricians' own words.

What follows is a selected group of stories and anecdotes—snapshots in time—about pediatricians in the last 75 years, including several accounts extracted from the rich treasury of the AAP Pediatric History Center Oral History Project. What was it like to be the only, or one of a few, female medical students? What was residency training like? What made the greatest teachers stand out? What was it like to make house calls? How did scientific and societal changes affect pediatric practices?

We have noted that more senior pediatricians have been more willing to share their experiences with us than the younger generation. Perhaps reflections on, and nostalgia about, personal experiences may be a function of age? Or perhaps younger pediatricians are filling out so many insurance forms they don't have any energy left over to write? Whatever the case, we will look forward to future AAP histories to look back at more of the equally poignant and compelling stories of the last 25 years.

GETTING INTO MEDICAL SCHOOL

The Only Woman in My Class

I originally got into medicine via the University of Missouri in Columbia. I was living with my family on a farm, driving to the university for my last 2 years of college. In my senior year, I had finished all my required courses except one. I thought, "What will I do with all my time?" I decided to go over to the medical school, which then was only a 2-year school, and said that I would like to take anatomy. They said, "OK." Tuition was very little because I lived there and also taught as a zoology instructor in the college in the mornings.

At the end of the year, I had finished a part of a year of medical school. Then my family moved to St Louis and I went with them. I decided to go over to the medical school there and see if they would let me in. They said, "Sure, come on and take the rest of the first-year courses that you missed." I never had an interview. I never gave them any documents, except transcripts of my grades. I was the only woman in my class and the only one that graduated.

Everybody kept telling me how hard it was, but medical school was not hard for me. In those days, if you were a man, you had to have a female around while you were examining a patient. When evening came around and my male classmates hadn't been able to get a nurse, I'd act as nurse for them. And then when I had trouble with an experiment in physiology, they'd give me a lift. They were always kind to me and I never had a feeling of being pushed around.

— *Katherine Bain, MD*
    (Adapted from the AAP oral history collection.)

Getting In Wasn't All That Easy

In the mid-1930s, getting into medical school as a Jew was not all that easy. You faced a very strict census. I went to Columbia University for 3 years and did very well. I remember being invited for a chat with the professor of physiology at Columbia, during which he defended the fact that there was a 10% cap on Jews and went on to explain that this was an attempt to have a more diverse student body. I didn't consider this to really be

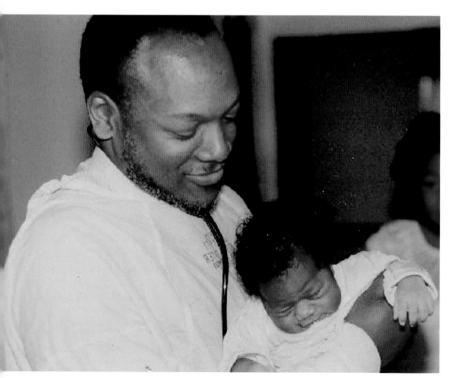

anti-Semitism; it was a way of life that I accepted. So, instead of New York, I was admitted to the St Louis University School of Medicine—a Jesuit school, no less! A professor at St Louis University knew and was devoted to my father because of their common interest in Judaism and Zionism. He spoke up for me with the dean of the medical school, so I really got into medical school because of a contact. I did very well and was elected to AOA [Alpha Omega Alpha, a medical honor society] in my senior year—there was a policy not to elect Jews into AOA until the fourth year. Did it bother me? Not at all. I thought that I was treated fairly.

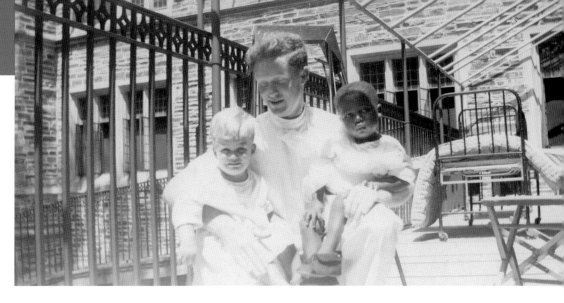

— *Joseph Dancis, MD*
   (Adapted from the AAP oral history collection.)

The Best-Laid Plans

As I planned my medical career, I was sure that I would attend Columbia University's College of Physicians and Surgeons [P & S] where, masquerading as a medical student during high school, I had often observed surgeries in the operating suites. My discussion with the admission panel at P & S seemed to go well until one of them asked, "Do you ever expect to make any major discoveries in medicine?" I responded, "Well, sir, from what little experience I have in reading about the great discoveries in medicine, I rather think that those who make them are building on the efforts of many who preceded them, but did not do the final thing that achieved success and fame. I would like to be the one who makes a major discovery, but I will be content to be a contributor to the process." I was then told, "We don't think that you've got the stuff that we are looking for at P & S." Soon after this discouragement, I went for an interview at Cornell University Medical College. After spending several hours interviewing in the New York Hospital, I met the Dean, who said graciously, "If you will accept it, Cornell would like to offer you a place in next year's entering class." [Editors' note: C. Everett Koop, MD, FAAP, went on to become the United States Surgeon General, 1982 to 1989.]

— *C. Everett Koop, MD*
   (Adapted from Koop CE. *Koop: The Memoirs of America's Family Doctor.* New York, NY: Random House; 1991. Copyright © 1991 by C. Everett Koop. Reprinted by permission of William Morris Agency, Inc., on behalf of the author.)

One of 10 Women at Columbia University's College of Physicians and Surgeons in the 1940s

When I decided to go into medicine despite my college major in history, I took the necessary premed sciences in my senior year. I only applied to Columbia P & S. The medical school application had to include a $50 fee. I called my father and told him that I wanted to talk to him in his office. He said that I could tell him what I wanted over the phone, but I insisted that I needed to see him face-to-face. I went to his office and told him that I wanted to go to medical school and needed $50 to apply. I think that he was very relieved to hear that was why I wanted to talk to him! He gave me the $50, but told me that it was best not to tell my mother.

Although I was accepted at P & S, I decided that I had to earn some money to help pay my own way. I remember going to see the dean, Dr [Aura E.] Severinghaus, and asked him to defer my admission so that I could save about $2,000 by teaching for a year while living at home. The dean said, "$2,000 should cover expenses for about a year; what will you do then?" I said, "If I'm no good, there will be no problems about future expenses, but if I'm any good, I'll come back to you for a scholarship." He smiled and said, "We will see you next year." I entered medical school in the fall of 1946—one of 10 women in a class of 110. I never felt uncomfortable or

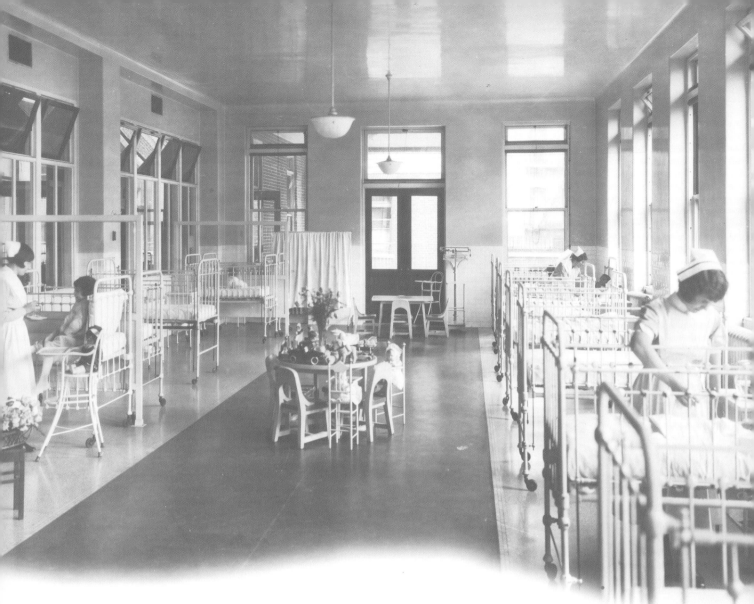

John Hopkins pediatric ward, Baltimore, MD, pre-1930s. Hospital design from the late 19th century often featured high ceilings and large windows to prevent airborne spread of infection.

out of place in medical school. I was proud and honored to be at P & S. All in all, I did well and was elected to AOA.

— *Audrey K. Brown, MD*
  (Adapted from the AAP oral history collection.)

"Don't Be a Woman Doctor, Be a Doctor Who Is a Woman"
Temple was the medical school that accepted me without delay, and Philadelphia was the least expensive city in which to live. Our family doctor,

of whom I was very fond, also suggested that I go to Temple. He gave me a gift of the best advice that I have ever had. He called me into his office and told me, "If you're going to succeed, take every test they offer and ask no quarter for your sex. Don't be a woman doctor, be a doctor who is a woman."

— *Murdina M. Desmond, MD*
  (Adapted from the AAP oral history collection.)

"It was remarkable that the dean, on the basis of a 15-minute interview, decided who would be in his first-year medical school class 3 years hence; and that was it."

HOWARD A. PEARSON, MD

"Why Don't You Apply to Harvard?"

I applied to about 5 medical schools, thinking that I would have the best chance of being accepted at one of the Philadelphia medical schools because they were close geographically as well as having outstanding reputations. Then my father said, "Why don't you apply to Harvard?" I told him that no Franklin and Marshall student had ever been accepted into Harvard. But at his insistence, I finally did apply to Harvard. I went to Boston and was interviewed by several people at the school. I never expected to be accepted. Only later did I realize that Harvard apparently had "state quotas," ostensibly to achieve geographic distribution and diversity, and they took 6 classmates and me as the Pennsylvania quota of 7. Whatever the reason, I felt very privileged to have been accepted.

— *Gerold L. Schiebler, MD*
  (Adapted from the AAP oral history collection.)

Acceptance to Medical School—Now and Then

I serve on the Admissions Committee at Yale now and we have a huge committee of 50 or 60 people. We receive more than 5,000 applications. We carefully review the Medical College Admission Test (MCAT) scores and grade point averages (GPAs), study letters of recommendation, look at activities outside of the classroom, and then select about 800 applicants for interviews. Two 1-hour interviews are conducted with each applicant, and we ultimately select 100 students for admission.

My own experiences on applying for medical school, on the other hand, were very different. I remember interviewing with Rolf C. Syvertsen, MD, the dean of Dartmouth Medical School, my first week in Hanover, NH. Dr Syvertsen would personally interview all the incoming freshmen who had declared for premed. It was remarkable that the dean, on the basis of a 15-minute interview, decided who would be in his first-year medical school class 3 years hence; and that was it. No MCATs, no letters of recommendation, no grades, but all 24 of us did all right. Several members of my class became professors and departmental chairs, one became a dean, and the rest were very successful, respected practitioners.

— *Howard A. Pearson, MD*

VIGNETTES OF MEMORABLE TEACHERS

John Howland, MD: Frugal to a Fault

As with the legendary Yankee, John Howland was frugal to a fault. A few examples of his cost-saving measures are illustrative. Howland never purchased an automobile, preferring to obtain rides to work with colleagues. He wore the same felt hat for 17 years and cleaned it annually by pouring gasoline through it. When asked why, he stated that gasoline at 17 cents a gallon was far cheaper than hat cleaning at $2.50 per year. At American Pediatric Society (APS) meetings in Atlantic City, he often ate lunch at a Childs Restaurant, whose menu listed the cost of food in one column and the calories of each item in another column. Always mindful of calories per dollar, he generally ate the same meal—pancakes, syrup, and sausage.

— *Russell W. Chesney, MD*
  (Adapted from Chesney RW. Who was John Howland and why was an award named after him 50 years ago? *Pediatr Res.* 2003;53:523-525. Used with permission.)

Cartoon of the very formal grand rounds of Kenneth D. Blackfan, MD, circa 1935.

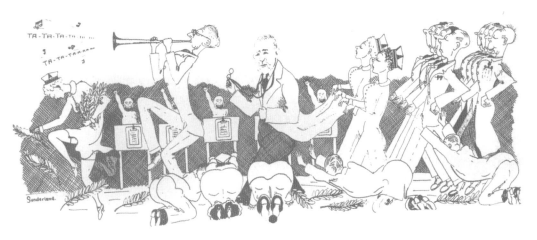

Kenneth D. Blackfan, MD: Rounds

Dr Kenneth Blackfan's frequent, usually daily, ward rounds were made in small, informal groups walking from bed to bed. However, his semi-weekly grand rounds, one day on the infant's

Paul Gaffney, MD, of the Children's Hospital of Pittsburgh holds an infant, circa 1965.

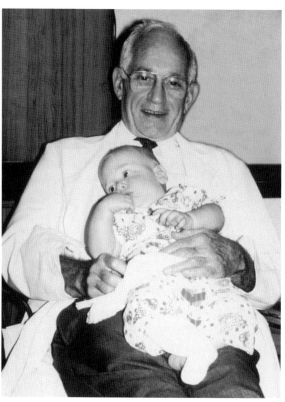

wards and another on the children's wards, were always attended by his whole staff and were large and just a bit formal— as a cartoon drawn by one of our pediatric students suggested. Even so, they were essentially teaching rounds with cases chosen for this purpose rather than for presenting unusual and rare diagnostic features.

— *Louis K. Diamond, MD*
(Adapted from Diamond LK. Acceptance of the Howland Award: reflections on pediatric care. *Pediatr Res.* 1973;7:858–862. Used with permission.)

Grover F. Powers, MD: Breakfast Rounds

On my first day as a third-year medical student assigned to pediatrics in 1942, Grover Powers, MD, greeted 4 of us new students saying, "Come with me." We dutifully followed him into a child's room. He stood silently looking at the child for several seconds, then abruptly turned on his heel and walked out. We had no choice but to follow him.

I inquired, "What's the matter? I thought we were going to examine the child."

He looked at me with a disapproving expression and commented, "That child is eating breakfast. You wouldn't expect me to interrupt his meal would you?"

Some years later, I had a conversation with J. Roswell (Ros) Gallagher, MD, who remembered this exact same scenario on his first day on pediatrics at Yale, 10 years earlier.

— *Morris A. Wessel, MD*

Bela Schick, MD: Humor on the Rounds

Bela Schick had a wonderful sense of humor and his rounds were extraordinary. I recall that once, when I presented a premature infant to him, that he said that he didn't like prematures to be closed up in incubators. He wished that I would get Dr Charlie Chapple in Philadelphia, who had invented the Isolette, to make one large enough for pediatricians to get into, so they would stop subjecting these babies to it.

— *Henry Barnett, MD*
(Adapted from the AAP oral history collection.)

Waldo Nelson, MD: That's Doctor to You

While deep sea fishing with half a dozen members of his department, Waldo Nelson insisted that they should call him "Bill" rather than "Dr Nelson." About 10 minutes later, Art (Mac) McElfresh, emboldened by this newfound informality and the conviviality of the occasion, said, "Bill, pass me a beer?" No response. He persisted, "Bill, will you pass me a beer?" Still no response. By this time, chagrined at his own temerity, Mac fairly whispered, "Dr Nelson, please pass me a beer." There was an immediate positive response.

— *Angelo DiGeorge, MD*
(Adapted from Pearson HA. *The Centennial History of the American Pediatric Society, 1888–1988.* New Haven, CT: American Pediatric Society; 1988. Used with permission.)

Ogden C. Bruton, MD: No Gamma Globulin!

In 1954 I had an appointment on the Pediatric Service of the Walter Reed Army Hospital in Washington. Colonel Ogden Bruton was the chief of the service, and he was a careful and caring pediatrician. I was there when he diagnosed the first case of agammaglobulinemia. Dr Bruton was treating, and agonizing about, a little boy who had multiple episodes of pneumonia, pneumococcal sepsis, and other serious bacterial infections. He had done every imaginable test and still had no answer. He knew that there were no abnormalities of the child's white blood cells and that the other major contributor to immunity was antibody. He sent his patient's serum to the Armed Forces Institute of Pathology where there was a Tiselius apparatus for protein electrophoresis. When the report came back that there was no gamma globulin peak, Dr Bruton could not believe it and sent more serum for analysis with the same result—no gamma globulin. He was still hesitant to make a definitive statement and wrote several letters to immunologists at the Children's Hospital Boston describing his findings and asking for their advice, but got no response. Shortly after Dr Bruton submitted an abstract for the annual meeting of the Society for Pediatric Research (SPR), he learned that the Boston group also had submitted an abstract describing 4 boys with similar findings, but no mention of Dr Bruton. I have been gratified that Dr Robert Good [a noted pediatrician and immunology researcher] in his writings, always refers to "Bruton's agammaglobulinemia."

— *Audrey K. Brown, MD*
  (Adapted from the AAP oral history collection.)

Richard L. Day, MD: Teaching by Example

When Richard Day, MD, was professor and chairman of the Department of Pediatrics at the University of Pittsburgh, he was known as a gentleman and a gentle man. He and his wife would take babies, who were hospitalized for failure to thrive, home for the weekend to nurture and parent them. He taught caring for patients by example and learning from him was fun. He required all students on pediatrics to spend 1 hour with their stethoscopes taped to the chest of a healthy newborn listening to the hearts adapting to extrauterine life.

In addition to taking in babies for weekends, he once appeared at the hospital in the middle of a severe snowstorm to take anyone who couldn't get home to his house for the night. Fifteen nurses welcomed the invitation and were treated to cookies and milk and a good night's sleep.

— *Lois Pounds Oliver, MD*

Rustin MacIntosh, MD: You Must Do It

During the early days of the retrolental fibroplasia, we were excited about our apparently successful use of adrenocorticotropic hormone (ACTH) to treat a small series of infants with the acute vascular changes of retinopathy of prematurity. However, 2 of the infants in our series, who had not received ACTH, recovered spontaneously. We decided that the question of efficacy could only be resolved by a comparative evaluation of ACTH using concurrent untreated controls. We went to our chief, Rustin (Rusty) McIntosh, MD, and asked for his permission to carry out a controlled clinical trial (this was years before institutional review boards). Rusty listened to our arguments without saying a word. He smoked a pipe in those days and I can remember

William A. Silverman, MD, as a resident.

151

that he didn't miss a puff as we told him of our agonizing fears about conducting a test of a treatment that, we were sure, prevented blindness but, equally, our concern about broadcasting claims of efficacy based on the weak evidence of our uncontrolled experience. After a few minutes of silence at the end of our impassioned presentation, Rusty said, "You must do it."

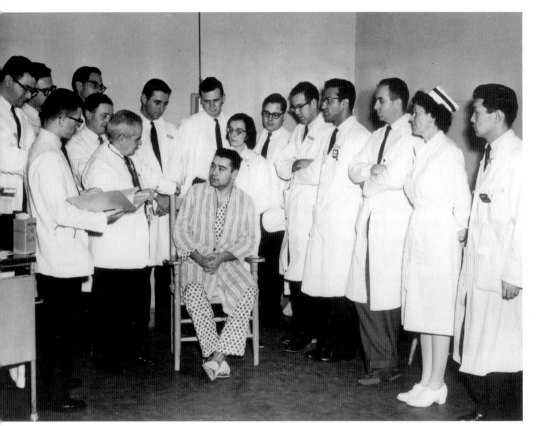

Maxwell Finland, MD, leading bedside teaching rounds in the 1960s.

I will always remember his courageous decision. The final responsibility for allowing what was at the time an unprecedented exercise involving newborn infants, rested solely on his shoulders. The results of the trial provided ample testimony to his wisdom in backing our view that rules of evidence must be rigidly observed. The controlled trial of ACTH treatment showed no benefit. In fact, it demonstrated an unexpected risk—fatal infections occurred more frequently in infants treated with ACTH than in controls! The incident was a wonderful example of Rusty McIntosh's insistence on the highest standards. He and his hospital service were synonymous with all that was best in medicine.

— *William A. Silverman, MD*

Alexander Nadas, MD: Until the Symphony Ends

Alexander Nadas, MD, came to the United States after a detour to England, where he studied pediatric cardiology. In 1940, he found a locum tenens doing general pediatrics in Greenfield, MA, in the office of Merritt Low, MD. Dr Low, later a president of the AAP, had been stricken with paralytic polio and Dr Nadas covered the practice during Dr Low's prolonged recuperation. Dr Nadas later recalled the difficulties he had making house calls. He would drive to the destined address and park his car outside, but would not move out of the car and away from its radio "until the symphony had ended." Finishing his medical business in the house, he would then return to his car and start out for the next call. If another symphony had begun, it made for a long day.

— *Benjamin K. Silverman, MD*

Charles Janeway, MD: Simple Habits

During the 1960s Dr Charles Janeway would drive from Boston to Atlantic City with some of the fellows and junior faculty from Children's Hospital. The latter were all booked at the Traymore Hotel, the site of the APS/SPR meetings. Dr Janeway would ask to be dropped off at one of the rather seedy boarding houses on a side street near the hotel where he would stay for the week, while his young faculty and fellows went on to the comparatively "magnificent" Traymore. In the same fashion, it was rumored that he took most of his meals in the local YMCA cafeteria, adjoining the boarding houses.

— *Samuel L. Katz, MD*
(Adapted from Pearson HA. *The Centennial History of the American Pediatric Society, 1888–1988*. New Haven, CT: American Pediatric Society; 1988. Used with permission.)

Learning by Doing

I graduated medical school in '38 and started my internship at Queen's General Hospital. What was medicine like in this municipal hospital? For one thing, it was the custom then to have a 2-year rotating internship. In the rotating internship, we took our periods in all of the major fields—medicine, surgery, and the subspecialties. It has fallen out of practice now, but it certainly did give you a feeling for the broad field of medicine. Then you entered specialization and pediatrics was usually an additional 2 years. All of the attendings were in practice. There were no full-time attendings. The house staff really ran the hospital and rarely thought of calling an attending for advice. We taught each other and we learned from experience. You learned by doing. There's a fallacy in that, but that's what it was. It was experience, and it was assumed you knew more if you saw or did more. This was at the very beginning of the controlled study. Controlled studies, of course, shook up this idea of experience and knowledge because so many things that people "knew" didn't stand up.

— *Joseph Dancis, MD*
    (Adapted from the AAP oral history collection.)

"Why Doesn't Somebody Call a Real Doctor?"

After my medical school training at Johns Hopkins, I began my residency at Morrisania City Hospital in New York City. On the first day I reported for my rotating internship, there were about 20 new interns gathered in something similar to an assembly hall—cold, impersonal, and bleak—for the necessary admission procedures.

It became immediately apparent that I was the only female in the group, which prompted a lot of more or less surreptitious glances in my direction, and sotto voce comments, inaudible to me, but predictably followed by grins and laughter by one and all.

We all underwent blood tests, and I remember that I was pleased that I made a lot less fuss about the venipuncture than my macho companions did. We were then informed that we had to have a urinalysis, and everyone was given a little bottle with a very narrow opening at the top. I accepted the container unflinchingly, but wondered whether I should ask for one more suitable to my anatomy. I quickly rejected the notion. After all, I was still in the state of mind where I felt I had to prove women and myself in general to be capable. "Anything you can do I can better" message was my signature at that time. (In my later, wiser years, I have learned that intense competition is counterproductive and a better policy is to emphasize and profit from the differences.) Off I went to the ladies' room with my little bottle, accompanied by curious glances and snickers from my colleagues. Fortunately, I had the area to myself and could engage in the embarrassing ritual in complete privacy. Head high, little bottle in hand, I returned to the assembly room. All eyes on me, I remained matter of fact and handed in my trophy without comment. No one ever commented, but it was a small step in my goal to be accepted as an equal. That notion was my main motivation at that time.

I then became a pediatric resident at the Mary Imogene Bassett Hospital in Cooperstown, NY. The hospital was situated on beautiful grounds and had fairly luxurious accommodations for patients and staff. The hospital even served very fine food, very different from my previous city experience. Good-quality laboratories were available down the hall, so different from the city lab where I had to send a request on an anonymous little laboratory slip to an invisible faraway lab in another building.

> *"When covering for the obstetrics resident, I dreaded hearing the crunch of the gravel in the circular driveway that led to the hospital that most likely meant that a patient in labor was probably going to deliver before morning."*
>
> BARBARA M. KORSCH, MD

As a pediatrician, with skill in gaining access even to the tiniest blood vessels, I was often summoned by internists and surgeons when they had trouble getting into a vein. Transfusions were a very complicated and tiresome process, especially in the middle of the night when I was wakened from much-needed sleep. We had few really effective interventions in those days, so we often used transfusions in the hope of increasing the patient's resistance. Quite often, when the baby had the same blood type as mine, I would do a cross match between the patient and me and give some of my blood. For babies, it was often just a couple of ounces. Once, as I was transfusing my blood into a baby, a colleague came to give me a hand. He looked up at the container, and indicated in some alarm that my blood cells were settling with great speed. "Why do you have such a fast ESR [erythrocyte sedimentation rate]?" he asked. When I checked my blood count the next day, I found out I was severely anemic! Little by little, I had depleted my system of iron.

There was only one qualified resident in pediatrics and one in obstetrics, so we made an arrangement to cover for one another every other night since we were trained in both specialties. When covering for the obstetrics resident, I dreaded hearing the crunch of the gravel in the circular driveway that led to the hospital that most likely meant that a patient in labor was probably going to deliver before morning. This meant getting up and doing the necessary examinations and preparations for labor and delivery. I would be scrubbed, standing by the patient waiting for the appearance of a male anesthetist who would make loud comments about the incompetence of young female physicians— "Why doesn't someone call a real doctor?" or "That's what you get when you start sending girls to do a man's job!" The diatribe was performed in front of the patient and the nursing staff, which undermined any confidence they might have had in me. Because of this, I became an expert at administering epidural local anesthesia, which was something I could administer all by myself in my own good time.

— *Barbara M. Korsch, MD*

Married to Pediatrics

My fiancé and I both went to medical school in New York City. We had interviews at Cornell. The person who interviewed me looked at me and said, "You don't look like our usual candidate. Don't you like men?" I answered him that I did like men and, in fact, was engaged. He said, "I hope it's not to one of our applicants." I unfortunately said that it was, and he said, "I have a suggestion. Here's my telephone number, and why don't you decide which of you should stay on our list." In the 1950s, women going on to medicine were considered to be very high-risk people who probably wouldn't continue in their careers. So he went to Cornell and I went to NYU medical school.

We were married the summer before we entered medical school. Four years later, we entered the intern matching plan, me for pediatrics and him for internal medicine. We were very concerned that we would not be in the same town. The matching plan was not as strict as it is today, and so when Dr L. Emmett Holt, Jr, called me and offered me a pediatric internship out of the matching plan, I was thrilled because my husband had been told that he had a good chance of also being accepted at Bellevue.

My pediatric residency was one of the most exciting times of my life. We had magnificent teachers. There were a number of women who were wonderful role models at Bellevue and NYU, where I think that it was nearly unique to have women who stood out in their fields. These women went into medicine because they loved medicine. During residency, my husband and I expected to see each other every other night, but for the first 6 months, we had opposite schedules and schedules were set in stone. For 4 years, there wasn't much of a social life because of schedules and tiredness. We both were paid $15 a month and needed financial help from our parents to get by.

— *Donna O'Hare, MD*
(Adapted from the AAP oral history collection.)

Training in Rochester

William Bradford, MD, was chairman of the department. He had a research laboratory that made significant contributions to our understanding of infectious diseases. In addition, he had a large general pediatric practice that he ran in his

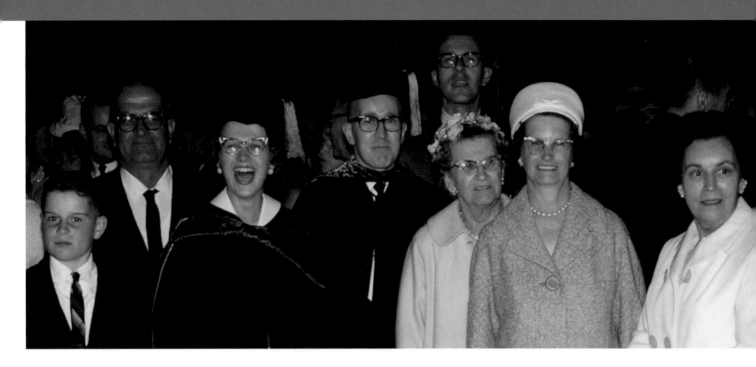

department office. This was not unusual in the 1950s because the era of full-time academicians had not yet arrived in many pediatric departments. There was reasonable supervision of interns on the wards, but almost none in the emergency room. (In those days, it was indeed a room and far from a department).

My first rotation was in the emergency room where I would see a seemingly endless number of children. At appropriate seasons, it seemed that most every febrile child had measles, and so a meticulous search for Koplik spots was always done. Another frequent diagnosis was impetigo, especially among the area's many migrant worker families. We had a small laboratory where we did our own blood counts and urinalyses. If we needed a chest X-ray, we had to wait until it was developed and then did a "wet reading" ourselves. Our therapeutic armamentaria were penicillin G, sulfadiazine, streptomycin, and chloramphenicol.

There were 3 age-related wards. The infant ward was divided by wood and glass partitions to reduce infection. An ultraviolet light was on all of the time that gave off an eerie glow at night. Many infants with diarrhea were treated with intravenous (IV) fluids. We had to mix the fluids ourselves in the treatment rooms. We carefully calculated the infant's extracellular volume and estimated the amount of fluid and electrolyte loss. From these, we the determined the right amount of D5W (dextrose 5% in water), normal saline, and lactated Ringer solution, and mixed them together in a burette. The burette was attached to IV tubing, and a sterile piece of gauze was taped on top to ward off infection. We never used gloves while mixing these concoctions. Needles were resterilized and used again and again, so they were often dull. It is a credit to the resiliency of the human species that so many infants not only survived, but also improved under our care.

— *Leon Chameides, MD*

Graduation day for pediatrician Phyllis Cavens, MD (third from left), from the University of Oregon Medical School in the 1960s. She was one of 4 women in her class of 80.

"*During residency, my husband and I expected to see each other every other night, but for the first 6 months, we had opposite schedules and schedules were set in stone. For 4 years, there wasn't much of a social life because of schedules and tiredness.*"

DONNA O'HARE, MD

155

Urban Pediatric Training in the Late 1960s

In 1968, I was rotating as a medical student at Albert Einstein College of Medicine at Lincoln Hospital in the South Bronx; at the time, arguably the worst slum in New York City. The hospital was so old that it still ran on direct current (DC) generated by a generator, possibly coal-fired, on-site, with only a small feeder line from the city-wide alternating current (AC) system. Each of our open wards was supposed to have 28 beds, but usually housed 36 patients. Each had only one AC outlet in the treatment rooms. Electrical appliances, like lamps, ran on DC, but none of the more modern pieces of medical equipment, such as cardiac monitors, defibrillators, and suction apparatus, had been converted to DC.

When a cardiac arrest occurred, the victim's bed had to be dragged into the treatment room where the resuscitation was done by a 3-person team of interns and medical students that were called the Three Ps: the Puffer, who used an Ambu bag; the Pumper, who did chest compressions (usually so vigorously that rib cracking was frequently heard); and the Plug Man, whose job it was to plug in and out, as needed, the various medical appliances. Since there was only one AC outlet, and since plugging in 2 devices at the same time would usually blow a fuse, only one device at a time could be used; ie, a cardiac monitor, or a defibrillator, or a Gomco suction, but not all 3, or even 2, at the same time. It was the Plug Man's job to plug the proper one in at the appropriate time, and be ready to rotate them quickly at critical moments during the resuscitation. The Plug Man was usually a medical student who had little experience with Puffing or Pumping at that stage of his education. All the Plug Man had to do was to keep up with the shouted orders of the other 2. It was always surprising to me that any patients ever survived this procedure, but a few actually did.

— *Walter M. Fierson, MD*

The Pediatrician as Intravenous Expert

Most of the first year of my residency in the mid-1950s was spent administering fluids and electrolytes to infants with severe dehydration and acidosis due to diarrhea. Diarrhea was a major cause of death during summer months in the South. Skill in initiating IV fluids to neonates and small infants belonged almost exclusively to pediatricians. Even surgeons called on us for this procedure. In small infants, the veins of the scalp were the most accessible. I can recall vividly strapping infants to restraint boards with adhesive tape, taking a 5 or 10 mL glass syringe with a 1.5", 22-gauge needle attached, and probing the scalp, desperately hoping to see a drop of blood in the syringe. As soon as blood appeared, the syringe would be gently disconnected and the needle would be attached to a heavy glass connector from a large rubber tube leading to the glass flask of fluid to be infused. Then came the tricky part—securing the needle, glass connector, and tubing in place with adhesive tape. These infusions rarely lasted more than a few hours before dislodgment or infiltration. Sometimes it was not possible to gain venous access even after many tries, so we had to resort to hypodermoclysis. This involved inserting needles into the subcutaneous tissue and starting an infusion drip, resulting in a huge swelling over the back

"There were so few women residents, many parents thought I was a nurse, and after I had examined their child, they would politely ask when the doctor would see them."

LOIS POUNDS OLIVER, MD

and sometimes further deranging fluid balance in these puffy babies.

A breakthrough occurred when we sawed the needle barrel into 2 halves and introduced a piece of plastic tubing to rejoin the cut ends, thus separating the heavy hub from the sharp end of the needle. Now, the needle was almost weightless and could be easily directed into the vein with a hemostat and secured for more than a day or so. For a year, we made our own reusable needles and kept the plastic tubing in jars of disinfectant. It wasn't long before entrepreneurs caught on and began to manufacture and sell sharp, sterile, and disposable scalp vein needles. Fluid and electrolyte therapy could now be more easily given. The mortality rate of diarrhea dropped significantly and hypodermoclysis was abandoned. The scalp vein needle is now standard and is used for IV access at all sites. This was only one of the many "unsung discoveries" from pediatrics that had a major impact on medical therapeutics.

— *Walter T. Hughes, MD*

Fluid and Electrolyte Therapy

In 1951, I went to Children's Hospital Boston to spend a post-residency year with William Wallace, MD, in the laboratory of James Gamble, MD. Dr Gamble was recently retired but came in regularly. A major focus of the laboratory was on the use of a flame photometer that Dr Wallace had built himself. It was being used for the first time to replace complex chemical methods for directly measuring serum sodium and potassium in metabolic conditions and other fluid and electrolyte problems.

There were already a number of research papers on these topics but they had been produced by laborious chemical analyses, dating back to the 1930s, for sodium, chloride, and potassium and, to 1924, for the volumetric analysis of total carbon dioxide. In most clinical situations, sodium levels were inferred from the measurement of chloride and bicarbonate. Bicarbonate was measured by the Van Slyke method. One of my first tasks was to master the Van Slyke apparatus to measure carbon dioxide. The Van Slyke apparatus consisted of a complex W-shaped piece of glassware with a manometer on one limb and a reservoir of mercury on the other limb, with several stopcocks in between. It was remarkably easy to break the equipment with 2 sequellae—cleaning up the mercury spilled on the floor, and building or repairing the glassware with a Bunsen burner and lots of patience. A number of lacerations resulted and the possible effect of inhalation of mercury remains unknown.

At that time, most of the pediatric subspecialties were essentially nonexistent, so we were referred to as the "salt and water" types. Other major figures in the salt and water field at that time included Daniel Darrow, MD, at Yale; Allan Butler, MD, at Massachusetts General Hospital; and Alex Hartmann, MD, in St Louis. Their disciples and trainees carried these changes throughout the country. The impact of the advances in fluid and electrolyte diagnosis and treatment on clinical pediatrics was rapid and dramatic. Children with diarrhea, diabetic ketoacidosis (DKA), and a variety of dehydration etiologies could be treated effectively, reducing both morbidity and mortality. Further in the future, the growing understanding of fluid and salt balance led to the use of oral rehydration fluids that have had a major impact on diarrheal disease in underdeveloped countries.

— *William B. Weil, MD*

Internship at Bellevue Hospital, 1952: The Joy of Learning

I decided on pediatrics as my career in my junior year of medical school. My choice was influenced by the wonderful teachers I had at Bellevue during medical school at New York University—L. Emmett Holt, Jr, MD; Edith Lincoln, MD; Saul Krugman, MD; Joseph Dancis, MD; and Jonathan T. Lanman, MD. For an intern, Bellevue was a Shangri La. I saw a lot and had a lot of responsibility. I was paid $50 a month and was on duty every other night and weekend. As interns, we had 4 meals a day, served in a huge dining hall with linen cloth-covered tables. The midnight meal (food was not eaten in the day) was actually a learning experience. We discussed patients and unique experiences of the day. The whole year flew by—I would have been an intern for life if they allowed it. I took care of my first infant with retrolental fibroplasia and participated in the first randomized trial done in premature infants. The high point of my internship was putting an IV into a 1,000-gram preemie with the lights out and my eyes closed! What I learned most at Bellevue was the sheer joy and excitement of learning.

— *Jerold F. Lucey, MD*

The Pay of a Pediatric Resident, 1955

Dr [Allan] Butler said to me in the first week of my pediatric training, "Gerry, we have a new policy at the Mass General now. We're going to pay you." I said, "Oh boy, what will the pay be?" He said, "$25 a month." As I was leaving, he asked, "Gerry, are you married?" When I said, "Yes, sir," he told me that there was a different pay scale for married house officers—$28 a month! It was hard to tell Audrey that she was worth $3 a month!

— *Gerold L. Schiebler, MD*
   (Adapted from the AAP oral history collection.)

Internship in the Mid-1950s

During my rotating internship in Bethesda, MD, in 1954 and 1955, our on-call schedule was every other night—34 hours on, 14 hours off, and every other weekend from Friday morning until late Monday afternoon. This was a hard time for my wife, Anne, who during that year, raised our 3 boys virtually single-handedly and was still washing diapers. I was so tired on my nights off that I usually fell asleep right after dinner. Once during that year, my parents came to Washington, DC, and invited us out for a nice dinner. Anne hadn't been out of the house for months and had a

Above right, Jerold F. Lucey, MD, longtime editor of *Pediatrics*, as a resident at 26 years of age, circa 1952; *below*, Howard A. Pearson, MD, past president of the American Academy of Pediatrics and coeditor of *Dedicated to the Health of All Children*, and a young patient with sickle cell anemia.

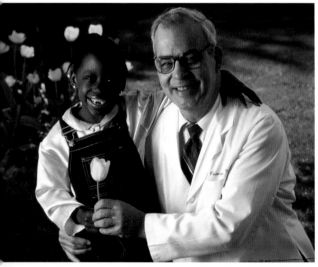
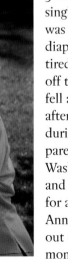

touch of cabin fever. We went to my parents' hotel room. I sat down and promptly went to sleep. My parents felt so sorry for me that they let me sleep and we never left their room. This was the nearest Anne ever came to divorcing me.

— *Howard A. Pearson, MD*

Pediatric Residency in the 1960s

I was a resident at the Children's Hospital of Philadelphia (CHOP) for 1 year, and at the Children's Hospital Boston for 2 years. My intern class at CHOP had 3 women. One of these women could afford an apartment, one was married, and I was the only single one. Housing was a most difficult issue. I was given a room on the third floor of an old funeral home across the street from CHOP, where the first 2 floors were offices. When space was needed for more offices, my monthly stipend of $75 was doubled, but I had to find my own housing. I found a furnished apartment for $95 a month, and I found out that the landlord's dog was being treated for heart failure with biweekly injections of mercuhydrin. I offered to give the dog injections for a $10 a month reduction in my rent. I prayed that the dog would live until June when I went to Boston.

   My interviewer at Children's Hospital Boston had told me that it was unlikely that the selection committee would take a woman resident. The Vietnam War must have changed their minds, as many men were being drafted. I went there with a salary of $150 a month. I was assigned a dormitory for my living quarters. The on-call situation was even worse. There were 2 rooms assigned for women on call, but the 3 women residents in the whole program had to compete with nurse anesthetists and operating room nurses for these 4 beds.

We also had to share a communal bathroom and shower room with the men. One resident went to Dr Janeway and told him that she was unable to take a shower under these circumstances. Since we were on duty from Saturday morning until Monday evening every other weekend, she pointed out that parents might not appreciate her lack of hygiene. Dr Janeway had a freestanding sheet metal shower installed for women only. It made a real racket when the shower was on, and we enjoyed annoying everyone who was still asleep by taking our showers very early.

There were so few women residents, many parents thought I was a nurse, and after I had examined their child, they would politely ask when the doctor would see them. Of course, this was an advantage with the children who tended to think of nurses as their friends and the doctors as their enemies. I think that pediatrics was more welcoming for women than many other specialties, making pediatrics a leader in integrating women into all areas of medicine.

— *Lois Pounds Oliver, MD*

Blackout in the Neonatal Intensive Care Unit, New York, NY, 2003

We were all just going about our day in the neonatal intensive care unit (NICU) with the usual rituals—checking labs and updating our flow sheets. Then, suddenly, the computers went black. Though only 4:10 pm on a midsummer day, the windowless pediatric resident conference room turned dark. The very first thought that ran through my mind was, "Bag the babies." As we ran to the NICU, I already knew which babies needed immediate attention. So was to begin my call on August 28, 2003—the day of the Blackout of 2003—in the NICU.

If it weren't for the silence, you almost would not have known the severity of the event at that moment. We had approximately 16 patients, but 5 of these were either on mechanical ventilation or receiving nasal continuous positive airway pressure (nCPAP). There was no electricity and the generators failed. Luckily, by the light of day, we were able to organize our missions. Attendings, residents, nurses, respiratory therapists, and fellows from every department rushed to help us. We alternated bagging the infants who needed it. We only had one pulse oximeter left that had enough battery charge and we moved that machine from patient to patient to check their oxygen saturations. However, we relied more on their color and clinical status. Then the pulse oximeter died.

After the initial commotion settled, we tried our best to continue normal activities. We did blood gases but, unfortunately, the laboratory was on the second floor and the NICU was on the eighth floor. Without elevators or lights, that was an experience in itself. Then, "the" phone rang, a direct line from the labor and delivery rooms to come immediately. I grabbed a gown and ran 5 flights down to labor and delivery. The distressed baby was born soon after my arrival. As I carried the newborn to the warmer, I felt blood trickling down my gown, then through my scrubs. The cord had not been clamped. A nurse twisted the umbilical cord like a hose to stop the flow of

"*The whole year flew by—
I would have been an intern for life if they allowed it.*"

JEROLD F. LUCEY, MD

blood. Labor and delivery had a working generator so, though dim, I could clearly see that there had been enough blood loss to warrant an admission to the now-dark NICU for observation.

Completely soaked with blood, I arrived back at the NICU, showered in the attending's dark call room, and borrowed clean scrubs. Then I ran back to the unit where a setup already had begun for placement of lines in our new admission. We had a nurse on a stool behind us pointing a flashlight onto the tiny umbilicus. As if it weren't already hard enough to get a line in the light, we were doing it in the dark!

Meanwhile we were transferring our sickest patients across the street to our nearby hospital, since its NICU had a working generator. We literally rolled the patients across the street in the Isolettes. I stopped traffic in the dark streets to let the Isolettes by. We rolled and bagged our way to the NICU across the street. Needless to say, it was an experience. The next morning, the new team came in for the day. They had no clue what we had been through. They didn't know we had no generator and that there was no light at all for hours. One intern had even slept through the whole thing since she was post call. During signout, it all seemed like a story—too crazy to be true. In retrospect, I'm happy that I was there to experience and survive the New York NICU Blackout of 2003.

— *Yvonne P. Giunta, MD*

How Technology Has Changed Pediatric Training
The training experience of pediatric house officers today is dramatically different from that of pediatricians who entered the field 75 years ago. Recent, rapid advances in technology have impacted the pediatrics training experience. As a house officer in the mid-1990s, I obtained my call schedules and other information from printed sheets distributed to my file folder "mailbox" in the departmental office across the street from the hospital. I documented progress notes in a paper chart and wrote medication orders in a book, taking great pains to write decimal points and dosage units clearly for fear that illegible handwriting might result in harm to a patient. Ordering radiological studies on a patient often involved locating the actual films after they were completed, combing through piles of films in the radiology department in a frenzied, and

occasionally futile, search, usually at the expense of time that could have been better spent elsewhere. During the morning's radiology rounds, we would crowd around the pediatric radiologist at a light box, straining to get a glimpse of any pertinent findings.

Today, working in a city hospital listed among the nation's "Most Wired," I marvel at the contributions made by technology in enhancing

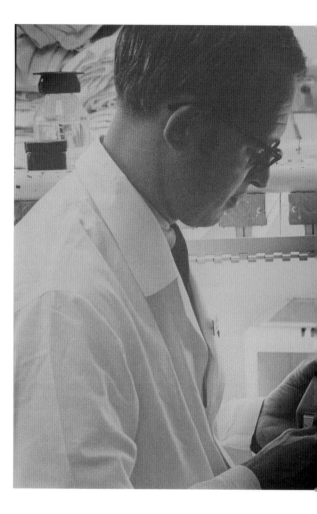

residency training. Residents no longer have to "round with the order book"; instead, they enter patient information into computers, and retrieve laboratory data electronically, including radiological, electroencephalogram (EEG), electrocardiogram (EKG), echocardiogram, and audiology results. Residents enter their sign-out sheets through the computer, and use electronic medical references. Thanks to our computerized radiology system, house officers no longer chase after "lost" films; patient studies are available for viewing at any workstation; and during x-ray rounds, the radiologist digitally highlights pertinent findings on a large-screen projection system. In clinic, patient information flows through an electronic medical record that automatically calculates growth percentiles. With multiple computers throughout the wards and in every examination room in clinic, residents have access not only to patient data, but also to the vast wealth of medical information on the Internet. Even the administrative aspects of training have been affected by technology, including the details of a house officer's daily life—residents obtain their on-call schedules and program information from our Web site. Nowadays, a resident "mailbox" refers perhaps more frequently to an e-mail inbox than to those file folders I recall from not too long ago.

— *Rachel J. Katz-Sidlow, MD*

PEDIATRIC PRACTICE AND CAREERS

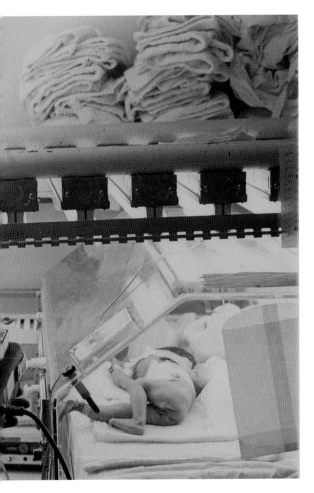

Desegregation in an Incubator

In 1927, when I went into practice in St Louis with my brother-in-law, Dr Park White, we became very involved in race relationships. My brother-in-law was very active in getting the hospital to become nonsegregated. The story is that they had 2 premature babies at the same time, one black, one white, and they only had one incubator. And he said, "Well, why not put them both in the same incubator?"; and from then on, they had no more trouble.

— *Katherine Bain, MD*
  (Adapted from the AAP oral history collection.)

House Calls in Rochester in the 1940s

After the end of World War II, I went into practice in Rochester, NY, with Burt Breese. It was not common at that point for doctors to practice together so this created quite a to-do in the pediatric community. While we had a general practice, we carried around materials in our little black bags so that we could obtain blood counts and throat cultures and take them back to our office where they would be run the next morning. This was a time that we did many house calls because it was not expected in those days that patients would come to the office when they were ill. The usual thing was for us to go out in the morning,

"Nowadays, a resident 'mailbox' refers perhaps more frequently to an e-mail inbox than to those file folders I recall from not too long ago."

RACHEL J. KATZ-SIDLOW, MD

after answering the telephone until 8:00 am, and make house calls. In this community, we could make about 2 ½ calls an hour. The mornings were not only for house calls but we also attended to newborns in the hospital. We returned to the office at about 1:00 pm and had an afternoon of office practice. When we finished, it was pretty close to dinnertime and we rotated as to which of us would take night call. We'd start right out after dinner and make house calls until about 11:00 pm. The one of us on call was available for house calls in the evening and all night. I worked 70 hours a week for as long as I was in practice, and I wouldn't have given it up for any reason at all.

With passing time, we began decreasing the number of house calls and began bringing more ill children to the office so that we could utilize laboratory studies—urines, blood smears, mononucleosis tests—things that helped in diagnosis. I'd like to say that the loss of house calls really made it a lot more difficult. When you would go to a house, you could get a better evaluation of that mother, her child, and their relationship. If you made a house call at 8:30 in the morning, and the house was all clean and the ashtrays were all emptied and polished and everything was in order, it told you something about the mother. So that when later the mother complained that she was having difficulty with discipline, you had a better understanding of why the child was having trouble with his mother. The whole parent-child relationship could often be cleared up by something you would note on a house call. It's difficult to replace this kind of information. House calls were a very time-wasteful activity, but they taught you a great deal.

— *Frank A. Disney, MD*
(Adapted from the AAP oral history collection.)

Practice in a Connecticut Village, 1941

My husband and I opened our medical office in the small rural town of Litchfield, CT, on Pearl Harbor Day, December 7, 1941. Within a year, my husband joined the Navy Medical Corps and was shipped out (and later was killed). I remained as the sole pediatrician in the area. My medical office was located in our modest colonial box-style home at the edge of the village common. The office space was limited. Patients would enter by the front door and wait on a big couch in the living room, facing the fireplace. Toys in the corner and under the piano kept the children busy. A door near the coat rack in the entry opened into a small examining room. A staircase led up stairs to the second-floor bedrooms. The biggest problem with this setup was trying to keep my own kids out of the way when patients came for an office visit. I often found my 2-year-old daughter sitting on the stairs next to the examining room, listening expectantly for the sudden cry of a child that I was immunizing. I worked alone with no regular staff. I kept my own records and did routine tests in a laboratory set up in the basement.

Bookkeeping was simple. Payments were in cash or in-kind—$3 for an office visit and $5 for a home visit. Laboratory tests and immunization were included. Most of my practice was office based and fairly standard—health and development checkups, immunizations, formula changes, and sometimes a rash or head cold. To my surprise, I found the need for hospitalization or specialty consultation to be rare. Having spent my pediatric training in urban medical centers where the patients were sick all the time, I had to get used to the realization that most of the patients I saw now were well most of the time and it was my job to keep them that way. Nevertheless, realizing that sometime, something might go wrong, I attempted to purchase liability insurance. The

> "Bookkeeping was simple.
> Payments were in cash or in-kind—$3 for an office visit
> and $5 for a home visit."
>
> ELINOR FOSDICK DOWNS, MD

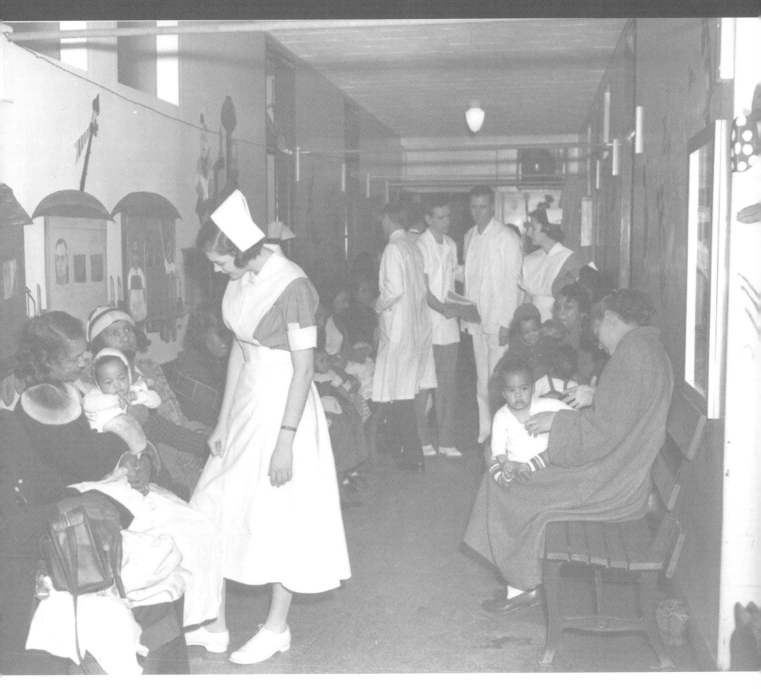

Hospital waiting room at Duke University, 1940s.

agents that I consulted in major insurance companies in Hartford, CT, were unfamiliar with this issue and contended that they didn't see that there was any need for it.

— *Elinor Fosdick Downs, MD*

House Calls in Baltimore in the 1950s
The practice of pediatrics at that time was very hard work because, in addition to the standard office hours, we made house calls, at least a couple a day. A thousand a year for me was not unusual. We had a large practice right in the middle of the city, so we had a large area to cover. We made a commitment that, once we took a family on, we would see them at home, so house calls were standard throughout the '50s. Our practice was mostly well-child care in the office and treating infections in the home. A parent wouldn't think of bringing a child into the office with a fever. There was fear too, because there were still people who remembered such illnesses as double pneumonia and also remembered that a child with otitis media could get mastoiditis. That's why they didn't bring children with fever out of the house.

We charged $7 for a house call no matter how far we traveled, but that was the nature of practice at the time and, indeed, you learned things in house calls. Almost always they were at the end of the day. You met the child's father. Often the mother would apologize about how the home looked and I'd say, "Madam, I didn't come to examine your habits, I came to examine your child." So it went. I frankly enjoyed practice, even including the house calls.

— *Milton Markowitz, MD*
   (Adapted from the AAP oral history collection.)

Practice in the 1950s: "Bless All the Nurses"

On completion of my residency in 1955 and entrance into pediatric practice, I recognized what I had learned was not the total body of knowledge. In those days, most grandmothers arrived with the diagnosis, and simply expected me to confirm their suspicion. My nurse, Faye, taught me the "gentle" things left out of my core curriculum. An example: A child came into my office sprayed from head to toe with paint. Her eyes peeked out from this red, sticky mess. The mother and I were in a panic, and Faye calmly stated that Dr Arnold would take care of the situation. I could not remember a course offered on removing paint, but beloved Faye took the child into the treatment room, later emerging with a beautiful youngster with normal skin and hair free of any vestige of her earlier adventure. Bless all the nurses.

— *Milton Arnold, MD*

Volunteer Clinics

Prior to the time that Medicaid and Medicare came in the 1960s, we had many volunteer physicians and we had in New York a good network of child health stations and clinics staffed largely by volunteer physicians that provided good clinical care and taught good parenting skills. The families felt comfortable there. Those volunteer physicians provided the best of care and they were concerned about the patients. They were dedicated. I remember some of them who would leave their private practices every week and come to the clinic at Bellevue to take care of those patients. They probably gave them more time than they gave their own private patients and they made certain that the interns, residents, and students that were working with them learned at the same time. There was no means test then, and anybody could walk into the clinics, which were located in areas of high risk in terms of low-income status families. I think that this was true, not only in the centers and clinics, but also in their offices. The climate then was that if a patient couldn't pay, most physicians did not really push them or send them to collection agencies. I think Medicaid and Medicare really changed medicine from a profession into a business and largely eliminated volunteerism, unfortunately.

— *Donna O'Hare, MD*
   (Adapted from the AAP oral history collection.)

Practice in the Rural South: Taking Time to Listen

As a solo pediatrician in a small town in northeast Alabama, I would use the excuse to "teach" medical students in Birmingham to take a break and get out of town. Inevitably, as one is ready to leave, a patient shows up in the emergency department. One summer day when I was running the usual 5 minutes late, with my preschool children and wife in the car, I was called to the emergency department on my way out of town. Standing before me was a very poor rural family with the father dressed in his unkempt overalls,

"*[M]ost grandmothers arrived with the diagnosis, and simply expected me to confirm their suspicion.*"

MILTON ARNOLD, MD

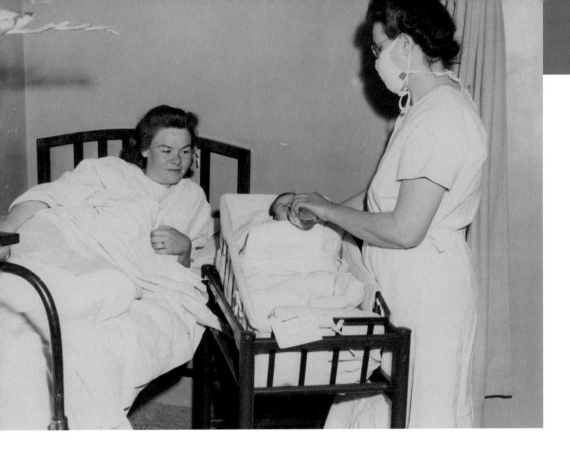

and his toothless wife in her dress stitched together from cloth from a sack of chicken feed, and their 1-year-old daughter, all without shoes and socks. The nurse was obviously indignant as to why they were there as the daughter did not appear in acute distress, was not malnourished, and seemed to be developing along her predicted milestones.

I hurriedly asked the father what was wrong. As the father stammered and stuttered and the mother was of little help, I am sure I radiated overt frustration in my tone and body language about his detaining my anticipated trip. They did seem to be concerned, although the child was not in acute distress, so I pushed the father again with the question, "Why in the world did you bring your child to the emergency department today?" This question also was met with some pauses and some frustration with his inability to conceptualize a response that would be helpful for his child. I felt sure I would be late with my session with the students.

At this point, I remembered some of the lessons from my professor, Tinsley Harrison, MD, who taught that, by listening to what the patient wanted to say, one could obtain a history sometimes more superior than one with directed questioning. I felt it was time to sit back, relax, and listen. After all, direct questioning was fruitless. The father thought for what seemed to me like a

long time. I was trying to reflect body language of being more receptive, supportive, and concerned. Brightness came to the father's eyes, some color to his face, as he had a thought. He asked me a question: "Doc...have you ever seen frog legs in hot grease?" It was the best description of a febrile seizure that I have ever obtained, either before or since.

— *Carden Johnston, MD*

Is There a Doctor in the House?!?
I wonder how many pediatricians shared my fear of being called from the audience attending a concert or theater to take care of an adult emergency. (Actually, it never happened.)

— *Sol Browdy, MD*

Right, Eskimo child with severe chickenpox, Alaska Native Medical Center, Anchorage, 1966.

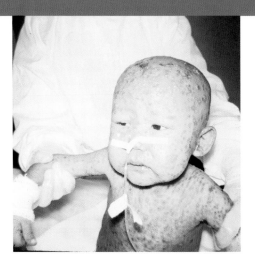

Pediatrics in Alaska

The beginnings of pediatrics in the 49th state occurred only about 50 years ago when, in 1953, Edward J. Powers, MD, with the Alaska Department of Maternal and Child Health, described some of the terrible problems of Alaskan children—rampant tuberculosis (TB), keratoconjunctivitis, measles, chronic bilateral draining otitis media, and many others. Tuberculosis was decimating the native population, in no small part because of the forced evacuation of the Aleuts from the Aleutian chain during World War II.

Helen Stoddard Whaley, MD, and I arrived almost simultaneously in the summer of 1954—me from a residency at Yale and she from a chief residency in Denver. We arrived in Anchorage, a dusty town with 2 paved streets and a population of about 30,000 men, women, and children, and probably a few dogs. We decided to be partners, but there was no office space available. We propelled ourselves to a local bank and, despite few financial resources, got a loan to buy an old, poorly insulated house that became our residences and offices for the next 3½ years. To our astonishment, delight, and relief, parents and children lined up at our front door within the week of our arrival; our first encounter with genuine Alaskans whose toughness, good nature, and lack of pretentiousness warmed us.

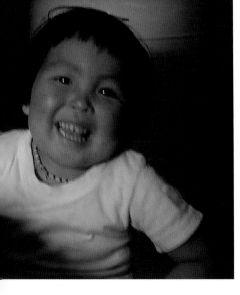

I made night house calls until a midnight call out for croup found me on an unmarked street (which turned out to be the wrong one!). When I knocked on the door, a sleeping woman arose, disrobed, and welcomed me to her portal! Thereafter, night calls were at the office. Parents would come by late at night and throw stones at my bedroom window to wake me to attend to their children's illness.

Early on, we dropped into the Bureau of Indian Affairs Hospital. The 2 doctors there, a surgeon and an internist, were overwhelmed by their census of 75 children with diseases such as acute rheumatic fever, TB, meningitis, otitic meningitis, mastoiditis, Pott disease, and glomerulonephritis. They were relieved when we made rounds in the evening to help them manage severely ill children delivered by bush planes in the late afternoon, who otherwise would have been dead by morning. Winters were long and cold. No one had a garage. Imagine house calls at 45°F below zero, car wheels frozen square, ice, fog, and the omnipresent worry about being stranded. So brief is the span of pediatrics in Alaska that it is hard to convey the sense of pioneering that led early pediatricians to the wondrous land, where they at first had to deal with neigh third-world pediatrics.

Once statehood was achieved in 1959, there was a slow but steady accretion of much-needed pediatricians to Alaska. At the same time, an expanding US Public Health Service addressed monumental problems, medical and social, in native Alaskan children. With the discovery of huge oil deposits at Prudhoe Bay and the opening of the Alaska pipeline in the mid-1970s, the formerly poor and sparsely settled territory became prosperous and both people and pediatricians moved to the state, vastly improving the welfare of Alaska's children.

— *John C. Tower, MD*

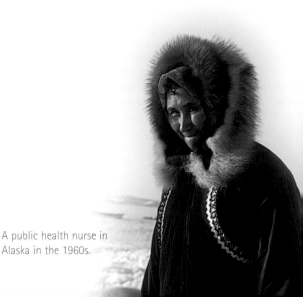

A public health nurse in Alaska in the 1960s.

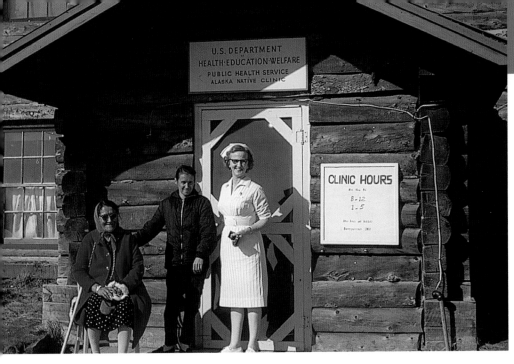

The Hudson Stuck clinic, Fort Yukon, AK, 1966.

Impact of Social Programs on Clinic Practice

I began working part-time with the New Orleans Health Department in 1988. Each of our 7 child health centers had a doctor for 4 hours each morning, and the clinics were jammed. Twenty patients were scheduled each morning, and nearly all came. Only a few private pediatricians took Medicaid children, so most came to us. Many children had little or no routine medical care. When the Early and Periodic Screening, Diagnostic, and Treatment (EPSDT) program came in 1989, more private doctors joined the program. By the time Kidmed came in 1991, almost all our local pediatricians were participating. In 1998, I was averaging 14 patients in a 7-hour day in the health department clinics, with time to read journals and do a study or 2 on the side.

With the advent of the Louisiana Children's Health Insurance Program (LaCHIP), many children with no insurance became eligible for full medical care. However, our clinic numbers did not increase, because these families now had access to private pediatricians. In fact, our clinics were getting a bit thin as time went on, as new pediatricians graduated into our community. In

September 2003, Louisiana's change to community care (primary care physician managed care) Medicaid reached New Orleans. Medicaid patients were assigned to private physicians, most of whom were eager to take them. Our clinics still offer medical care to the uninsured and to those whose insurance doesn't cover preventive care. Our clinics have become community care providers, and some families have come back to us, despite our austere circumstances. But it is wonderful to know that all our children can be well cared for, at least for now.

— *Mary C. Darken, MD*

J. Roswell Gallagher, MD: Father of Adolescent Medicine

In the mid-1950s, Ros [Dr J. Roswell Gallagher] came to the Children's Hospital Boston from Phillips Academy Andover where he had been very successful for many years treating and counseling prep school students. After the war, he came to see Charlie Janeway about getting an examining room, to open what he said would be an "adolescent clinic." This was the genesis of the whole adolescent medicine movement.

> "Adolescence, a stage of development which normally lasts for some 6 to 7 years— but for many, a lifetime."
>
> BILLY F. ANDREWS, MD

At that time, his patients were mostly upper- and upper-middle-class adolescents from the suburbs. The parents would bring in their teenaged kids because of things like acne, or because their boy was not growing as fast as classmates. The parents would come in and say, "He only got a C in History. He got a B+ before; tell me what's wrong with him." This kind of practice was fine for Ros because he was used to privileged prep school students. He believed that you should never have a parent around when you examine adolescents and that you shouldn't sit behind a desk when talking to them. Ros would have been surprised at the practice of adolescent medicine at Children's Hospital today. Most of the patients do not come from the affluent suburbs. They are now seeing kids with truancy, drug addiction, alcoholism, teenage pregnancies, delinquencies, sexually transmitted disease, and even AIDS.

— *Thomas E. Cone, Jr, MD*
   (Adapted from the AAP oral history collection.)

Serendipity: Adolescent Medicine and the American Academy of Pediatrics Annual Meeting
I attended my first AAP Annual Meeting (now the National Conference & Exhibition [NCE]) in 1969. Well into my second year of pediatric residency, I was still unclear as to where my professional career would lead me.

The 1969 Annual Meeting was held at the Palmer House in Chicago, IL. In those days a banquet was held on the last day of the meeting. Being a resident, I could not afford to take my wife to the meeting, so my dinner partner was a gentleman who was at the time a bachelor. We introduced ourselves and made small talk about who we were and what we did. He was Bill Long, MD, a pediatrician who had just completed a fellowship in adolescent medicine at the University of Colorado and had gone back to Jackson, MS, to set up his practice. I had never heard of adolescent medicine as a component of pediatrics but quickly realized that my favorite patients tended to be the older kids. I invited Bill to have a beer at the bar with me after dinner to pick his brain further about this new subspecialty. I was a bit taken aback when at the

Program from the 1969 American Academy of Pediatrics Annual Meeting in Chicago, IL, a meeting that proved serendipitous for Joe M. Sanders, Jr, MD.

bar Bill ordered a glass of milk, but I was intrigued when he explained what he was doing and how much satisfaction he had gained by doing it.

When I went home I did further research and found that the AAP had a policy statement that was issued in 1938, which stated, "The practice of pediatrics begins at birth and should extend through the adolescent period. In most instances, the termination of pediatric practice would be between the sixteenth and eighteenth years of life." I learned that in the 1950s Dr J. Roswell Gallagher described the medical plight of adolescents and later started the first medical service to deliver care to this group. Dr Gallagher believed adolescents were too old for the pediatrician and not yet old enough to be cared for by the internist. In the early 1960s a number of prominent pediatricians had become interested in the health care for this group, including C. Henry Kempe, MD. A new organization had started and was called the Society for Adolescent Medicine (SAM) (founded in 1968).

The rest, as they say, is history. I applied for fellowship training at 2 programs, one in San Francisco, CA, and the other in Denver, CO. Because I was a "freebie," in that the US Army had agreed to pay my salary while gaining this training, I would train at the institution at no cost to them. I elected to take my training in San Francisco under the tutelage of John J. Piel, MD, and then pursued an active academic career in the subspecialty.

Serendipity is often more productive than careful planning. Thank goodness my program director sent me to the AAP 1969 Annual Meeting; otherwise, who knows where my career may have led me. Incidentally, I have never missed an AAP Annual Meeting (NCE) since 1969!

— *Joe M. Sanders, Jr, MD*
   (Editors' note: Dr Sanders served as the executive director of the AAP from 1993 to 2004.)

Private Practice of Adolescent Medicine in the 1970s
About the time I was finishing my fellowship in adolescent medicine in Denver in 1976, an article appeared in the *Wall Street Journal*, estimating that there were about a dozen adolescent medicine people in private practice in the United

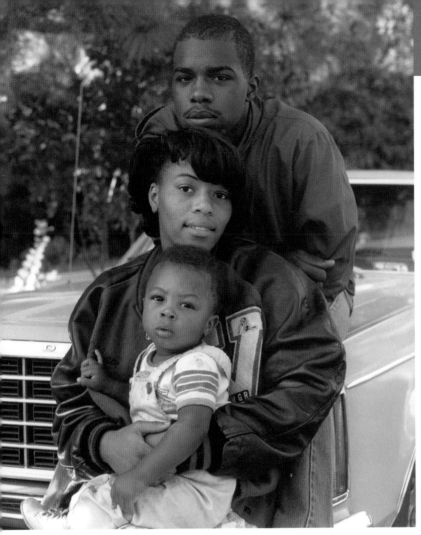

adolescents. Actually, things have not changed appreciably since then, except we're busier. I'm seeing fewer kids with drug problems and a lot more with obesity and ADHD. Zits have remained stable.

In the late 1970s, having been unsatisfied in keeping the Georgia Chapter of the AAP Committee on Adolescence going for lack of members, Alan Sievert, MD; Eduardo Montana, MD; and I decided to try to establish a Regional Chapter of SAM. There had not been a previous attempt to involve a large geographic area. The requirement for a chapter, however, was a request by 10 members of SAM. So, out of necessity, the Southeastern Regional Chapter of SAM was formed, stretching from Louisiana to Virginia, with 10 signatory members. At the founding meeting in Stone Mountain, GA, we decided we had sufficient signatures, and that we didn't have to include Missouri, which we all thought was a stretch to include in "the Southeast."

— *Edward M. Gotlieb, MD*

Gender Issues and the Balance of Career and Family

During my chief pediatric residency in 1960, a child development fellowship was offered to me. In one of the discussions with the fellowship director, she asked the question, "Are you going to use birth control?" I was 5 months pregnant at

States. Since I was about to become the thirteenth, my program directors encouraged me to stop off at the office of Dr Bill Long in Jackson, because they were sure he could tell me how to get started in private practice. Bill invited me to spend a day in his office, and by the time I left, had given me every form he had developed, explained what I was likely to see in practice, and told me how to bill for my services and how to carve out a practice with referrals from other pediatricians who did not want to be bothered with such stuff.

So my wife, Jackie Gotlieb, MD, and I hung up a shingle in suburban Atlanta, GA, and started seeing patients—she, younger kids; me,

> *"I'm seeing fewer kids with drug problems and a lot more with obesity and ADHD. Zits have remained stable."*
>
> EDWARD M. GOTLIEB, MD

that time. Needless to say, my enthusiasm for that fellowship waned and I accepted another professional opportunity. After a few years, I became the director of the diagnostic center at a residential facility. On a personal note, I was employed half-time with limited night or weekend call, since medical students moonlighted at the facility. Three of our 4 children were born during this 5-year period of employment.

— *Antoinette Parisi Eaton, MD*
    (Editors' note: Dr Eaton later became the first woman president of the American Academy of Pediatrics.)

Women in Academic Pediatrics

It is my own impression, not subject to any statistical control at all, that the qualities of generosity and graciousness towards others, and of a certain serenity of spirit, which, in the mature human being are peculiarly the hallmark of inner gratification of the soul, are no less prevalent among the women who have made their careers within the field of academic pediatrics than they are among women in other spheres of life. Whether or not women in academic pediatrics are, on the average, as productive in their research or as scintillating in their teaching and writing as are their male colleagues really does not seem of paramount importance. The fact is that there have been and there are, in the field of academic pediatrics, enough outstanding women, married and unmarried, with and without children, so that pediatrics would have been the poorer without their contributions; and the fact is also that several generations of women in this field have led not only useful but enjoyable and satisfying lives. This realization should provide sufficient encouragement for our younger would-be colleagues.

— *Margaret H. D. Smith, MD*
    (Adapted from Waring WW, Washington L. *Pro Parvulis: On Behalf of the Little Ones. A History of the Department of Pediatrics, Tulane Medical School, 1834–2003.* New Orleans, LA: Tulane Medical School; 2003. Used with permission.)

Helen Taussig Chooses a "Subspecialty"

Edwards Park was famous for choosing and guiding young members of his staff into new subspecialties where they gained great eminence, for which he denied all responsibility. On his staff was a tall, young woman named Helen Taussig. At Park's suggestion, she had spent some time looking after "blue babies" and other children with congenital heart disease. In 1930, Park suggested to her that she might consider making this her career. Soon thereafter, on a visit to her home in Cambridge, she consulted with her father, an eminent economics professor at Harvard. She told her father about the nature of the work and the problems involved. Professor Taussig responded, "Helen, for a woman, recognition will only come through specialization." Incidentally, despite her father's lofty position, Helen Taussig had been denied admission to Harvard Medical School because she was a woman, so she enrolled at Johns Hopkins instead.

— *Fred Richardson, MD*
    (Adapted from Pearson HA. *The Centennial History of the American Pediatric Society, 1888–1988.* New Haven, CT: American Pediatric Society; 1988. Used with permission.)

You've Come a Long Way, Baby Doctor

Kathaleen (Kay) Perkins, MD, graduated from Albany Medical School in the early 1950s and was 1 of only 2 female medical students in a class size of 40. Although the male students were reluctant to be a female student's cadaver partner, she was able to gain the respect of her fellow students and was elected president of her class, the first woman in the country to be president of a medical school class. She completed her pediatric residency at Albany and eventually went on to a fellowship in adolescent medicine at University of Rochester. Kay never married and once commented when asked about marriage, "You just couldn't do that easily back then...you had to pick a career or your family...and I chose the career." Although Kay never gave birth to any children, she cared for thousands of other people's children, and in her early practice, she often worked every day and night of the week.

Jump ahead to 40 years later to my own experiences. I graduated from Dartmouth Medical School in 1990 as one of a class of roughly 60 students, of which nearly half were women. I married my husband Tim that same year and am now raising 2 young children. I have the luxury of being able to work part-time as both an academic and private practice pediatrician. In the 21st century, it is much easier for a woman pediatrician to be able to enjoy both family and career.

— *Linda S. Nield, MD*

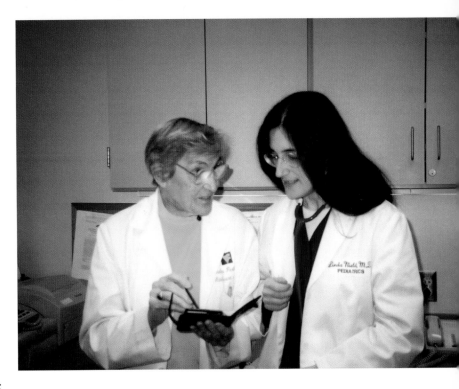

Two generations of woman pediatricians, Kathaleen Perkins, MD (left), and Linda S. Nield, MD (right), 2003.

Pediatrics and the Media—A New Way of Healing

It's 4:00 am. The phone rings. I stumble out of bed, shower and dress, grab a cup of coffee, and am out the door. I can barely see the road up the windy hill through the fog and blackness. As I park the car, I look ahead at the familiar building. I stride through the side door, greet the producer and head to the set. Camera rolls, and, in 3 minutes, I demystify the flu epidemic and encourage parents to vaccinate their children on KEYT, Santa Barbara, CA, morning news. For the last year, I have served as an on-camera health expert for a local morning news show and a columnist for *LA Family* magazine. I have experienced, first-hand, the influence a pediatrician in the media can have.

"So that's what the hooks in the back of my minivan are for," one of my nurses said after reading my car seat safety article. She then went outside to reinstall her car seats using the LATCH

> *"In the 21st century, it is much easier for a woman pediatrician to be able to enjoy both family and career."*
>
> LINDA S. NIELD, MD

171

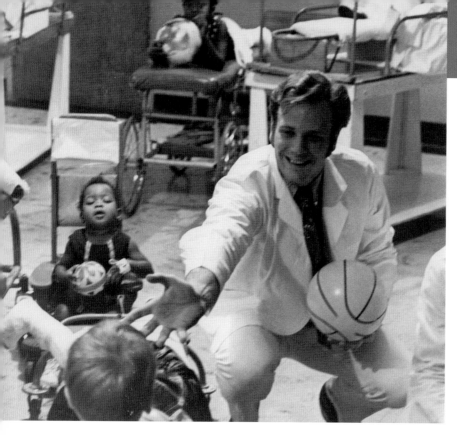

system already in her car. Later, a dad stopped me in the hall to tell me that he bought a booster seat for his 7-year-old daughter after reading my article.

Just last week, a mom I had never seen before brought her healthy, 10-year-old son into my office for a physical examination. He hadn't been seen for a complete examination since kindergarten, so I asked her what brought them in today. She said that my news segment on the importance of back-to-school physical examinations convinced her to schedule an appointment for her son and her 2 daughters who I would see later that week.

As a pediatrician, my days and, often, my nights are spent caring for sick infants, children, adolescents, and young adults. Through media, I have found that I can, in a few minutes, encourage many more parents to take a proactive role in their child's health than I can in a 10-hour day at the office. So the next time my phone rings early in the morning, I know I'm making a difference whether in one child's life or 1 million viewers.

— *Tanya Remer Altmann, MD*

"Reflected Glory": A Spouse's Perspective on Pediatricians

When my husband Bob [Robert E. Hannemann, MD] began his practice, we had behind us a year in the army, 4 years of medical school, a year of internship, and a residency in pediatrics.

I remember vividly those first few months of practice—the middle-of-the-night phone calls, his rising from the warm covers, and my pledge to be the dutiful wife. I thought I should get up with him, make him a warm cup of something, and wait for his return, whether it was an hour later or at dawn. This lasted about 1 week. After that, I perfunctorily awakened with the phone calls, sat up for a brief moment, and then cowardly slithered down under the covers so the light did not disturb my sleep. Did Bob ever complain about my lack of cooperation when he had to carry out his late-night obligation to his patients? No. I wish he had, sort of, because then I might not have felt so guilty. Upon his return from his nighttime forays, and if I was awake enough to be coherent, he chatted about little so-and-so who he had gone to see.

Most of his patients came with ordinary colds, fever, and earaches, but some had serious problems, though I was not usually privy to these illnesses. Once, I was included in the saddest time for one of Bob's patients, but it was not from Bob that I heard of a little girl's losing battle with leukemia. Our son was in first grade with this child and he brought me the bad news: "Angela is real sick, Mom. She may die." I could read on Bob's face that this was the worst part of pediatrics—losing a patient but, even more, losing a neighbor and friend of the family. All of Bob's medical school education could not prepare him for this pain, nor could he muster enough comfort for our son and me.

Even today, now that he has retired from practice, it seems that every week we have chance encounters with his former patients. Recently, while we were in a restaurant, "Hi, Dr Hannemann!" echoed across the room. Here was a former patient who was just as bubbly and petite at 40 as she had been at 5 years of age. She said she wished he lived somewhere where he could take over the care of her children. "I knew I would never find another doctor just like you," she said with a smile. Then she included me in her conversation. "Eleanor, I want you to know that I appreciated the phone calls I made to your home." She went on to remind me that, at age 12, she had frequently called Bob at home at all hours, to either confide something or to discuss personal problems. He usually remembers, is gracious and kind to, and is still as interested in his former patients as he was before the retirement mode took over.

I value the affection of his former patients and love to stand in the reflected glory of my pediatrician-husband.

— *Eleanor A. Hannemann*

WARTIME STORIES

As they did with most facets of American society, World War II and the military actions in Korea, Vietnam, and the Persian Gulf had profound effects on pediatrics and changed the lives of all who experienced them. During World War II, there was a doctor draft and most medical students and residents enlisted in the Army or Navy Medical Corps Reserves. Medical school was shortened by one third to 3 years, and internships were also only 9 months long. Very few dependents were sent overseas. Dependent children at home usually received pediatric care from private pediatricians, often subsidized by the Emergency Maternity and Infant Care Act. Pediatricians, or physicians who would later become pediatricians, served in the medical corps of the army and navy and had wartime experiences in many theaters of operation. The institution of the Berry Plan in the late 1950s enabled physicians to defer entering the military until they had completed their residencies. Many pediatricians were assigned to facilities that cared for service dependents in the United States and overseas, giving them an opportunity to experience general ambulatory pediatrics. In the Korean, Vietnam, and Persian Gulf conflicts, pediatricians—often from the Medical Corps or National Guard—served in combat areas. It has been said that the most frequent specialty represented in advanced combat areas was pediatrics. Pediatricians were especially appreciated because they were used to adolescents, which many of the soldiers were, and because they knew how to start IVs!

US military officer during humanitarian assistance operations in Al Faw, Iraq, October 2003.

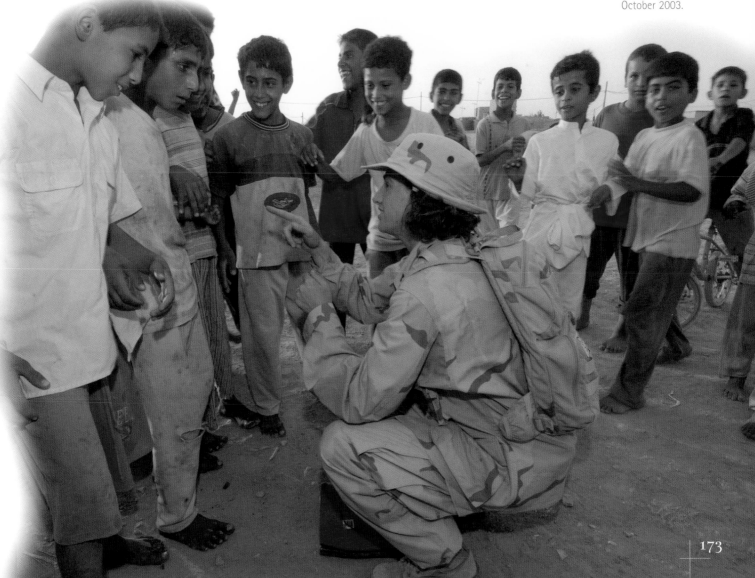

Some good things did occur as a consequence of the wars. The use of penicillin during World War II led to the use of the antibiotic in the rest of society, with wonderful results. Countless physicians became skilled in the surgical treatment of trauma, greatly enhancing treatment in civilian emergency departments. Blood transfusion therapy advanced markedly and national programs for obtaining and distributing blood were set up.

Because the wars of the 20th century have been so defining for the nation and for pediatricians, it seems appropriate to record some tales of their wartime experiences.

The Liberation of Dachau

V-E Day occurred on May 8, 1945. The Dachau camp had fallen about a week earlier. As an Army Medical Corps officer, I was sent there on May 10. Dachau had been put under strict quarantine because of an estimated 4,000 cases of typhus fever among its inmates. I was dispatched from Vittel, near Nancy, and my trip went through a victorious France, through little towns with children dancing through the streets waving the tricolor, cheering any American vehicle that passed.

Dachau is a little town about 12 miles above Munich. In March 1933, Heinrich Himmler, who was police commissioner of Munich, announced the establishment of a concentration camp at Dachau for imprisoning "enemies of National Socialism." A total of about 250,000 prisoners were ultimately processed through Dachau; 40,000 to 50,000 of them died.

Camp conditions as we found them were almost indescribable. Dachau had been built to house 10,000 people, jam-packed. When we arrived, there were 32,600 people. In the blocks or barracks, the men slept in shifts day and night. The bunks were slats covered with burlap and were tiered up to the low ceilings. The stench at Dachau was something that I never will forget, something that doesn't show in photographs.

There were many diseases including scabies, TB, typhoid and, of course, typhus. One hundred or more inmates died each day from typhus alone. The medical program for freeing the camp from typhus included weekly dustings with DDT powder. I, myself, had frequent liberal dustings before going on the infested wards. In recent years, it has made me a little angry to follow a car with a bumper sticker that says "To Hell with DDT."

DDT was a great lifesaver at Dachau and I believe that DDT saved my life.

We set up a ward of 60 beds for treating active cases using para-aminobenzoic acid and hyperimmune rabbit serum. Uninfected inmates were immunized against typhus with the Cox vaccine. The prisoners were vaccinated, deloused, put into sterilized clothes, and isolated for 14 days before being allowed to return to their homes. We were successful and the epidemic ended. We saved literally thousands of men with only food, sanitation, and simple medications.

It is difficult for me to fully describe this extraordinary experience. At Dachau, we found thousands of men, resigned to an inevitable death. They were depressed and withdrawn; they were skin and bones and they were filthy dirty. Suddenly their world was turned around. There was a chance and a hope of survival. There was food. Suddenly they were going to live "not for just a day, not for just a year, but always," as Irving Berlin once wrote.

— *David H. Clement, MD*

Piloting a Navy Bomber in World War II

Of all the combat missions that I flew, the one for which I received the Distinguished Flying Cross was particularly memorable. Our Navy B24 was attacking a Japanese airfield in Malaysia, a little above Singapore, and making passes at about 150 feet. I didn't notice that we were taking fire until I saw gas streaming out of our starboard wing. It was clear we had been hit in a very vulnerable spot. One wounded crewman had the tip of his nose scratched by shrapnel. We spent several weeks persuading him into accepting a Purple Heart.

We were about 1,000 miles from our home base in Palawan, the southernmost Philippine Island, and there was no nearer alternative. Realizing we had used a large amount of gasoline on our low-level attacks as well as from the ruptured tank, I knew it would be a tight squeeze on available fuel, so we dumped our guns, ammunition, and empty gas tanks to reduce our weight.

It was dark by the time we were halfway home, and we needed to take the most direct route home. As embarrassing as it was for us in the navy, we radioed a base in Borneo and asked the army to send out a Black Widow Night Fighter with its sophisticated radar equipment to give us a firm location fix. We finally arrived back at Palawan after a flight of 16.1 hours.

In preparing for our landing on the 50-foot-wide runway, I realized the starboard tire might be blown and stationed our chief ordnanceman in the port hatch with a carbine and gave him instructions to shoot out the good tire if the starboard tire was blown, only if and when I gave him the order. I also ordered our copilot to be ready to pull full throttle on the starboard outboard engine if the tire was blown, but only if I gave him the order. During the landing, all hell broke loose because, indeed, the tire was blown! Before the plane could swerve off the runway, the men took matters into their own hands and performed their assignments admirably and without my orders. Their prompt actions probably saved our lives! We bounced straight ahead to a screeching halt in about 200 feet as the vibration from those flat tires rocked the entire plane. I was so shaken I could hardly stand up to make my way out to claim a dollop of Old Overholt from our flight surgeon. Our plane was full of holes and was subsequently junked. When we measured the remaining gasoline, there were only 250 gallons left.

We usually flew a B24 Privateer that had been modified by removing 2 auxiliary wing tip gas tanks, each holding 200 gallons of fuel. On that particular day, our usual plane had been grounded for maintenance so we were assigned an older B24 Liberator that still had the auxiliary tanks. Fortunate for us! If we had been flying our usual plane that day, we would have wound up with our feet wet!

— *Thomas C. Peebles, MD*
(Adapted from the AAP oral history collection.)

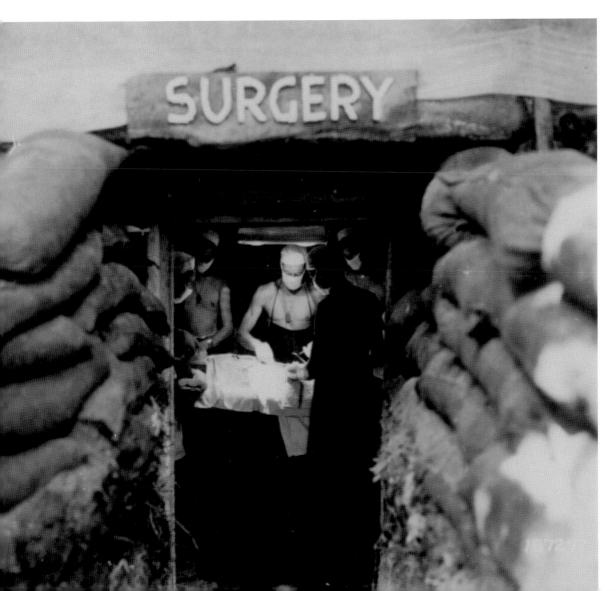

An underground surgery room at Bougainville (an island in the Pacific Ocean), December 1943.

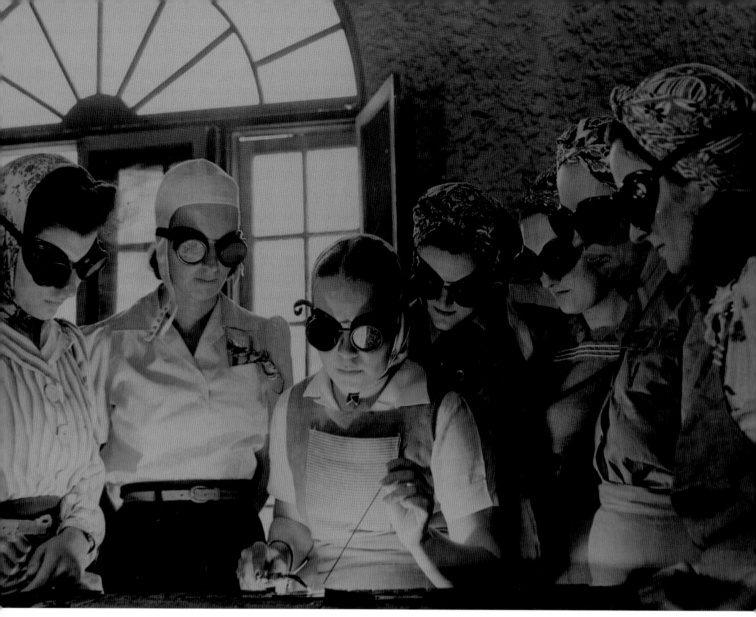

Women attending vocational school to learn war work, Daytona Beach, FL, 1942.

I Was Stationed 10,000 Feet From the Bomb

I finished my residency in 1943 and had applied for a commission in the army when I got an order telling me to report to an address in Santa Fe, NM. My wife and I were sent from there to an isolated location on top of a mesa where there was a laboratory and a lot of houses in what we learned was Los Alamos. It was a fairly sizeable community, mostly of physicists. A lot of them were young with young children so they needed a pediatrician. It was the only real practice I had done before or have done since. It was all very secret. We were closely watched; our mail was censored. I had thought that being a doctor was pretty high on the totem pole, but not there. Many of the physicists looked down on doctors—particularly army doctors. At first, I told everybody who called, "I'll come over to see you." And after a while, the physicists were telling other families not to call me because I was too busy. It was a wonderful practice with very challenging parents who wanted to know every step I was taking, and why.

I was at the test shot at Alamogordo, NM, when the first atomic bomb was set off. I was stationed 10,000 feet from the bomb. When it went off, we knew it worked because of the tremendous blast. After Hiroshima and Nagasaki, I was sent with a group to go to these cities to see if it would be safe for occupying troops, but we sat in Okinawa for a month because General MacArthur felt that there would be a risk. When we finally got in, there was no significant radiation, although we found some radiation in the rubble of hospitals due to medical radium. We then went to Washington for 6 months to write a report. It was quite an experience.

— *Henry L. Barnett, MD*
(Adapted from the AAP oral history collection)

Left at Home in the United States

In 1943, World War II had an impact on all aspects of life, including the practice of medicine and the medical school environment. I was a lieutenant, junior grade, in the Naval Reserve, but I was one of the few medical students who were not accepted to active duty status. I was very disappointed in being rejected by the US military. I asked Dean Davison [Dr Wilburt C. Davison] to arrange another physical examination for me. This did not work out as well as I had hoped.

When I arrived at Fort Bragg, I was sent to a large tent with other inductees. We were all naked and I, weighing 125 pounds, was the smallest male being examined. The word "SPECIAL" had been written in red paint on my chest indicating that I had been rejected before because of a large cavernous hemangioma on my right hip. I got by the first examining doctor by holding my hand over the hemangioma, but when I went into an adjoining tent, a psychiatrist wanted to know why I always kept my hand on my hip. When I showed him the hemangioma, he palpated the area vigorously and his fingernails were so sharp that my leg started bleeding. No water was available so he tried to clean the area with a paper towel, but this only smeared the blood widely. He quickly sent me to the next tent where a navy officer was sitting. He asked the naked group if anyone would like to be in the Navy. I held up my hand, stepped forward. He glanced at this 125-lb boy with a bloody leg and picked up a large rubber stamp. With some gusto he stamped a large, red rejection on my record. I felt as if I had been stabbed in the chest by the stamp.

When I tried to leave the base to return to Duke, the MPs at the gate took me off the bus and placed me in a guard building. I showed them the word "SPECIAL" on my chest but they were not impressed. In a few hours, I was released. I doubt if many medical students were ever in a similar predicament, when at the same time, they could neither get in nor get out of military service.

Eleven years later, I was drafted and was on active duty in the US Air Force for 2 years. I was stationed in Nassau County, NY, where there were more pediatricians than in my entire state of North Carolina. I enjoyed my tour of duty, but I was happy to return to my own practice.

— *George E. Prince, MD*

A Pediatrician in the Persian Gulf War

It was late evening on the 23rd of February 1991, when the Third Battalion/Ninth Marines began to push north across the sand berms marking the border between Kuwait and Saudi Arabia. Their mission was to secure an opening in the first of 2 belts of mines that the occupying Iraqi army had placed in southern Kuwait. I was riding in a Humvee ambulance in a long procession of amphibious assault vehicles (AAVs), tanks, and other vehicles. As battalion surgeon, I, along with one other physician and 62 corpsmen, was responsible for the medical care of the 1,200 men of the battalion. In my mind that night, I reviewed the assault plans that had predicted 30% casualties in the first 24 hours of the invasion.

Fortunately, there was no resistance as the battalion made its way across the first band of mines, so we pushed on, and within hours, were crossing the second minefield. After securing the trenches beyond the mines, and as the marines began rounding up prisoners, mortars began to rain down on them, and the first marine casualties fell. The wounded men were quickly brought to the battalion aid station where we stabilized them for evacuation by helicopter to definitive surgical care. At break of day, a group of Iraqi soldiers who had hidden through the night inside the perimeter began to attack. Their assault was

"When the cheering Kuwaiti residents learned I was a pediatrician, they brought their children out for me to examine."

GORDON SCHUELLER NAYLOR, MD

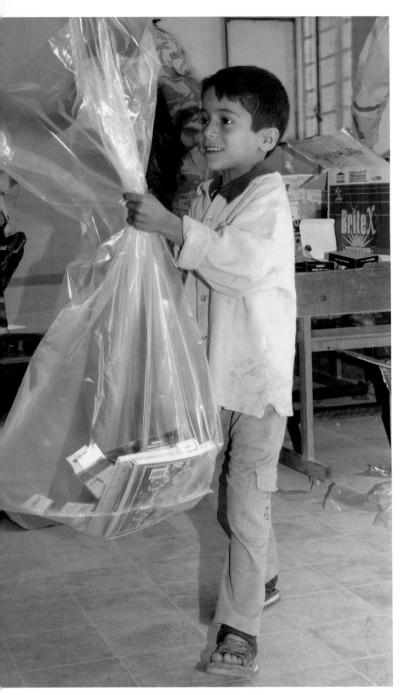

A child from Umm Qasr, Iraq, collects school supplies provided by US naval forces, February 2004.

quickly put down without any American casualties, but as the day went on, a major tank battle ensued. My colleague and I, along with our corpsmen, were busy throughout the next day caring for numerous Iraqi casualties from the fighting. I treated 12 wounded Iraqis that day and I still remember vividly the face of a teenaged Iraqi soldier who was killed in combat. I slept that night in a foxhole wearing my helmet and flak jacket, as well as my pistol.

As the following day broke, preparations were made for the final phase of the operation. The battalion was to lead the assault on Kuwait International Airport on the outskirts of Kuwait City. Two corpsmen and I in an AAV accompanied the main combat elements of the battalion that would make the primary assault, a fast and aggressive attack. As we approached the airport, a fierce ambush erupted in an orchard. In the midst of this fight, an American tank from another battalion mistook our AAV for an Iraqi vehicle, and began to fire at us with its main gun. Two shots barely missed us. We swerved to and fro frantically before finally escaping the "friendly" tank by hiding behind a sand berm. Within hours, the airport was captured and the war was essentially over. I had become the first American physician to enter Kuwait City.

After a base was established at the airport, I had the opportunity over the next few days to visit neighborhoods and the main hospital in the city. When the cheering Kuwaiti residents learned I was a pediatrician, they brought their children out for me to examine. Their care had been excellent before the Iraqi invasion, so I saw mostly acute problems such as sore throats and minor skin infections. I made rounds on the pediatric ward at the hospital where there were no basic services such as clean water and electricity, and I gave them medical supplies. I talked to Kuwaiti pediatricians about their wartime experiences.

"Our medical assets were 2 army pediatricians, a nurse, a medic, and a supply of medicines. We all carried weapons and wore Kevlar helmets and body armor."

RICHARD S. K. YOUNG, MD

They told of Iraqi soldiers who had stolen incubators and other equipment from the nurseries. Within a few weeks, my unit returned home to California, and I returned to my family and pediatric clinic at the Naval Hospital. It is evident that the many pediatricians who served on the front lines of this and other wars, have proven repeatedly that their skills in visual diagnosis, airway management and shock recognition and treatment are ideally suited for treating wounded young soldiers on the modern battlefield.

— *Gordon Schueller Naylor, MD*

An Army Pediatrician in Iraq

We had been encouraged by the army to conduct "humanitarian medical exercises" for Iraqi civilians. "Mount up; let's roll," was our order that morning. Our convoy rolled toward a village located a few miles from the gates of Baghdad, Iraq. Our medical assets were 2 army pediatricians, a nurse, a medic, and a supply of medicines. We all carried weapons and wore Kevlar helmets and body armor.

"Have we advertised the humanitarian exercise?" "No," replied our civil affairs commander. "We can't, because of the terrorists. Besides, everyone will invite 10 relatives from Baghdad." We pulled into the village and posted guards. Groups of curious children appeared as MPs and Iraqi police protected the vehicles from theft. Within 30 minutes of our arrival, a crowd of 400 had formed a long queue.

The patients were triaged into the dental and medical suites. Dental services were limited, as our equipment would not operate on the 220 V Iraqi power. Patients streamed into the medical room. More than half of the patients were children, reflecting the fact that men may have multiple wives.

Some of the children had easily treated pediatric disorders—ringworm, eczema, coughs, colds—and we dispensed medication from our medical chests. Others were more problematic. One child had amblyopia. Another was stigmatized by saliva on her bib due to bulbar palsy. A mother attributed her child's deafness and mutism to "the Americans." Our sole interpreter

Gordon Schueller Naylor, MD, with Kuwaiti children during the first Gulf War, 1991.

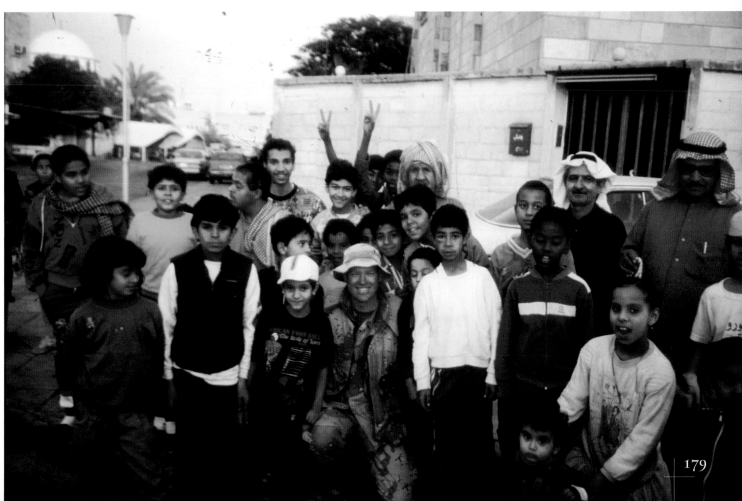

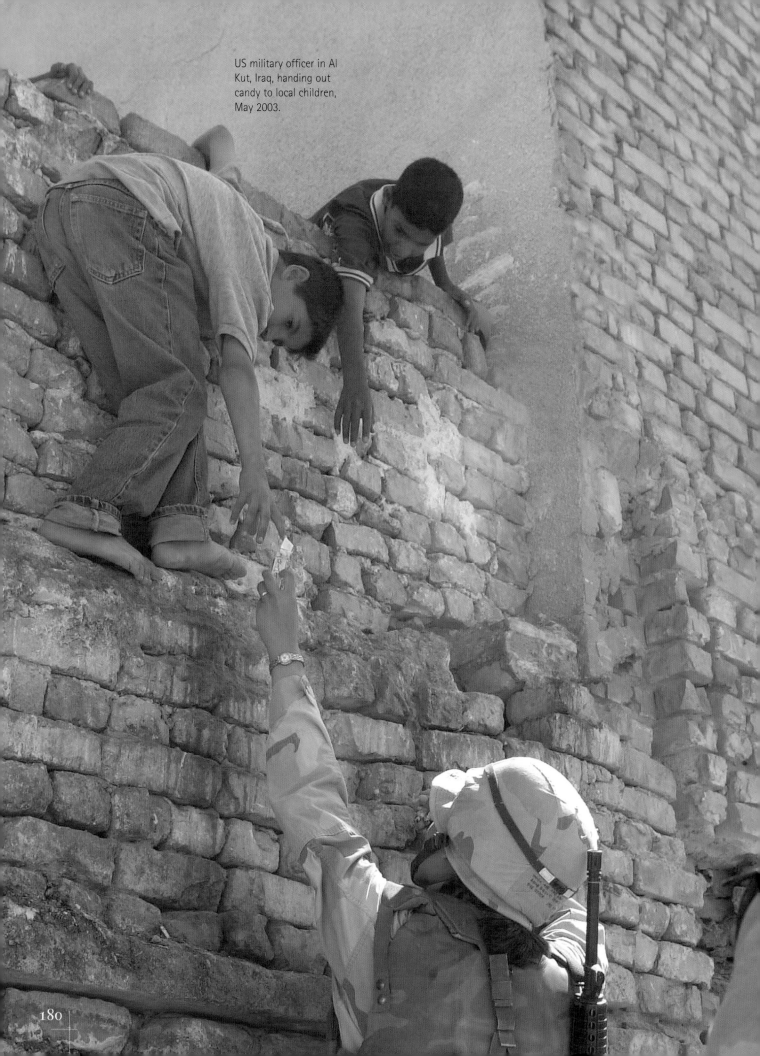

US military officer in Al Kut, Iraq, handing out candy to local children, May 2003.

gamely spent a minute or so with each provider. While we waited, the traditional language of medicine, holding of hands, a smile, and gestures must suffice.

I was summoned by the medic. A 13-year-old was depressed. We were uncertain about mental health resources. The shortcomings of Iraqi health care are attributable to the 10-year oil embargo, repression by Saddam Hussein, and the resulting "brain drain." The medic summoned me again. A former Iraqi soldier lifted up his gown, disclosing a suppurating wound in his hip where shrapnel has resulted in osteomyelitis. We provided him a month's worth of Keflex, realizing that he required debridement and IV antibiotics. It's noon. "Time to go!" called out the civil affairs commander. There are still more patients waiting.

Our humanitarian exercise is a microcosm of the American experience in Iraq. The Iraqis want us to go, but want us to stay. We're on a tight timetable....We're competing with the man-in-the-moon metaphor, "You Americans can put a man on the moon, why can't you give me a job? Why can't you snap your fingers and produce 24-hour power? Why can't you fix depression or esotropia or osteomyelitis?"

— *Richard S. K. Young, MD*
(Editors' note: Dr Young is a lieutenant colonel in the 118th National Guard Reserve Medical Battalion and submitted this account from the war zone in Iraq in early 2004.)

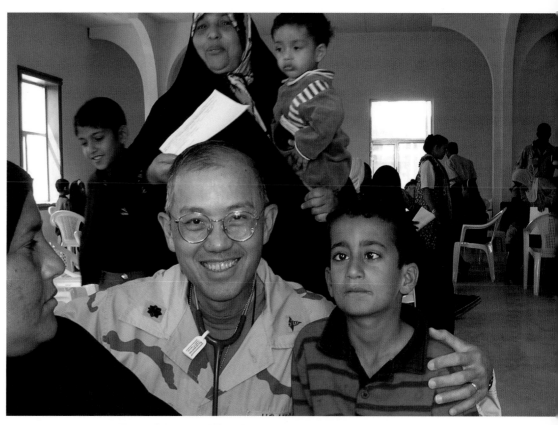

Richard S. K. Young, MD, with Iraqi child, 2004.

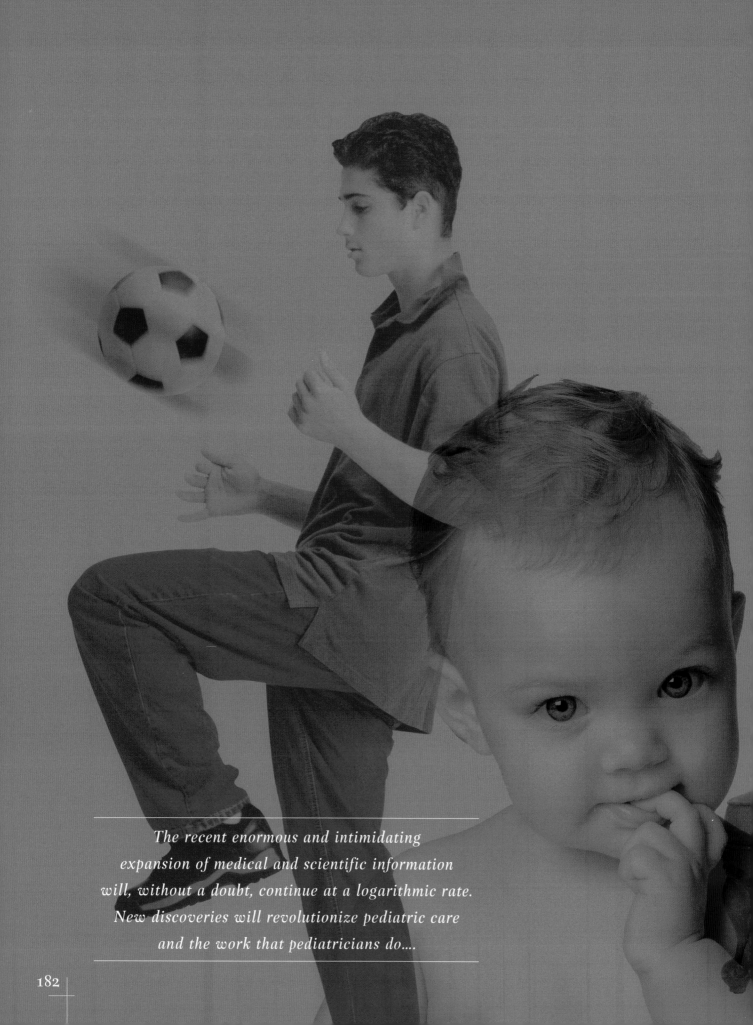

*The recent enormous and intimidating
expansion of medical and scientific information
will, without a doubt, continue at a logarithmic rate.
New discoveries will revolutionize pediatric care
and the work that pediatricians do....*

182

Chapter 8
Child Health in the 21st Century

A Look Ahead

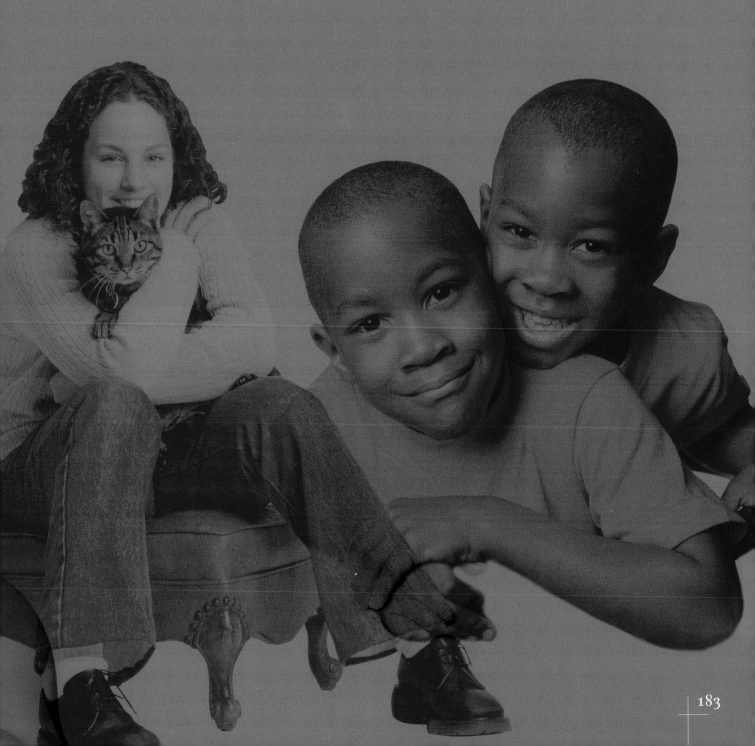

Even more difficult than describing the history and accomplishments of the American Academy of Pediatrics (AAP) in the past 75 years is predicting what may happen in its second 75 years. The recent enormous and intimidating expansion of medical and scientific information will, without a doubt, continue at a logarithmic rate. New discoveries will revolutionize pediatric care and the work that pediatricians do.

Some predictions can be made with near certainty. Today's medical school classes are equally divided between men and women and the challenges and rewards of a pediatric career are particularly attractive to women. Before too long, an increasing majority of AAP members and most of its leaders will be women. One would hope that a second prediction will come true as well—namely, that the United States would finally commit sufficient resources to guarantee every child access to health care.

The following prognostications of what may occur in a few selected areas give a tantalizing snapshot of what could happen in the future, although we all realize that crystal balls are often cloudy.

"WHAT'S PAST IS PROLOGUE"*—SOME HISTORICAL MUSINGS ON THE FUTURE OF AMERICAN PEDIATRICS

In looking back on the history of American pediatrics over the past century, we can be proud of a long tradition of aggressive advocacy for child welfare and the prevention of disease. Because children can't always speak for themselves, it is essential for pediatricians to protect their patients' interests. When the field of public health first gained steam as a social force in improving the lives of Americans during the 19th and early 20th centuries, pediatricians were at the head of the line as vociferous activists on behalf of children. They helped provide clean milk for infants and developed the well-child examination to discover and treat problems before they became serious. Other pediatric leaders lobbied for stringent child labor reforms and safer schools.

As has been recounted earlier in this volume, this commitment to social activism led to a rift with the American Medical Association during the 1920s that set forces into motion, eventually leading to the founding of the AAP in 1930. Although federal child health programs during the New Deal and Second World War generated heated debate among the AAP rank and file, by the 1960s the AAP had clearly embraced a vision of child advocacy going far beyond professional interests. The contributions of AAP members to child welfare range from promoting immunization to ensuring access to care, and are far too numerous to recount here. Even Benjamin M. Spock, MD, whose gentle advice did so much to shape the raising of the baby boom generation, became a very different kind of symbol through his opposition to the Vietnam War and nuclear weapons—social issues that he construed as threats to children.

Pediatricians can be proud of their many contributions to child health. A little more than a century ago, 20% of American babies died before their first birthdays—usually of now wholly preventable maladies such as smallpox, diphtheria, whooping cough, and dehydration. In 2004, the infant mortality rate is less than 1%—most typically related to premature births. Yet the continuing relevance of social activism to pediatrics has been illustrated by the emergence of several new and deadly problems in recent years. An epidemic of obesity has struck children with a vengeance. There are no single villains in this morality play, but it does not take a rocket scientist to figure out that the widespread sales of junk food in our schools, the prevalence of fast-food meals eaten by all Americans, the hours spent on television viewing and video game playing, the types of foods advertised in the media, and the concomitant lack of physical activity is something we pediatricians need to become exercised about. Similar claims could be made about the incidence of cigarette smoking by our youths, substance abuse, and exposure to environmental toxins ranging from polluted air and the rise of asthma to childhood lead poisoning, to name only a few serious issues we must help address in the years to come.

*Quote is from William Shakespeare's *The Tempest*.

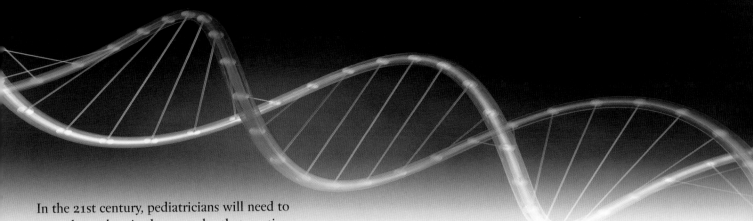

In the 21st century, pediatricians will need to reassert themselves in the struggles that continue to thrive surrounding food safety, child protection, environmental health and disease prevention—every bit as fervently as our predecessors. It will take a form of activism that may seem out of place within the confines of the clinic or hospital but is, nevertheless, just as vital. The good news, as we contemplate the future of pediatrics, is that the history of our proud organization (not to mention the AAP membership certificates hanging in all of our offices) proves that we are more than able to be active in, as the AAP constitution states, "all aspects of the work for the welfare of children."

— Howard Markel, MD

GENETICS IN PEDIATRICS IN THE NEW MILLENNIUM

The AAP was the first organization of its type to create a Committee on Genetics and to recognize that the knowledge and technologies of genetics could serve patients, families, and society safely and with benefit to health. As the importance of environmental causes of diseases continues to decrease because of effective immunizations, antibiotics, and public health, the relative contribution of genetic causes to diseases in the population will inevitably increase. A century after Mendel's laws of inheritance were seen to apply to humankind, and 50 years after the molecular nature of the DNA molecule was discovered, it is apparent that DNA in the germline is "the eternal molecule." Genes are digital information—they are copied, they function in cells and bodies, and they are the vehicles for inheritance. Every person reading this sentence has ancestors who passed on their genes to her or him.

Pediatrics is concerned with the health and diseases of children. Some children are born with conditions whose principal causes lie in their genome. However, mutant genes are not the equivalent of illness or an unhappy destiny; destiny can sometimes be altered. Genetic disease (even Mendelian disorders) is never "simple"; it is complex and subversive. Mutant genes are not rare; they are everywhere among us. Five percent of young adults have a fully declared condition attributable to genetic variation, while 60% of people will experience a genetic illness during their lifetime. Genetic variation in the genome of Homo sapiens is normal; it causes "disease" only when it is perceived as "illness."

The Human Genome Project, completed in 2003, is revealing more than we anticipated, and it is a beginning rather than an ending of our inquiries into the genome. In the decades to come, there will be a fuller understanding of the number of genes we actually have and of their function.

While we learn more about the biology of our health and disease, to know only the mutant gene will never totally explain disease. It soon will be possible, using rapid and accurate technologies, to analyze the genome of an individual patient. This ability has ethical implications that have yet to be defined. However, to know the person who has a genetic disease, to listen and to observe carefully and compassionately, and to examine expertly will remain the essence of clinical practice in spite of the advances at the DNA level. It will always be as important, perhaps more important, to know even more about the child than the disease the child may have.

— Charles R. Scriver, MD

THE FUTURE OF NEONATOLOGY

Important changes in the care of newborns occurred in the past 40 to 50 years, much of it triggered by advances in technology. So what can we expect in the coming years? Some advances will build on partial successes of the past decade; others will take methods developed in the laboratory and move them to the bedside (incubatorside), while others are still at the "idea" stage.

More than a decade has passed since the introduction of liquid ventilation, using perfluorocarbons, into neonatology. I anticipate that it will become an established alternative for management of neonatal ventilatory failure. Gene therapy should also find a place in the standard therapy for neonates who are identified with a single gene defect. The polymerase chain reaction (PCR) methodology has already been applied to diagnose several viral, and some bacterial, illnesses. Screening neonates with suspected infection with PCR for a wide range of pathogenic organisms will be possible.

Although not yet widely available, the establishment of simulated delivery rooms and neonatal intensive care units (NICUs) will enable pediatric residents to practice resuscitation and respond to other emergencies before they are exposed to actual "live" situations. Heart rate, respiration rate, and oxygen saturation monitors can be programmed to simulate emergency situations, to which the learner can respond under videotape surveillance. Programs such as these may ultimately replace traditional methods of training.

Both genes and cells can be labeled with light-emitting enzymes (luciferases). Such internal light sources can be detected externally and become "biological reporters," and bioluminescent imaging is likely to have clinical application. The ability to take fetal cells and grow them selectively has significant therapeutic potential. Such "tissue engineering" has already occurred for skin grafts and will continue to expand. On another front,

vaccines have been developed against individual subtypes of group B streptococcus (GBS), and it will soon be possible to immunize pregnant women against GBS, replacing the current widespread use of intrapartum antibiotics.

Trying to imagine what ideas will find their way into clinical neonatology is fraught with difficulty, but one old idea that is unlikely to be translated into reality is the "artificial placenta." I think it is probable that blood substitutes will emerge and that skin surface electrodes for measuring glucose, electrolytes, and other biochemical determinations will become available, reducing the need for phlebotomy. Most importantly, we will gain knowledge through clinical and basic investigation to address neonatology's greatest challenge—how to prevent prematurity.

— *Alistair G. S. Philip, MD*

PEDIATRIC INFECTIOUS DISEASES IN THE 21st CENTURY

Despite remarkable progress for the past several decades, considerable challenges remain for the discipline of pediatric infectious diseases. Looking forward into the 21st century, these include conquering illnesses that affect many millions of children of the developing world, especially human immunodeficiency virus (HIV) infection, tuberculosis, malaria, and parasitic disorders. Improved health for children of the developed world will include enhanced prevention of infection in the immunocompromised host as well as many new vaccines targeting a broad variety of infectious disorders.

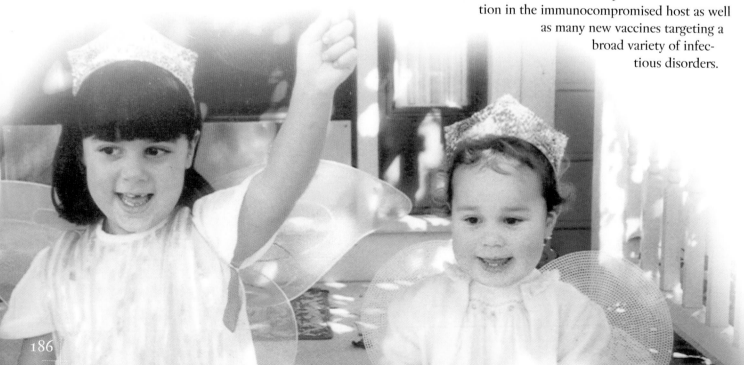

The genomic era of medicine has arrived, and the quantity and quality of available genomic data, both microbial and mammalian, will continue to increase at a remarkable pace. This will impact the field of pediatric infectious diseases profoundly. Well over 100 bacterial genomes have been sequenced since the *Haemophilus influenzae* genome in 1995, including many other important human pathogens. Information about microbial genomes will lead to improved understanding of mechanisms of virulence, identification of new targets for antimicrobial therapy and development of more effective antimicrobials, improved and more rapid diagnostic methods, and many new and increasingly effective vaccines. The results of the Human Genome Project also will facilitate significant advances related to the pathogenesis of infections, new insights into the host-parasite relationship, and elucidation of mechanisms and determinants of host susceptibility and resistance to specific infections. Utilization of DNA microarray analysis and newer proteonomic methodologies to understand gene expression and the role of specific proteins involved in the pathogenesis of infections will facilitate these advances.

It is highly probable that the 21st century will see the identification of currently unrecognized pathogens, some of which may be associated with important chronic disorders that are not now known to be related to infection. Spread of pathogens from animals to man, perhaps even pathogens from other planets, as well as enhanced global spread of new and old pathogens may occur. Emergence of challenging new microbes with dramatic patterns of antimicrobial resistance is likely. The threat of bioterrorism and the public health response thereto also will likely impact the field of pediatric infectious diseases.

Therapeutic advances in the 21st century will capitalize on both the genomic information noted previously and computer-designed agents directed at new targets. These likely will include drugs

Children, Terrorism & Disasters Toolkit
www.aap.org/terrorism

Disaster Preparedness to Meet Children's Needs

American Academy of Pediatrics
DEDICATED TO THE HEALTH OF ALL CHILDREN

that modulate the immune response to infection as well as impacting the infectious agents directly. Hopefully, advances also will be made in the delivery of existing vaccines and other preventive and therapeutic measures to areas of the world where children still succumb to infections for which effective preventive and/or therapeutic measures now exist.

Finally, the 21st century should see remarkable progress in vaccine development and technologies, possibly including DNA-based vaccines, effective HIV vaccines, even edible vaccines. It is hoped that the remarkable benefits of vaccines can be more widely disseminated, and unscientifically based opposition to immunizations can be overcome more effectively.

All the advances suggested here, and others that are as yet unforeseen, should directly and indirectly contribute substantially to the health of children throughout the world.

— *Stanford T. Shulman, MD*

CHILDREN AND TERRORISM: WHAT LIES AHEAD?

The events of September 11, 2001, the growing numbers of large-scale terrorist attacks abroad, and the international media's coverage of world events in real-time and of unprecedented scope and immediacy have raised our consciousness and concerns about our own safety, and that of our children. Some even have warned that terrorists may target children in future attacks. When crises occur, pediatricians will be the first responders to children's health concerns and will be a trusted source of health information. Pediatricians must be able to identify physical symptoms caused by a terrorist event, deliver initial treatment, and interface with and support local and regional responses. Because primary care has become the de facto mental health care system in the United States, in the setting of a crisis, pediatricians will need to detect somatization, screen for adjustment problems, perform timely and effective triage, provide supportive

Left, Children, Terrorism & Disasters Toolkit, published in 2002 by the American Academy of Pediatrics.

Peds-21: Pediatrics for the 21st Century

In November 2003, the American Academy of Pediatrics held the first in a planned series of symposia to address key issues expected to impact the future of pediatrics. Following are a few of the conclusions that emerged from those discussions:

- An affordable and practical Web-based electronic medical record system that is started at birth should be a top priority.
- Evidence-based research and consensus recommendations, as well as health supervision schedules and forms, should be linked to the electronic medical record.
- Child health investigators and child economists should be encouraged to conduct studies of child health–oriented health services. This research should be conducted in the various venues where children receive care.
- Racial, ethnic, and language differences need to be considered in child health–oriented research.
- Medical students and pediatric residents need to be taught about the importance of identifying and using community resources with an emphasis on the entire family. Standards of care for community pediatrics need to be developed and integrated into training programs and continuing physician education.
- The core knowledge base of pediatrics, including core subspecialty knowledge, needs to be defined. General pediatricians should be able to take care of most clinical problems seen in their offices. Suggestions for referral of specific conditions to subspecialists should be developed.
- Insurance companies and the federal and state governments should be convinced of the long-term health benefits and cost-effectiveness of preventive health care services.
- Efforts should be undertaken to address disparities in health care, the provision of culturally effective care, and enhancing the diversity of the pediatric workforce.

interventions, and make appropriate referrals for mental health support and counseling. Because many pediatricians do not feel adequately prepared to fulfill these roles, there will be an increased emphasis placed on these areas in pediatric trainee and continuing medical education. These efforts to ensure all pediatricians have the skills to address physical and mental health needs of children in the setting of a crisis will have the added—and not incidental—benefit of enabling them to address more effectively the medical needs and mental health needs of children, even in the absence of a crisis.

Pediatricians will help design and implement crisis preparedness plans that address the needs of all members of the community, including children, even as we hope that we will never have to implement the plans we are developing—but all the time realizing that the process has already enhanced our ability to deliver quality pediatric care every day.

— David J. Schonfeld, MD

NUTRITION IN THE 21st CENTURY

Nutrition has been an important component of pediatrics from its very beginnings. Attempting to guess what may happen in the years ahead is problematic, but some things occur to me. I think that the whole area involving so-called "alternative" or natural substances is going to be scrutinized carefully by orthodox medicine. Some of the many alternative substances, herbs, and antioxidants may, in fact, have nutritional value that we are missing. It is difficult to judge them now because they are almost totally unregulated. In the near future, I think that they are going to be put under the umbrella of the Food and Drug Administration and standardized. We then will know what and how much is being sold; today you cannot tell by the labels. It also will be possible to conduct controlled studies concerning their possible value. I think that we will find that there are more vitamins than we know today and that there are necessary nutritional factors being taken out of our diets because of the use of more and more refined foods. Many of our foods will be preserved by radiation; more of our food will be genetically modified. Before much of the public will freely accept radiated and genetically modified foods in their diets, their safety must be definitively proven.

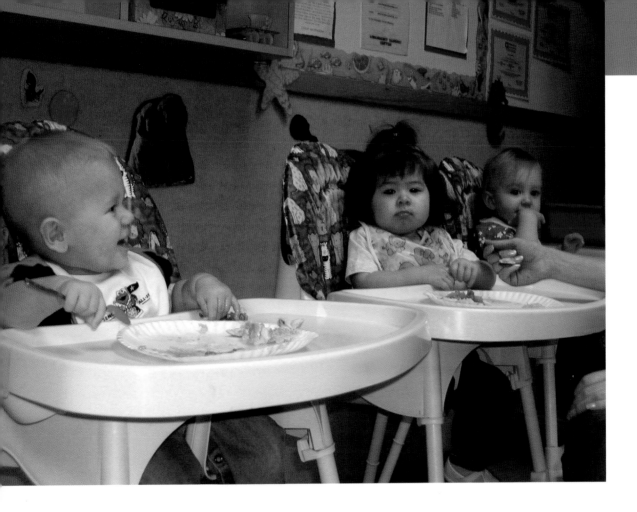

Infant formulas must continue to be scrutinized carefully because they may be the sole foods that an infant consumes. During the 20th century, a number of mini-epidemics of nutritional diseases occurred in infants because of depletion of important substances (such as pyridoxine and chloride) during formula processing. With increasing numbers of formulas and special formulas, recurrence of these kinds of misadventures are likely. Obviously, most could be avoided by breastfeeding; however, the possible transmission of environmental toxins to infants through breast milk must continue to be closely monitored.

In the United States and much of the developed world, caloric overnutrition resulting in obesity has become an epidemic disease accompanied by complications such as type 2 diabetes mellitus. Reduction of caloric intake, more attention to balanced intake of foods, and increased physical activity are social as well as nutritional issues that are not being well addressed today. It is possible that new approaches—pharmacological and hormonal—may provide physicians of the 21st century with new and innovative approaches to obesity, but their safety and effectiveness in children will need to be demonstrated.

Paradoxically, in much of the rest of the world, undernutrition, starvation, and malnutrition remain a rampant problem. One hopes that in the new millennium the global socioeconomic imbalances that lead to preventable malnutrition can be solved.

— *Lewis A. Barness, MD*
(Adapted from the AAP oral history collection.)

HEALTH PROMOTION AND PREVENTION

What does the explosion of new knowledge in genetics, neuroscience, behavior, and environmental science, combined with technological advances, pose for the health promotion and prevention aspects of pediatric practice of the 21st century? The partnership between pediatricians, patients, and parents to promote the health and optimal development of each child remains at the heart of pediatric practice. The greatest opportunity is to focus the use of the new technologies and knowledge to improve health outcomes for all children, especially those with special health care needs. The biggest challenge will be to do it in a manner that strengthens and supports these

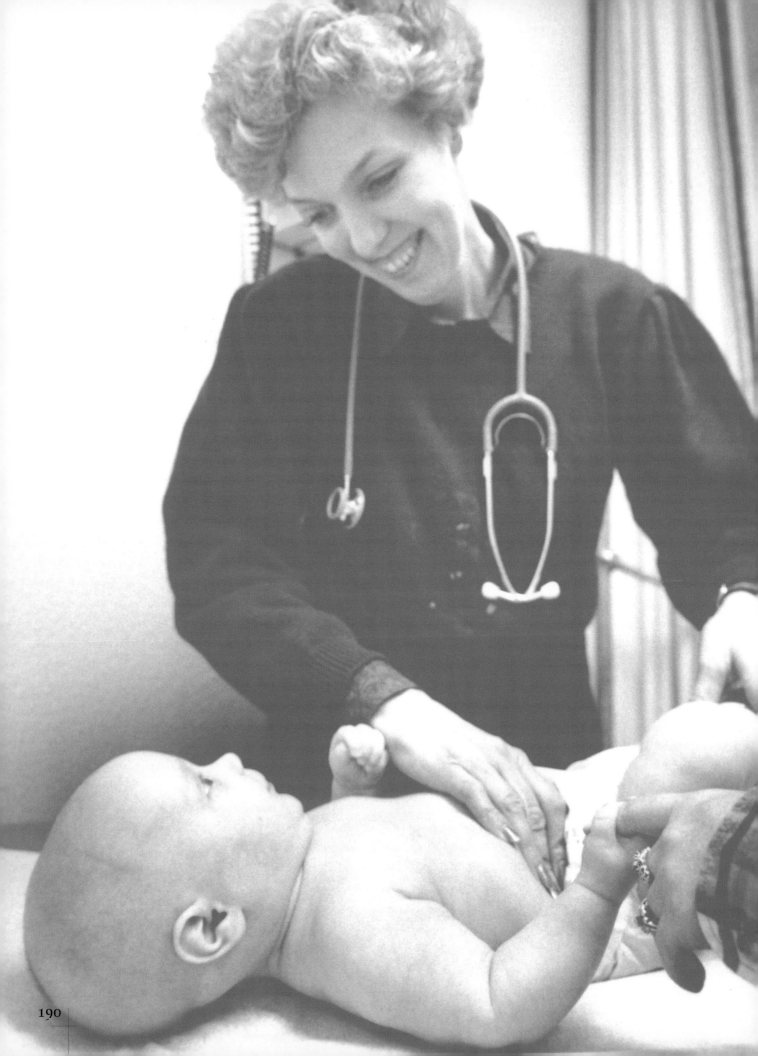

partnerships and relationships so important to parents and children.

Among the areas of special relevance to the well-child visit of the 21st century are new knowledge and technologies, the importance of healthy behavior choices, and the medical home and community pediatrics.

New Knowledge and Technologies

Genomics will result in a well-defined understanding of the individual risk and disease treatment. Parents will have access to conflicting Internet information and will need navigation and interpretative skills of the pediatrician in applying them for optimal outcomes in their children. Neuroscience is expanding our knowledge of the dramatic effects of chemicals in the brain. Even more interesting is the effect of positive and harmful childhood experiences (eg, neglect, understimulation, violence) on the actual chemical makeup and neuronal connections of the child's brain. Chemical influences of the environment will require expertise about the potential effects of and protections from the many toxins and allergens in the physical environment.

Pediatricians in practice also will be able to benefit from new knowledge not developed in the health care sector—advances in systems improvement in business and engineering have lessons for office and hospital settings. With the use of patient registries for children with chronic conditions, screening tools, and organized office and community team approaches, provision of high-quality comprehensive care improves. The electronic medical record will make it easier for practices to collect data to document and continue to improve the systematic supports that ensure that quality care is delivered. Even communication with patients and parents may change. Phone and e-mail communications may add to or

substitute for some office visits in the context of a solid ongoing physician-patient relationship. To have time to deliver the necessary care, practices will be invited to make the best use of technology in all the other areas of data management, billing, and communication with other health, education, and early care professionals, as well as the parents and children themselves.

Healthy Behavior Choices

While pediatricians continue to update their knowledge to treat the results of unhealthy behavior choices—obesity, type 2 diabetes,

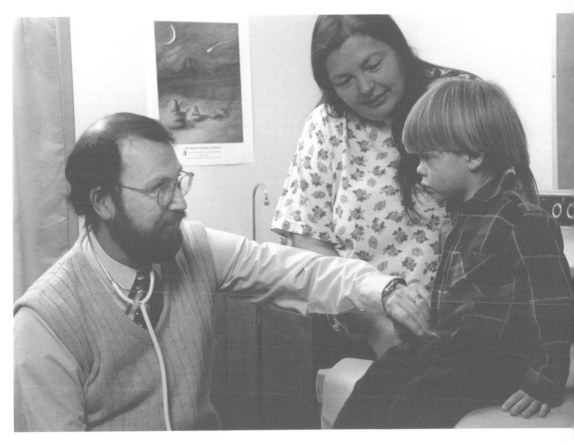

substance abuse, sexually transmitted infections, and traumatic brain injury—the need for deepening their expertise in the promotion of healthy behaviors among children, youth, and parents will emerge. The demand for these services will only grow as more people realize the dramatic effects that healthy behaviors established during childhood and adolescence have on adult morbidity and mortality.

Pediatricians combine their existing skills as health advisors with newly emerging information to help parents understand what specific

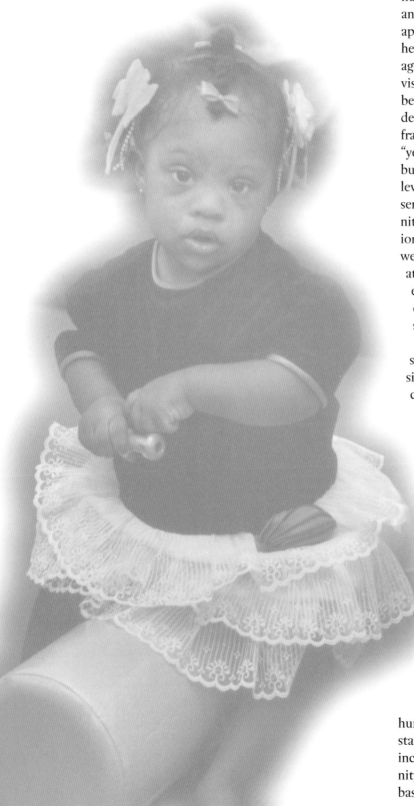

approaches they can use at home and advocate for in their schools and communities to promote their adoption of healthy behaviors related to nutrition, physical activity, emotional well-being, and safety. The explicit use of strength-based approaches adds an important dimension to the health supervision visit. The parent and school-aged child or youth leave the health supervision visit with an understanding of not only the risk behaviors to be avoided but also of the positive developmental assets to be encouraged. This framework that describes what kids need to say "yes" to constitutes the platform from which to build protective factors. Youth who report higher levels of mastery in school and life and a strong sense of belonging with their family and community are less likely to participate in risky behaviors. As assessment and promotion of emotional well-being remain a major component of pediatric health care, increased physician skill and experience with behavioral health issues will contribute to patient, family, and physician satisfaction.

When unhealthy behaviors already exist, skill at "motivational interviewing," shared decision making, and knowledge of appropriate community resources are involved so that individualized approaches can be developed collaboratively with the child and parent.

Medical Home and Partnership With the Community

A medical home remains the best approach for all children and especially those with special health care needs, where the care is continuous, comprehensive, compassionate, culturally effective, coordinated, family centered, and accessible. The medical home of the future might also be characterized by parent and youth advisory groups; collaborative practice with nurse practitioners and physician assistants; colocation of mental health professionals, public health, human services, and developmental specialists; a staff member whose contribution to the practice includes a comprehensive knowledge of community resources; group well-child visits; or data-based partnerships with payers to match quality care for families with more significant needs with fair reimbursement.

All of the health promotion goals discussed in the office setting can only be achieved when the school and community offer diverse opportunities for children and their parents to eat well; participate in vigorous, safe physical activity; volunteer, mentor, or be mentored; and master recreational and academic skills. The fact that a majority of preschool children spend part of their day in early care and education settings offers another venue for implementation of health promotion activities. Access to high-quality health care, dental care, and mental health and substance abuse treatment is a requirement in this equation. This is where community pediatrics comes in. As the understanding of the power of coordinated approaches in changing health and educational outcomes for kids becomes more apparent, more pediatricians will spend part of their time working at the community and state level with parents, youth, other professionals, payers, and policy makers making change happen.

— *Paula M. Duncan, MD*

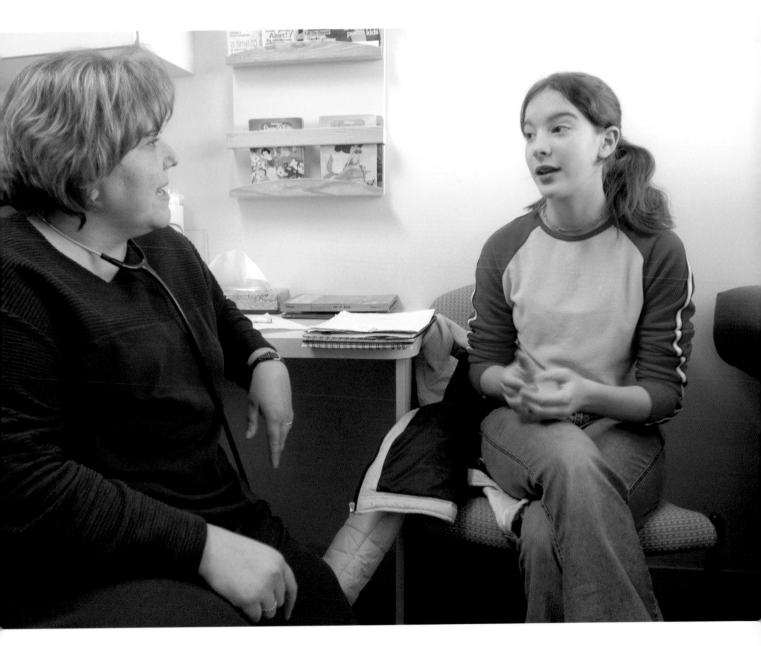

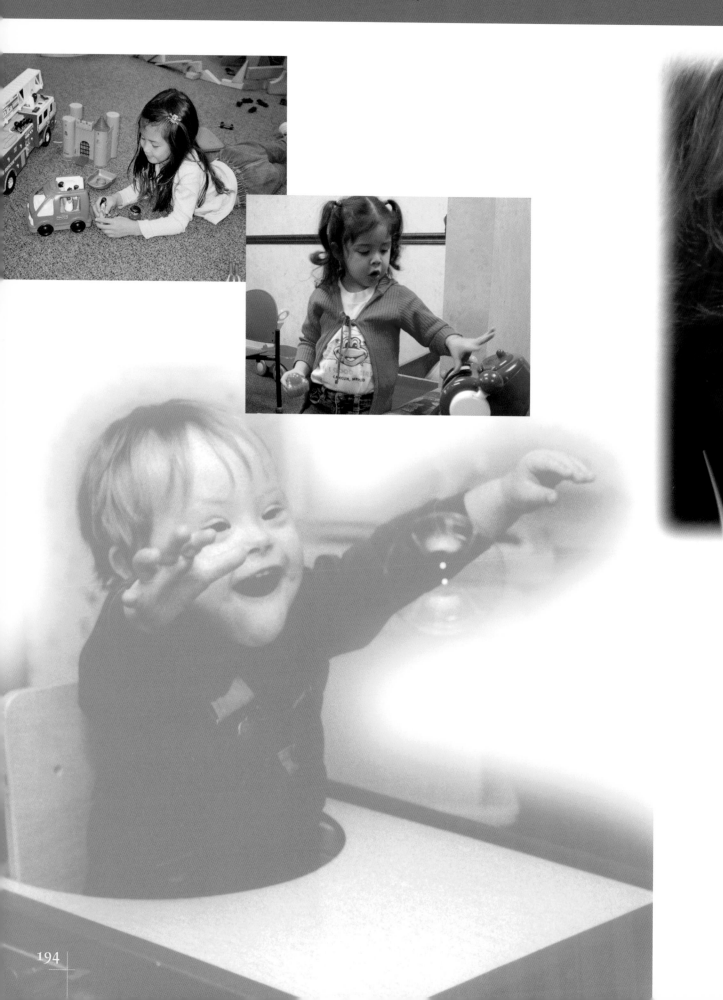

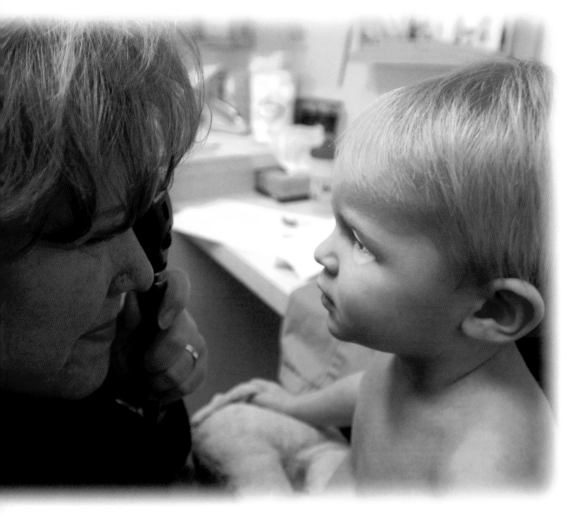

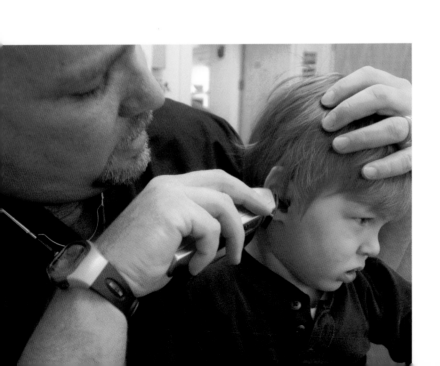

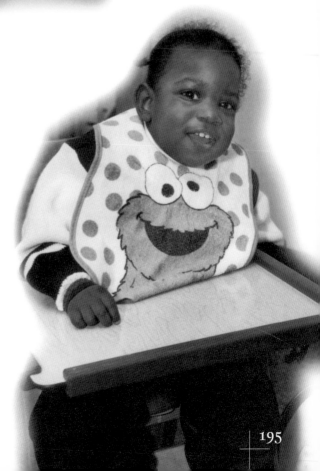

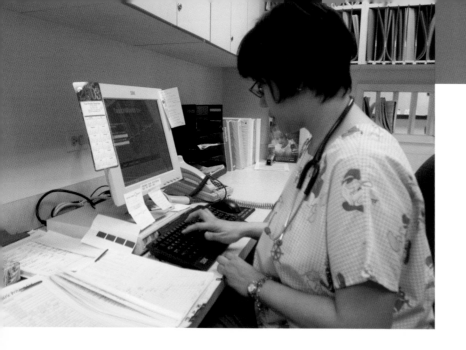

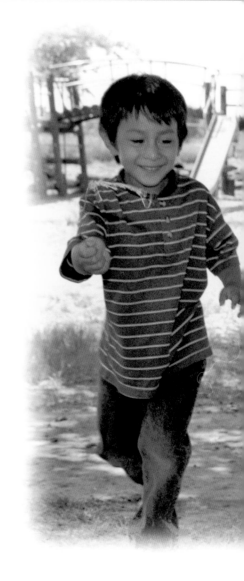

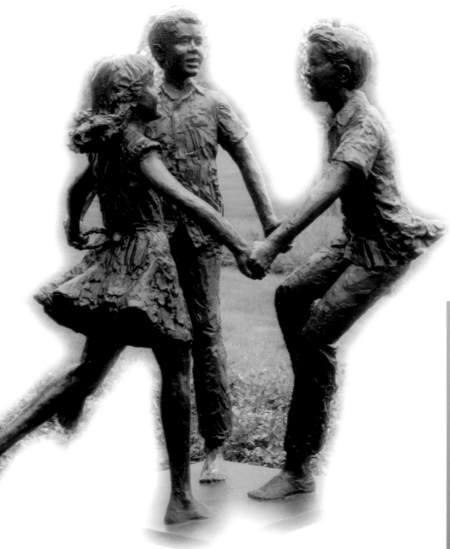

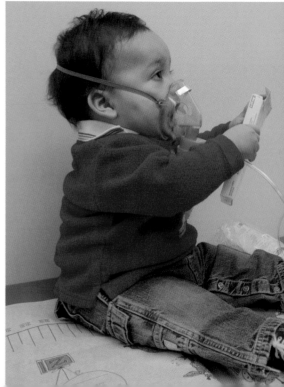

"Together," a statue that was dedicated to Joe M. Sanders, Jr, MD, on May 20, 2004, on his retirement as executive director of the American Academy of Pediatrics (AAP). The statue is located on the grounds of the AAP headquarters in Elk Grove Village, IL.

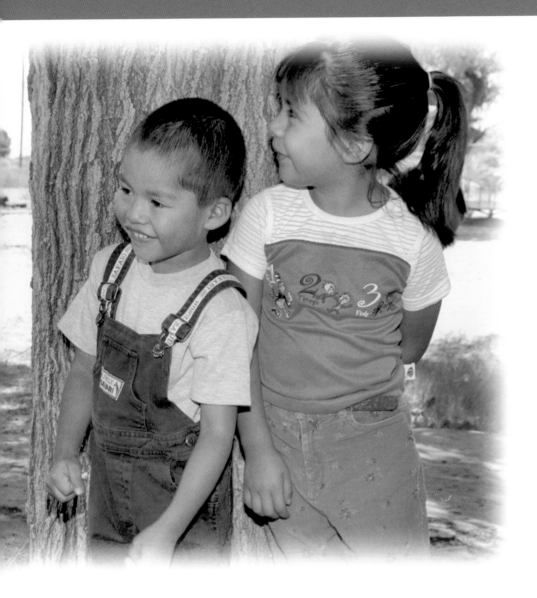

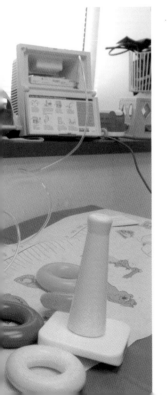

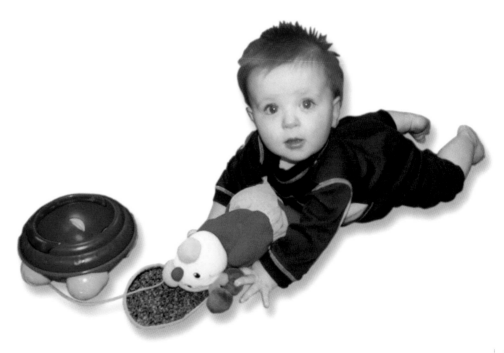

APPENDIX

1930-1931 Isaac A. Abt, MD	1947-1948 John A. Toomey, MD	1964-1965 Harry A. Towsley, MD
1931-1932 John L. Morse, MD	1948-1949 Warren R. Sisson, MD	1965-1966 James G. Hughes, MD
1932-1933 Samuel McC. Hamill, MD	1949-1950 Edward B. Shaw, MD	1966-1967 William S. Anderson, MD
1933-1934 John Ruhrah, MD	1950-1951 Paul W. Beaven, MD	1967-1968 George B. Logan, MD
1934-1935 Thomas B. Cooley, MD	1951-1952 Warren W. Quillian, MD	1968-1969 Hugh C. Thompson, MD
1935-1936 Henry Dietrich, MD	1952-1953 Philip S. Barba, MD	1969-1970 Russell W. Mapes, MD
1936-1937 Laurence R. DeBuys, MD	1953-1954 Roger L. J. Kennedy, MD	1970-1971 R. James McKay, Jr, MD
1937-1938 Philip Van Ingen, MD	1954-1955 Crawford Bost, MD	1971-1972 Jay M. Arena, MD
1938-1939 Henry F. Helmholz, MD	1955-1956 Harry Bakwin, MD	1972-1973 Robert M. Heavenrich, MD
1939-1940 Joseph B. Bilderback, MD	1956-1957 Edgar E. Martmer, MD	1973-1974 James B. Gillespie, MD
1940-1941 Richard M. Smith, MD	1957-1958 Stewart H. Clifford, MD	1974-1975 John C. MacQueen, MD
1941-1942 Edward C. Mitchell, MD	1958-1959 James C. Overall, MD	1975-1976 Merritt B. Low, MD
1942-1943 Borden S. Veeder, MD	1959-1960 William W. Belford, MD	1976-1977 David W. Van Gelder, MD
1943-1944 Franklin P. Gengenback, MD	1960-1961 George M. Wheatley, MD	1977-1978 Saul J. Robinson, MD
1944-1945 Joseph S. Wall, MD	1961-1962 Carl C. Fischer, MD	1978-1979 Edwin L. Kendig, Jr, MD
1945-1946 Jay I. Durand, MD	1962-1963 Clarence H. Webb, MD	1979-1980 Bruce D. Graham, MD
1946-1947 Lee Forrest Hill, MD	1963-1964 Frank H. Douglass, MD	1980-1981 R. Don Blim, MD

1981–1982
Glenn Austin, MD

1982–1983
James E. Strain, MD

1983–1984
Paul F. Wehrle, MD

1984–1985
Robert J. Haggerty, MD

1985–1986
Martin H. Smith, MD

1986–1987
William C. Montgomery, MD

1987–1988
Richard M. Narkewicz, MD

1988–1989
Donald W. Schiff, MD

1989–1990
Birt Harvey, MD

1990–1991
Antoinette P. Eaton, MD

1991–1992
Daniel W. Shea, MD

1992–1993
Howard A. Pearson, MD

1993–1994
Betty A. Lowe, MD

1994–1995
George D. Comerci, MD

1995–1996
Maurice E. Keenan, MD

1996–1997
Robert E. Hannemann, MD

1997–1998
Joseph R. Zanga, MD

1998–1999
Joel J. Alpert, MD

1999–2000
Donald E. Cook, MD

2000–2001
Steve Berman, MD

2001–2002
Louis Z. Cooper, MD

2002–2003
E. Stephen Edwards, MD

2003–2004
Carden Johnston, MD

2004–2005
Carol D. Berkowitz, MD
(president-elect at time of
publication)

American Academy of Pediatrics
Executive Secretaries/
Executive Directors/CEOs

1930–1951
Clifford G. Grulee, MD

1951–1967
E. H. Christopherson, MD

1967–1980
Robert G. Frazier, MD

1980–1986
M. Harry Jennison, MD

1986–1993
James E. Strain, MD

1993–2004
Joe M. Sanders, Jr, MD

2004–
Errol R. Alden, MD

SELECTED READING

In writing their portions of this history, the editors acknowledge their debt to a wide range of works in the history of pediatrics and child health. The American Academy of Pediatrics (AAP) itself has commissioned 2 histories, beginning with the opinionated but elegantly written *The American Academy of Pediatrics: June 1930–June 1951* by Marshall Carleton Pease, MD. For accounts on later developments and legislation by the AAP the reader should consult *American Academy of Pediatrics: The First 50 Years* by James G. Hughes, MD.

Among the sources consulted for the early history of pediatrics and child health in the United States, 3 deserve to be especially singled out. *History of American Pediatrics* by the late Thomas E. Cone, Jr, MD, offers a wealth of material on the history of childhood diseases, infant feeding, and the first medical pioneers of pediatrics. Historian Richard A. Meckel's *Save the Babies: American Public Health Reform and the Prevention of Infant Mortality, 1850–1929* provides perhaps the best overall account of the early 20th-century "baby saving" crusades that are so important to the background of American pediatrics. Our accounts of how childhood itself has changed over the course of the 20th century draws particularly upon Joseph E. Illick's concise *American Childhoods*.

Many other sources that have influenced this history are cited below, and the reader is encouraged to seek those of particular interest.

CHAPTER 1

Apple RD. *Mothers and Medicine: A Social History of Infant Feeding, 1890–1950.* Madison, WI: University of Wisconsin Press; 1987

Cone TE Jr. *History of American Pediatrics.* Boston, MA: Little, Brown, and Co; 1979

Cone TE Jr. *200 Years of Feeding Infants in America.* Columbus, OH: Ross Laboratories; 1976

Golden J. *A Social History of Wet Nursing in America: From Breast to Bottle.* New York, NY: Cambridge University Press; 1996

Grant J. *Raising Baby by the Book: The Education of American Mothers.* New Haven, CT: Yale University Press; 1998

Halpern SA. *American Pediatrics: The Social Dynamics of Professionalism, 1880–1980.* Berkeley, CA: University of California Press; 1988

Holt LE. *The Diseases of Infancy and Childhood.* New York, NY: D. Appleton and Company; 1897

Meckel RA. *Save the Babies: American Public Health Reform and the Prevention of Infant Mortality, 1850–1929.* Baltimore, MD: Johns Hopkins University Press; 1990

Scott AF. *Natural Allies: Women's Associations in American History.* Urbana, IL: University of Illinois Press; 1993

Stern AM, Markel H, eds. *Formative Years: Children's Health in the United States 1880–2000.* Ann Arbor, MI: University of Michigan Press; 2002

Veeder BS. *Pediatric Profiles.* St Louis, MO: C. V. Mosby; 1957

CHAPTER 2

Brownlee RC. The American Board of Pediatrics: its origin and early history. *Pediatrics.* 1994;94:732–735

Hughes JG. *American Academy of Pediatrics: The First 50 Years.* Evanston, IL: American Academy of Pediatrics; 1980

Pearson HA. *The Centennial History of the American Pediatric Society 1888–1988.* New Haven, CT: American Pediatric Society; 1988

Pease MC. *The American Academy of Pediatrics: June 1930–June 1951.* Evanston, IL: American Academy of Pediatrics; 1952

Strain JE. The birth and evolution of *Pediatrics. Pediatrics.* 1998;102(suppl):163–167

CHAPTER 3

Hunt M. Extraordinarily interesting and happy years. Martha M. Eliot and pediatrics at Yale, 1921–1935. *Yale J Biol Med.* 1995;68:159–170

Pease MC. *The American Academy of Pediatrics: June 1930–June 1951.* Evanston, IL: American Academy of Pediatrics; 1952

Starr P. *The Social Transformation of American Medicine.* New York, NY: Basic Books; 1984

Strain JE. The birth and evolution of *Pediatrics*. *Pediatrics*. 1998;102(suppl):163–167

Wegman ME. The American Pediatric Society, the American Academy of Pediatrics and the Children's Bureau: 1944–1945. In: Pearson HA. *The Centennial History of the American Pediatric Society, 1888–1988*. New Haven, CT: American Pediatric Society; 1988:86–89

CHAPTER 4

Chafe WH. *The Unfinished Journey: America Since World War II*. 5th ed. New York, NY: Oxford University Press; 2003

Coles R. *Children of Crisis: Selections from the Pulitzer Prize–Winning Five-Volume Children of Crisis Series*. Boston, MA: Little Brown and Company; 2003

Halpern SA. *American Pediatrics: The Social Dynamics of Professionalism, 1880–1980*. Berkeley, CA: University of California Press; 1988

Helfer RK, Kempe CH, eds. *The Battered Child*. Chicago, IL: University of Chicago Press; 1968

Hughes JG. *American Academy of Pediatrics: the First 50 Years*. Evanston, IL: American Academy of Pediatrics; 1980

Illick J. *American Childhoods*. Philadelphia, PA: University of Pennsylvania Press; 2002

Kempe CH, Silverman FN, Steele BF, Droegemueller W, Silver HK. The battered-child syndrome. *JAMA*. 1962;181:17–24

Pawluch D. *The New Pediatrics: A Profession in Transition*. Hawthorne, NY: Aldine De Gruyter; 1996

Pleck E. *Domestic Tyranny: The Making of Social Policy Against Family Violence from Colonial Times to the Present*. New York, NY: Oxford University Press; 1987

Prescott HM. *A Doctor of Their Own: The History of Adolescent Medicine*. Cambridge, MA: Harvard University Press; 1998

Richmond JB. A report on Project Head Start. *Pediatrics*. 1966;37:905–912

CHAPTER 6

Baker JP. *The Machine in the Nursery: Incubator Technology and the Origins of Newborn Intensive Care*. Baltimore, MD: Johns Hopkins University Press; 1996

Cone TE Jr. *History of the Care and Feeding of the Premature Infant*. Boston, MA: Little Brown; 1985

Desmond MM. *Newborn Medicine and Society: European Background and American Practice (1750–1975)*. Austin, TX: Eakin Press; 1998

Diamond LK. Replacement transfusion as a treatment for erythroblastosis fetalis. *Pediatrics*. 1948;2:520–524

Fass B. Brief history of the *Red Book*. 2001 Tales From the *Red Book* presented at: 43rd Pediatric Symposium; November 10, 2001; Long Beach, CA. 19–24

Holder AR. *Legal Issues in Pediatrics and Adolescent Medicine*. 2nd ed. New Haven, CT: Yale University Press; 1985:88–101

Koop CE. *Koop: The Memoirs of America's Family Doctor*. New York, NY: Random House; 1991

Miller GW. *The Work of Human Hands: Hardy Hendren and Surgical Wonder at Children's Hospital*. New York, NY: Random House; 1993

Pearson HA, Diamond LK, Philip AGS. The rise and fall of exchange transfusion. *NeoReviews*. 2003;4:e169–e174

Pickles MM. *Haemolytic Disease of the Newborn*. Oxford, England: Blackwell Scientific Publications; 1949

Randolph J. History of the Section of Surgery, the American Academy of Pediatrics: the first 25 years. *J Pediatr Surg*. 1999;34(suppl 1):3–18

Randolph J. The first of the best. *J Pediatr Surg*. 1985;20:580–591

Silverman WA. *Retrolental Fibroplasia: A Modern Parable*. New York, NY: Grune & Stratton; 1980

PHOTO CREDITS

All photos not included in the following list are courtesy of the American Academy of Pediatrics.

Front Cover

Left: The Maryland Historical Society, Baltimore, MD

Lower right: March of Dimes Birth Defects Foundation

Chapter 1

Page 1: Yale-New Haven Hospital Archives

Page 2/top: Museum of the City of New York

Page 2/middle: Chicago Historical Society (DN-0004502; Chicago Daily News)

Page 2/bottom: Chicago Historical Society (DN-0004619; Chicago Daily News)

Page 3/top left: Denver Public Library

Page 3/top middle: Library of Congress, Prints and Photographs Division, LC-USZ62-120168

Page 3/top right: Library of Congress, Prints and Photographs Division, LC-USZ62-106989

Page 3/bottom: Denver Public Library

Page 4/top left: Colorado Historical Society (CHS-B489; Harry H. Buckwalter)

Page 4/top right: Denver Public Library

Page 4/middle: Library of Congress, Prints and Photographs Division, LC-DIG-nclc-00715

Page 4/bottom: George Eastman House

Page 5/top: Wollstein M. The Babies' Hospital of the city of New York. *Arch Pediatr.* October 1896

Page 5/middle: Library of Congress, Prints and Photographs Division, LC-USZ62-72475

Page 5/bottom: West JP. A case of congenital cretinism. Arch Pediatr. 1895

Page 6/top left: US National Archives & Records Administration

Page 6/top right: Library of Congress, Prints and Photographs Division, LC-USZ62-77635

Page 6/bottom left: Library of Congress, Prints and Photographs Division, LC-DIG-nclc-00616

Page 7/upper left: Library of Congress, Prints and Photographs Division, LC-USZ62-107658

Page 7/upper right: Holt LE. *The Diseases of Infancy and Childhood.* New York, NY: D. Appleton and Co; 1897

Page 7/right: Library of Congress, Prints and Photographs Division, LC-USZ62-76989

Page 8/top: Library of Congress, Prints and Photographs Division, LC-USZ62-69050

Page 8/bottom: Chicago Historical Society (DN-0003885; Chicago Daily News)

Page 9/top: Archives of the Boston Floating Hospital

Page 9/middle: Library of Congress, Prints and Photographs Division, LC-USZ62-72012

Page 9/bottom: Yale-New Haven Hospital Archives

Page 10/middle: Countway Library of Medicine

Page 10/lower left: Caulfield E. *A True History of the Terrible Epidemic Vulgarly Called the Throat Distemper Which Occurred in His Majesty's New England Colonies Between the Years 1735 and 1740.* New Haven, CT: Yale Journal of Biology & Medicine; 1939

Page 10/lower right: Yale University Library

Page 11/top: College of Medicine and Surgery, Philadelphia

Page 11/bottom left: Williams SW. *American Medical Biography.* Greenfield; 1845

Page 12/bottom left: Yale University Art Library

Page 12/bottom center: Yale University, Harvey Cushing/John Hay Whitney Medical Library

Page 12/bottom right: College of Medicine and Surgery, Philadelphia

Page 13/top left: American Pediatric Society

Page 13/top middle: American Pediatric Society

Page 13/top right: American Pediatric Society

Page 14/bottom: Alan Mason Chesney Medical Archives of the Johns Hopkins Medical Institutions

Page 16/left: Strauss LG. *Diseases in Milk.* 2nd ed. New York, NY: Dutton; 1917

Page 16/right: *Rotch's Pediatrics.* 4th ed. Philadelphia, PA: Lippincott; 1903

Page 17: Children's Hospital Boston

Page 18: Chicago Historical Society (DN-0000806; Chicago Daily News)

Page 19: Yale-New Haven Hospital Archives

Page 20: Yale-New Haven Hospital Archives

Pages 22 and 23: Darroll J. Erickson, MD

Page 24: Library of Congress, Prints and Photographs Division, LC-DIG-nclc-04836

Page 25: US National Library of Medicine, National Institutes of Health

Pages 26 and 27: Library of Congress, Prints and Photographs Division, LC-USZ62-112839

Page 27/top: William A. Silverman, MD

Page 28: Yale-New Haven Hospital Archives

Page 196/lower left: Oscar Einzig
Pages 196 and 197/top: Indian Health Service,
    US Department of Health and Human Services

Back Cover
Top: William A. Silverman, MD
Middle right: Library of Congress, Prints and
    Photographs Division, FSA-OWI Collection,
    LC-USF35-276
Bottom right: Mark Battrell

INDEX

213